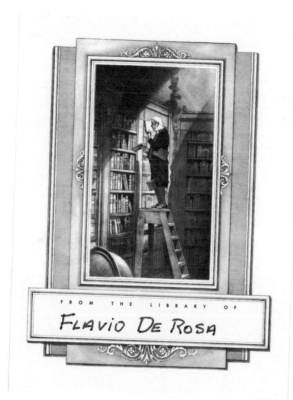

INTENSIVE CARE
FOR NEUROLOGICAL
TRAUMA AND DISEASE

INTENSIVE CARE FOR NEUROLOGICAL TRAUMA AND DISEASE

Edited by

Barth A. Green, M.D.

Chief, Acute Spinal Cord Injury
Associate Professor, Department of Neurological Surgery
University of Miami School of Medicine, Miami, Florida

Lawrence F. Marshall, M.D.

Associate Professor of Surgery/Neurological Surgery
University of California, San Diego, California

T. J. Gallagher, M.D.

Associate Professor of Surgery and Anesthesiology
University of Florida College of Medicine
Gainesville, Florida

1982

ACADEMIC PRESS
A Subsidiary of Harcourt Brace Jovanovich, Publishers
New York   London   Paris
San Diego   San Francisco   São Paulo   Sydney   Tokyo   Toronto

ACADEMIC PRESS, INC.
111 Fifth Avenue, New York, New York 10003

United Kingdom Edition published by
ACADEMIC PRESS, INC. (LONDON) LTD.
24/28 Oval Road, London NW1 7DX

LIBRARY OF CONGRESS CATALOG CARD NUMBER: 82-11358

ISBN: 0-12-788284-7

PRINTED IN THE UNITED STATES OF AMERICA

82 83 84 85   9 8 7 6 5 4 3 2 1

Contents

Foreword

Among the earliest antecedents to our modern intensive care units was a three-bed neurosurgical postoperative recovery unit formed by Dandy in 1923 at the Johns Hopkins Hospital.* This unit was based on the need for continuous observation and nursing management directed toward airway-ventilation maintenance in postoperative patients. Dandy's unit opened because he recognized that care of the neurosurgical patient required more than a good operation. As increasingly complex surgical procedures emerged, the need for close postoperative observation was substantiated. Postanesthesia recovery rooms were established. Soon a cadre of recovery room nurses developed. It was only a matter of time before their talents were put to use in patients requiring prolonged periods of intensive "recovery room care."

World War II created the need to develop specialized shock units for battlefield and civilian mass casualties. Thus, the concept that the sickest patients should be isolated under the care of more expert nurses was established.† Following this concept, victims of the poliomyelitis epidemics of the early 1950s were placed in centralized units. There followed rapid development of respiratory care techniques, which form the foundations of modern intensive care.* Soon thereafter, coronary care units came into being and by the end of that decade, evidence accrued indicating that respiratory and cardiac intensive care lessened mortality from life-threatening diseases.

These results inevitably led to the opening of other intensive care facilities such as the neonatal intensive care nursery, dialysis and burn units, trauma centers and neurologic intensive care units. Unfortunately, such balkanization of intensive care is

---

*Hilberman, M.: The evolution of intensive care units. *Critical Care Medicine* 3:159-165, 1975.

†Shoemaker, W.C.: The changing ICU. *Critical Care Medicine* 1:92, 1973.

often dictated more by local hospital politics than by the efficient delivery of safe care. These isolated pockets of intensive care expertise may actually inhibit progress in intensive care delivery and research. This course and volume are major steps in redirecting the care of the acutely ill neurosurgical patient into coordinated multidisciplinary pathways. Rather than isolate these patients and their problems, the organizers of the course sought input from general surgeons, internists, neurologists, neurosurgeons, anesthesiologists and nurses. As the following brief history of the development of neurologic intensive care will show, progress in this field has occurred most rapidly where multidisciplinary input has been amalgamated into patient care.

One of the cornerstones of progress in intensive care has been based upon technological development on life-support and monitoring systems. Enhanced monitoring capabilities, coupled with physician input, have done much to facilitate the recruitment of expert nursing personnel to the neurologic intensive care unit. Retention of these specialized nurses is central to running a neurologic intensive care facility. In fact, it was the shortage of adequately prepared nurses in community hospitals that gave the greatest postwar impetus to the growth of the modern intensive care unit. In order to keep up with the demand for nurses knowledgeable in complex technological and monitoring developments, the sickest patients were concentrated into a central facility. Only belatedly did the large teaching hospitals recognize the success of the intensive care unit in community hospitals.*

The modern neurologic intensive care environment is based upon developments in other specialized care units. These efforts have given us mechanical ventilation techniques, blood gas measurement and cardiovascular support protocols. Based upon these therapeutic modalities, the neuro-intensivists have introduced their specialized techniques: (1) intracranial pressure (ICP) monitoring; (2) cerebral blood flow-metabolism determination; (3) continuous EEG assessment; (4) multimodal evoked potential measurement; and (5) computed transmission and emission tomography. The basics of the application and use of these powerful tools in life-threatening neurologic diseases are critically discussed in this volume.

---

*Shoemaker, op. cit.

These methods now permit rational application of therapies based upon manipulations of ICP and cerebral blood flow-metabolism. In the absence of the specialized neurologic intensive care environments, novel concepts, such as the use of barbiturates for ICP and metabolic control, could not be safely or critically evaluated. Experience with barbiturates thus far has led some to believe that some CNS depression may actually be of benefit during acute intracranial disease. This goes against the old concepts that these CNS drug depressants should never be given to patients with neurologic dysfunction. Current neurologic monitoring techniques have also improved the margin of safety, as well as the rational base for application of osmotherapy, hyperventilation, positive-end-expiratory pressure (PEEP), diuretics and muscle relaxants. Older concepts concerning optimal patient positioning have only recently been confirmed. The danger of administering repetitive noxious stimulation in order to perform neurologic evaluation in comatose patients has been demonstrated. Less dangerous electroneurophysiologic techniques are emerging which can be substituted for the former. These advances are only the tip of the iceberg in terms of improved therapeutic specificity for patients with acute neurologic dysfunction.

Delivery of intensive care is exceedingly expensive and control of these costs is complex. Identification of patients who will not benefit from intensive care will increase the cost effectiveness. Along these lines, we have witnessed development of prognostic indices such as the Glasgow Coma Scale. This clinical scale, in combination with modern neurologic monitoring techniques, should greatly improve selection of patients who would benefit most from modern neurological intensive care techniques.

I look toward a future filled with challenges for neurointensivists. We will be called upon to initially evaluate a large number of drugs with putative specific neuroresuscitative actions. We will have to be selective in evaluating new neurodiagnostic and monitoring modalities. Presently the spectrum of gadgets offered to us is dazzling. Only through careful selection can we protect the neuro-ICU from becoming a storehouse for mounds of electronic gear. Our goal of improved cost-effective care can be achieved only by active communica-

tion among those with diverse backgrounds and a shared
interest in patients with acute neurologic disease.

Harvey Shapiro, M.D.

Preface

As the discipline of Critical Care Medicine developed as a unique specialty, it became apparent to these co-editors that a significant gap of knowledge existed with regard to information related to neurological disorders. The result of these discussions was the first conference on Intensive Care for Neurological Disease and Trauma held in Miami, Florida. Following a most positive response from attendees including physicians from many related disciplines and from critical care nurses, it was decided to continue this concept as an annual course with both the East Coast and West Coast seminars. This volume is the result of requests to the editors to make available a text based on information provided at the first course. Those who were present at that meeting will recognize that each lecturer has completely revised and expanded his presentation to include a more comprehensive analysis of his subject matter. This material is not being presented as a complete and final authority on the subject of Neuro-ICU but rather as a contemporary overview of this rapidly developing area of science and patient care. It is the opinion of these editors that the multidisciplinary team approach to the critical care of neurologically afflicted patients has resulted in and will continue to effect an improved patient outcome as reflected by a decrease in morbidity and mortality.

Barth A. Green, M.D.
Lawrence F. Marshall, M.D.
T. J. Gallagher, M.D.

Acknowledgments

The editors are grateful to the authors for the time and care invested in the preparation of their papers and are especially grateful to Dr. Harvey Shapiro, an internationally recognized authority on this subject, for his efforts in the preparation of the foreword of this volume. Recognition must be given to Dr. H. L. Rosomoff, a pioneer in neurological critical care, for his support of these seminars and the preparation of this volume. The person primarily responsible for the success of this course was Mrs. Betty Howard, Director of Continuing Medical Education at the University of Miami. A special thank you to Mrs. Elinor O'Neil, senior staff coordinator of the Department of Neurosurgery, who spent many hours dealing with the countless details associated with the preparation and review of these manuscripts. Gratitude also goes to Mimi Hochberg, who has shown a degree of patience, persistence and understanding far beyond the call of duty. Finally, we the editors will dedicate this text to our main energy source, our wives and children, without whose indulgence and support this publication would remain "just a good idea"!

Emergency Medical Services and the Pre-Hospital Care of Spinal Cord Injuries

Barth A. Green, M.D., K. John Klose, Ph.D. and James T. O'Heir

Objectives

1. To present an introduction to the general concept and constitution of Emergency Medical Services in the United States.
2. To present a brief overview of the problem of neurological trauma.
3. To present the accident scene management protocol for acute spinal cord injury as a model to other forms of trauma system pre-hospital care.
4. To present pre-hospital assessment forms for spinal cord and head injury.

Introduction

Modern Emergency Medical Services in the United States evolved as a result of the now-classic white paper, "Accidental Death and Disability — The Neglected Disease of Modern Society," released by the National Academy of Sciences — National Research Council Committee on Shock and Committee on Trauma in 1966. This document drew attention to the severe deficiencies existing in emergency medical care and served as a catalyst for a series of events directed toward the improvement of the care of trauma victims. It stimulated pas-

Barth A. Green, M.D., K. John Klose, Ph.D. and James T. O'Heir, Department of Neurological Surgery, University of Miami School of Medicine, Fla.

This work is supported in part by the National Institutes of Health, NINCDS #NS14468 and Rehabilitative Services Administration #13-P-59258.

1

sage of the National Highway Safety Act of 1966 and the Emergency Medical Services Systems Act of 1973.

By far, the most important legislation regarding Emergency Medical Services was the Emergency Medical Services Act of 1973 (PL 93-154) and the amendment of 1976 (PL94-573). This statute, as amended, instructed the Department of Health, Education and Welfare (DHEW) to designate a lead agency, the Division of Emergency Medical Services (DEMS), to provide program administration, technical assistance, informational programs, award grants and coordinate an interagency committee on Emergency Medical Services. Further, it provided the mechanism and funding for communities to develop their own Regional Emergency Medical Services delivery systems.

Emergency Medical Services Systems center around the 15 components identified by Congress in the Emergency Medical Services Systems Act. These components are:

1. Manpower
2. Training
3. Communication Systems
4. Transportation
5. Facilities
6. Critical Care Units
7. Public Safety Agency Utilization
8. Consumer Participation
9. Accessibility
10. Patient Transfer Mechanisms
11. Coordinated Medical Record Keeping
12. Public Information & Education
13. Independent Review & Evaluation
14. Disaster Planning
15. Mutual Aid Agreements

These components, therefore, provide Emergency Medical Services physicians, planners and administrators with specific organizational structures and evaluation mechanisms. In addition to these components, seven critical patient groups have been identified and include:

1. Major Trauma
2. Burn Injuries
3. Spinal Cord Injuries

4. Poisoning & Overdoses
5. High-Risk Infants
6. Acute Cardiac Emergencies
7. Behavioral & Psychiatric Emergencies

These seven groups were selected, since they represent the major categories of emergency medical problems. They are also easily identified and useful in planning operational and evaluation models. These "most critical" patients benefit from a systems approach that addresses their specific requirements. The systems care developed for these categories may then be applied to other emergency patients with injuries or illnesses of a less severe nature or those more difficult to identify.

As for the future, it has been proposed that ten centers be established, one in each of the major DHEW regions. These "centers of excellence" typically would be situated in a major medical center and would be responsible to:

1. Describe and establish the dimension and parameters of EMS problems in a variety of settings: rural, metropolitan, wilderness.
2. Establish a commitment by the health care delivery and academic community to better understand the EMS problem.
3. Provide input as to better utilization of technology and limited resources.
4. Provide input for improved system development.
5. Provide input into the development of model programs of public education and prevention — the ultimate goal.

The necessity of a continued emphasis on Emergency Medical Services is best described by the following tables:

1976

| Motor Vehicle Deaths | 46,700 | All Accidental Deaths | 100,000 |

1977

| Motor Vehicle Deaths | 49,510 | All Accidental Deaths | 103,202 |

1978

| Motor Vehicle Deaths | 51,500 | All Accidental Deaths | 104,500 |

During the period of August 1964 to January 1973, there were 46,572 combat deaths reported in Viet Nam. Annually, by vehicular fatalities alone, we exceed 8½ years of combat fatalities. Accidental injuries in 1978 resulted in $19.3 billion in lost wages, $9.9 billion of which were vehicular-related injuries.

There were 7,560,000 head injuries reported in the United States during the calendar year 1976. Of these, 1,255,000 were classified as major head injuries. One quarter of all trauma deaths occur as a result of head injury, and brain injury has been demonstrated in 75% of the victims of fatal road accidents.

The National Data Center for Spinal Cord Injuries reports upon data received from 14 spinal cord injury centers throughout the United States. Based upon these data, extrapolations indicate an approximate incidence rate of 35 spinal cord injuries per million population. The data also indicate that approximately 13% of these spinal cord injury victims also sustain head injury.

Spinal cord injury system care, including pre-hospital management, is relatively advanced when compared to other categories of EMS programs. For this reason, these programs have served as a model for other forms of trauma and will be presented in great detail in the remainder of this paper. The majority of principles of identification and accident scene management of these injuries can be applied to head injuries, since they are often associated with one another and cannot be easily recognized, especially in the comatose patient. Further discussion of pre-hospital management of head injuries will be presented in Marshall's paper on head injury elsewhere in this volume.

All hospital physicians and allied health personnel dealing with spinal cord injuries should realize the important role that their pre-hospital colleagues play in the health care delivery system with regard to the spinal cord injury victim. The following treatment protocol includes the diagnosis and stabilization of the spinal cord injury victim at the accident scene and transport to the hospital. Many of the concepts presented hereafter are considered controversial and represent the opinions and experience of these authors.

Accident Scene Management and Emergency Medical Services

At the scene of an accident, the initial consideration is recognition of the patient with a spinal cord injury. The following list includes the most significant signs seen with acute spinal cord injuries.

1. Motor signs: weakness or paralysis of extremities and/or trunk muscles.

2. Sensory signs: absence or alteration of sensation of trunk and/or extremities.

3. Incontinence: loss of control of bladder and/or bowels.

4. Superficial signs: abrasians, lacerations or deformities of the spine, neck or head regions.

5. Pain: tenderness or pain on palpation of the spine or neck. The patient's neck or back should not be moved to determine if it is painful, it should only be palpated.

6. Any unconscious patient must be considered to have a spinal cord or spinal column injury until proven otherwise.

7. An injury to other systems (e.g., head injury) may mask a spinal cord injury; conversely, a spinal cord injury can mask other system injuries (e.g., visceral rupture or fracture of long bones).

Once the accident victim has been identified as a possible spinal column or spinal cord injury, the following priorities should be followed:

Respiratory

A. *Placement of an appropriate, secure airway.*

In an awake patient, to prevent gagging use a bite stick, i.e., a cut-off standard oral airway or a tongue blade wrapped in tape. In an unconscious patient, a full standard oral airway should be inserted or, optimally, an EOA (esophageal obturator) should be utilized. The airway should always be taped to prevent loss in case of emesis or seizure or a combative patient. If emesis occurs, an infant bulb syringe with the tip cut off is of benefit for removing stomach contents or blood clots. Standard suction tubing is still necessary for deeper respiratory tree toilet. The neck should never be moved out of a neutral position in order to establish an airway in any patient suspected of having a spinal injury.

If the insertion of an airway does not by itself result in effective ventilation, as determined by bilateral auscultation of the lungs, then the patient should be intubated. If intubation is necessary, the use of an EOA (i.e., pharyngeal intubation) is preferable at the accident scene because of the comparative ease of placement without the need to hyperextend the head or neck. Such equipment is now standard in all paramedic rescue kits.

B. *Artificial assistance.*

If the patient for any reason has insufficient respiratory excursions, then ambu-bagging should be immediately initiated. Such insufficient respiration commonly occurs because of paralysis of intercostal muscles and/or diaphragmatic muscles, or from direct trauma to the rib cage or lungs. Other signs of respiratory distress may include cyanosis or excessive retraction of accessory neck muscles associated with respiratory efforts.

C. *Proper environment.*

Patients with spinal cord injuries should receive oxygen supplementation at all times during the accident scene management and transportation. This should be administered via nasal cannula or O_2 mask. Often, a patient with a spinal cord injury may appear to be breathing adequately, but on admission to a hospital baseline arterial blood gases may be far below acceptable levels. An arterial blood gas PO_2 in the 60 to 70 range or a PCO_2 of 50 may be acceptable in a patient with a chronic spinal cord injury, but in the acutely injured individual, one should maintain a minimum PO_2 value of at least 100 and a PCO_2 of less than 45. These levels should be maintained because of the compromised blood supply and disrupted tissue metabolism well documented in acutely traumatized spinal cords. The presence of smoke or noxious gases at the accident scene further necessitates the immediate use of such a controlled environment.

Cardiovascular

A. *Stop active hemorrhage.*

Significant bleeding points should be treated with appropriate pressure dressings. Penetrating objects to the neck or spinal region should not be removed until the patient is in the hospital and blood transfusions and ORs are available. If objects are too long or too large to allow effective patient handling, they may be shortened to a length of several inches from the point of entry. Control of hemorrhage from spinal or neck bleeding sites should be by "localized pressure" rather than any form of circumferential dressing. A large bore intravenous line should be started on all spinal cord injury patients and Ringer's lactate solution infused.

B. *External cardiac massage when necessary.*

Immediate reestablishment of circulation to the neural structures is of critical importance in any effort directed toward salvage of neurological function. In certain cases, defibrillation is necessary as determined by the EKG tracing obtained by the paramedic and by ongoing consultation with the ER physician. Various cardiogenic drugs may be administered when indicated, depending upon the EKG and other cardiovascular parameters.

C. *Treat shock.*

Spinal cord injured patients may present with neurogenic shock, hemorrhagic shock or a combination of both. In most cases one or the other type is clinically predominant. In either case there is a low blood pressure and a relatively low body temperature. The key to the differential diagnosis is the brady-cardia (usually a pulse below 60) in neurogenic shock and the relative tachycardia (usually a pulse above 100) in hemorrhagic shock. The nature of the pulse is usually slow and regular in neurogenic shock patients, in contrast to the rapid irregular pulse noted in cases of hemorrhagic shock. Neurogenic shock is associated with a loss of sympathetic nervous system control of the peripheral vascular tone in the extremities resulting in pooling of blood and inadequate central blood return to maintain sufficient cardiovascular function. The bradycardia is due to the loss of sympathetic inhibition of the parasympathetic effects of the vagus nerve. Patients in neurogenic shock usually present with a systolic blood pressure of approximately 70 mm Hg or lower and a pulse below 60. The quickest and most effective treatment for either type of shock is placing the patient in a Trendelenburg position of 30 to 40 degrees which immediately decreases the lower extremity blood pooling and increases the central return of blood. The effect of the Tren-

delenburg position may be complemented by use of a MAST
suit to collapse the lower extremity and abdominal vasculature.
These suits must be used with caution in cases of suspected
lumbar or thoracolumbar junction fractures, because they may
aggravate the neurological injury in cases of severe spinal disruption and instability. Shock suits are not only being carried in
ambulances, but are also being used in many ICUs across the
country. The more specific treatment for hemorrhagic shock is
fluid replacement utilizing blood and volume expanders.
Specific treatment of neurogenic shock at the accident scene
after decreasing peripheral pooling by positioning and/or the
use of a shock suit should include the administration of 0.4 mg
of atropine intravenously to help block the dominant vagal
effect (i.e., bradycardia). This is only a temporary measure, but
most often will result in an increase in the pulse rate, resulting
in an increased cardiac output during the brief period it takes a
patient to arrive at a hospital where cardiac index parameters
can be monitored with the use of a Swan-Ganz catheter. The
overriding consideration must be to maintain perfusion of vital
organs including the spinal cord during the early minutes and
hours following injury. Caution must be used in delivering fluids
to patients in neurogenic shock in contrast to patients in hypovolemic or hemorrhagic shock. In neurogenic shock there is
usually sufficient blood volume, but a problem exists in distribution of fluids. Large increases in volume may cause the
patient to develop cardiogenic failure, i.e., trading off one
problem for another.

Splinting the Patient

Regardless of the posture in which they are found following
injury, all patients should be placed in a neutral supine position
and splinted from the top of the head to the bottom of the
buttocks. This can often be accomplished simultaneously with
assessment and stabilization of respiratory and cardiovascular
parameters by accident scene personnel working together on all
priorities. It has been estimated that as many as 20% of spinal
injuries involve multiple levels which is why the entire spinal
column must be immobilized. The best method for splinting is
using plywood half- and full-length boards. Three-inch tape
should be placed over the forehead with sandbags on either side
of the head and neck. The tape over the forehead minimizes the

chances of cervical displacement. If sandbags are not available, rolled towels or blankets may be used. If tape is not available, ropes or belts may be substituted. If plywood boards are not available, a door from a nearby house or a seat removed from a car may be substituted.

A new air vacuum splint developed in France is now available and is an excellent immobilizing device. It is capable of immobilizing the patient supine, with versatility for individual characteristics of anatomy, i.e., kyphoscoliosis or other deformities, that in rare cases make the use of a standard spine board difficult and ineffective.

The use of scoop stretchers is prohibited because they are open in the center at a point where the spine requires the most support. Towels, blankets or pillows should not be placed below the neck or back because they can further aggravate spinal column deformity and result in secondary injury. If patients are found in the prone position or on their side, it is best to use a log roll maneuver to attain the desired neutral supine position.

Other methods, although less preferable, include a lift accomplished by a minimum of four persons or a scooting maneuver which can be used for sliding a patient up onto a cart when a board is not available. In both cases, at least one rescuer should be primarily responsible for immobilizing the head and neck in a neutral position, i.e., neither flexed, extended or rotated. It should be emphasized, again, that the log roll maneuver causes the least distortion of the spinal column. If a patient is already supine and must be placed on a splint, they may be log rolled on their side, and then back down onto the splint.

Once the patient is on a board or appropriate splint in a neutral position, the hands and feet must be tethered together to prevent them from falling off the board or cart and suffering injury. A strap or tape should be placed loosely over the chest (to prevent compromise of respirations) and more firmly around the pelvis, knees and ankles. If possible, a foot board is applied and, if not, the feet are taped to prevent sliding towards the foot of the board. The sandbags prevent slippage toward the head.

Extrication and Transportation

When moving a patient to a neutral position, the head must not be left in flexion, extension or rotation. With very gentle traction with hands locked under the jaw and neck, the patient's head and neck should be placed in alignment with the axis of the body. As long as the neutral position is not surpassed, no further damage to the spinal cord will occur with this maneuver. Traction with weights should never be applied at the accident scene. There is the danger of overdistraction in cases of severe spinal column disruption, which could result in secondary injury with aggravation of neurological deficit. Chin straps are discouraged because of problems with airway access, especially in cases of emesis when a patient with mouth held tightly shut might be at high risk for aspiration.

The use of soft or rigid cervical collars in the immobilization of these patients should be avoided. These devices can give the rescuer and the victim a false sense of security. If stressed, they allow extension, flexion or rotation of the neck with only minimal movement restriction. In addition, a relatively inelastic collar may act as a tourniquet to the neck which inevitably responds to trauma with swelling. Such constriction may compromise blood and air flow. The collars may also shield from view a previously unidentified site of venous or arterial hemorrhage, i.e., an expanding hematoma, or mask a ruptured trachea and the development of subcutaneous emphysema. In addition, the application of these devices may result in a greater deformity of the neck associated with increased neurological deficit.

Emergency medical care should be administered to any significant associated injury for temporary stabilization before a patient is moved.

The two most frequent causes of death in the pre-hospital phase are *aspiration* and *shock*. In extricating and transporting patients with spinal cord injuries or at high risk for such, all of the above described priorities must be adhered to, but are ineffective without the most important ingredient, *common sense*. No two patients present with identical symptoms or injury characteristics and rarely are two extrication problems the same. We have found that the combination of personnel with good training plus common sense gives any rescue attempt the most merit.

In order to minimize the chances of aspiration or shock regardless of etiology, we recommend that all spinal cord injury patients (or head injury patients with possible spinal cord injuries) be transported splinted supine in a Trendelenburg (head down) position with 30 to 40 degrees of tilt. The more extreme tilt should be used only if the systolic blood pressure drops below 70 mm Hg. If a patient vomits while at this angle, the emesis will more likely follow gravity and come out of the nose and mouth. (This is why it is imperative to keep the airway accessible and clear at all times.) In cases of interhospital transfer of spinal cord injuries, a nasogastric (sump) tube should be inserted and stomach contents emptied. During transportation, the nasogastric tubing should be left open to gravity drainage. These steps can often prevent the dire consequences of aspiration in spinal cord injured patients who often have associated respiratory system compromise. It must be noted that there is a significant incidence of vomiting in patients transported by ambulance and an even higher incidence in patients transported by either helicopter or fixed wing aircraft.

It is imperative that a specially trained paramedic attend each patient at the accident scene and in transit to the hospital to insure that all high priority measures are employed with these critically injured victims. Although speed of extrication and transportation are important factors, they must not be placed as a priority above the principles discussed in the preceding paragraphs. The emphasis must be placed on getting an *alive* patient to the ER with all systems stabilized to permit the potential for maximum neurological recovery. The choice of ambulance, helicopter or fixed wing transportation must depend upon availability of equipment, distance to be covered, geographical location, time of day, traffic, weather and the general physical and neurological status of the patient. Often, a combination of these vehicles in a well-coordinated effort provides an optimal emergency evacuation.

Equally important is a refined communications system allowing consultation between the primary accident scene rescue crew and the nearest trauma center and/or spinal cord injury center. It is almost impossible to monitor vital signs in an ambulance and even more difficult with the noise and vibrations of a helicopter or fixed wing aircraft. Recent development of small portable Doppler stethoscopes makes the monitoring of both the blood pressure and pulse feasible during transportation.

Communications between accident scene personnel and in-hospital team members allows the mobilization of appropriate ER equipment and staff, as well as radiological, surgical and intensive care facilities required for optimal diagnostic and therapeutic regimens. In most cases, it is desirable to transport the patient to the nearest designated ER, where appropriate first aid, diagnosis and further stabilization can be accomplished. Then, when appropriate, a timely secondary transfer to a spinal cord injury center should be initiated. If a spinal cord injury center is readily accessible, the patient should be transported directly to the center.

These authors recommend timely transfer to a spinal cord injury center because of the multidisciplinary team of physicians and allied health personnel who staff such a center. These teams are committed to provide a comprehensive systems approach (i.e., beginning at the accident scene including acute care, rehabilitation and, finally, lifelong follow-up). It is also these authors' opinion that such a system (because of their volume experience and total commitment) can provide optimal care for the spinal cord injured.

Pre-hospital assessment forms for spinal cord and head injury are presented in Figures 1-4.

Summary

These authors have presented specific guidelines for the identification and management of spinal cord injuries from the moment of trauma until the arrival at the first receiving hospital. Rarely have pre-hospital interventions in any disease or traumatic state been considered to play such an important role as in the acute spinal cord injured patient. It has been well documented that the first moments, minutes and hours are most significant in the eventual neurological outcome of each patient. It is these authors' hope that further research in this phase of care will continue. All neurosurgeons, neurologists, orthopedic surgeons and other physicians and allied health personnel dealing with these injuries should give the EMS systems the greatest degree of support, locally and nationally, with regard to participation in personnel training as well as in programs of public education and safety. Such efforts will result in an optimal patient care experience in which pre-hospital treat-

UNIVERSITY OF MIAMI
DEPARTMENT OF NEUROLOGICAL SURGERY
CNS TRAUMA RESEARCH

SITE OF INJURY MOTOR ASSESSMENT

NAME_____

EXAMINER_____

DATE OF ASSESSMENT_____

    CODE - Present = 3 Normal strength & range of motion
            Abnormal= 2 Weak strength, flicker of muscle or loss of range of motion
            Absent = 1 No motion

This exam is to be done only with the patient in a neutral supine position!!

                                                      L   R

SHOULDER ELEVATION..(Shrug shoulders)..................................... (10-11)

ELBOW FLEXORS.......(Bend elbow).. (12-13)

ELBOW EXTENSORS.....(Straighten elbow).................................... (14-15)

WRIST EXTENSORS.....(As though raising hand to stop traffic).............. (16-17)

INTEROSSEI..........(With hand & fingers flat spread and close fingers)... (18-19)

UPPER ABDOMINALS....(Ask patient to tighten stomach muscles, then feel)... (20-21)

LOWER ABDOMINALS....(Ask patient to tighten stomach muscles, then feel)... (22-23)

HIP FLEXORS.........(Raise knee to chest)................................. (24-25)

KNEE FLEXORS........(Tester raise thigh, ask patient to bend knee)........ (26-27)

KNEE EXTENSORS......(Tester raise thigh, ask patient to straighten knee).. (28-29)

FOOT FLEXORS........(Point toe as in stepping on gas).................... (30-31)

FOOT DORSI-FLEXORS..(Opposite of above; ankle up)........................ (32-33)

FOR OFFICE USE ONLY

CARD #'s... (1-2)........ (1-2)

                           Assessment #_____

HOSPITAL ID........................(both cards)...... (3-4)

PATIENT #..........................(both cards)...... (5-9)

FIGURE 1.

UNIVERSITY OF MIAMI
DEPARTMENT OF NEUROLOGICAL SURGERY
CNS TRAUMA RESEARCH

SITE OF INJURY SENSORY ASSESSMENT

NAME_____
EXAMINER_____
DATE OF ASSESSMENT_____

This exam is to be done only with the
patient in a neutral supine position!
USE A PIN PRICK

(CODE: 0=Absent 1=Present)

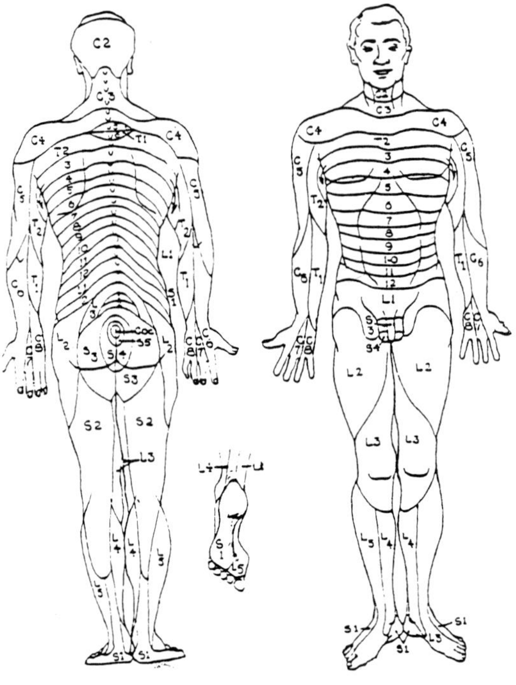

	Left	Right	
-C2			(16-17)
-C3			(18-19)
-C4			(20-21)
-C5			(22-23)
-C6			(24-25)
-C7			(26-27)
-C8			(28-29)
-T1			(30-31)
-T2			(32-33)
-T3			(34-35)
-T4			(36-37)
-T5			(38-39)
-T6			(40-41)
-T7			(42-43)
-T8			(44-45)
-T9			(46-47)
-T10			(48-49)
-T11			(50-51)
-T12			(52-53)
-L1			(54-55)
-L2			(56-57)
-L3			(58-59)
-L4			(60-61)
-L5			(62-63)
-S1			(64-65)
-S2			(66-67)
-S3			(68-69)
-S4			(70-71)
-S5			(72-73)
-C01			(74-75)

FOR OFFICE USE ONLY

CARD #'s.. (1-2)........ (1-2)
Assessment #_____

HOSPITAL ID...........................(both cards)...... (3-4)
PATIENT #.............................(both cards)...... (5-9)

FIGURE 2.

HEAD INJURY ASSESSMENT
UNIVERSITY OF MIAMI
DEPARTMENT OF NEUROLOGICAL SURGERY
CNS TRAUMA RESEARCH

GLASCOW COMA SCALE

(FOR CATEGORIES I, II AND III - CIRCLE 1 RESPONSE)

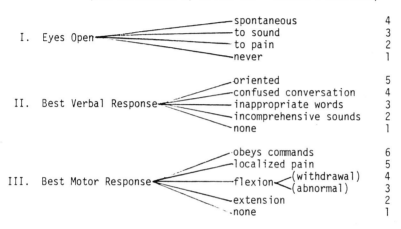

I.	Eyes Open	spontaneous	4
		to sound	3
		to pain	2
		never	1
II.	Best Verbal Response	oriented	5
		confused conversation	4
		inappropriate words	3
		incomprehensive sounds	2
		none	1
III.	Best Motor Response	obeys commands	6
		localized pain	5
		flexion (withdrawal)	4
		(abnormal)	3
		extension	2
		none	1

P U P I L S

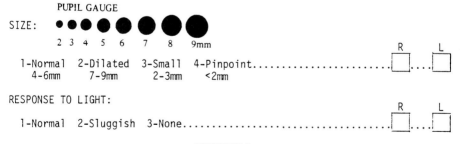

PUPIL GAUGE

SIZE: ● ● ● ● ● ● ●
        2 3 4 5 6 7 8 9mm

1-Normal   2-Dilated   3-Small   4-Pinpoint....................... R   L
 4-6mm   7-9mm   2-3mm   <2mm

RESPONSE TO LIGHT: R   L

1-Normal   2-Sluggish   3-None.................................

FIGURE 3.

GLASCOW COMA SCALE

To assess a patient by use of the Glascow Coma Scale proceed according to the following definitions:

I. Eye Opening

    A. <u>Spontaneous</u> - sleep/wake rhythms present, arousal does not imply awareness. Scored as 4 points (pts)

    B. <u>To Sound</u> - response to any verbal approach, not necessarily command to open eyes. (3 pts.)

    C. <u>To Pain</u> - tested by stimulus to limbs. (2 pts.)

    D. <u>Never</u> - (1 pt.)

II. Best Verbal Response

    A. <u>Oriented</u> - patient knows name, place, why he is there, month and year. (5 pts)

    B. <u>Confused Conversation</u> - patient's attention can be held, he responds in a conversational manner but shows confusion or disorientation. (4 pts.)

    C. <u>Inappropriate Words</u> - no sustained conversation, speech is exclamatory, random, usually swearing or shouting. (3 pts.)

    D. <u>Incomprehensible Speech</u> - moaning, groaning - no recognizable words. (2 pts.)

    E. <u>None</u> - (1 pt.)

III. Best Motor Response

    A. <u>Obeys Commands</u> - self-explanatory (do not use hand grasp due to possible misinterpretation of grasp reflex). As patient to "stick out tongue", "left arm", "open, close eyes." (6 pts.)

    B. <u>Localizes Pain</u> - apply pain to arms not legs. (It is possible to elecit reflexive responses in the legs). Apply pain to nail beds, if arm flexes, then apply a series of stimuli to head and neck area. If patient attempts to remove stimulus he is localizing the pain. (5 pts.)

    C. <u>Flexion Withdrawal</u> - a rapid, more appropriate response to pain associated adduction of the shoulder. (4 pts.)

    D. <u>Flexion Abnormal</u> - a slower response to pain with adduction of the shoulder including decorticate posturing. (3 pts.)

    E. <u>Extension</u> - an obviously abnormal response to pain associated with adduction and internal rotation of shoulder and pronation of the forearm. Included at this level would be decerebrate posturing as a response to pain. (2 pts.)

    F. <u>None</u> - (1 pt.)

FIGURE 4.

ment will complement acute medical and surgical care, rehabilitation and the lifelong follow-up components of the systems.

Bibliography

Benes, V.: Spinal Cord Injury. Baltimore, Williams and Wilkens, 1978.

Ducker, T.B. and Perot, P.L.: National Spinal Cord Injury Registry. Charleston, S.C.:Division of Neurosurgery , Med. University of South Carolina.

Hall, W.J., Green, B.A. and Colandonato, J.P.: Spinal cord injury: Emergency management. Emergency Medical Services 5: May-June 1976.

Young, J.S. and Northrup, N.E.: Statistical information pertaining to some of the most commonly asked questions about spinal cord injury. SCI Dig. 1:11-33, 1979.

Self-Evaluation Quiz

1. Signs of a potential spinal cord injury at the accident scene include the following:
   1. Motor deficit
   2. Sensory deficit
   3. Incontinence of bowel and/or bladder
   4. Unconscious patient
   5. Superficial abrasions, lacerations and/or deformities of neck or spinal area
   a) 1 and 3
   b) 1, 2 and 3
   c) 2 and 5
   d) All of the above
   e) None of the above

2. The three major priorities in accident scene management of a possible spinal cord injury include:
   1. Respiratory system stabilization
   2. Cardiovascular system stabilization
   3. Urological system stabilization
   4. Spinal column immobilization
   5. Splinting distal extremity fractures
   a) 1, 2 and 5
   b) 1, 2 and 3
   c) 1, 3 and 5
   d) 2, 4 and 5
   e) 1, 2 and 4

3. The two major causes of death in the pre-hospital phase of managing a spinal cord injury victim are:
   1. Fat emboli and atelectasis
   2. Pneumothorax and hemothorax
   3. Aspiration and shock
   4. Shock and arrhythmia
   5. Pulmonary emboli and hypoxia
   a) 1
   b) 2
   c) 3
   d) 4
   e) 5

4. Neurogenic shock is characterized by:
   1. Tachycardia, hypotension, hypothermia
   2. Bradycardia, hypothermia, hypotension
   3. Bradycardia, hyperthermia, hypotension
   4. Tachycardia, hyperthermia, hypotension
   5. Bradycardia, hypertension, hypothermia
   a) 1
   b) 2
   c) 3
   d) 4
   e) 5

5. Neurogenic shock results from loss of:
   1. Sympathetic system control mechanism
   2. Parasympathetic system control mechanism
   3. Cervical or upper thoracic spinal cord injury
   4. Mid to lower thoracic spinal cord injury
   5. Peripheral nerve control mechanism
   a) 1 and 3
   b) 2 and 3
   c) 1 and 4
   d) 2 and 4
   e) 4 and 5

6. Appropriate accident scene management of neurogenic shock may include:
   1. MAST suit
   2. Atropine
   3. Digitalis
   4. Trendelenburg position
   5. Reverse Trendelenburg position

a) 1, 3 and 4
b) 2, 3 and 4
c) 1, 2 and 5
d) 1, 2 and 4
e) 1, 3 and 5

7. Patients suspected of sustaining a spinal cord injury should be moved by:
1. Dead man's lift
2. Potato sack lift
3. Log roll maneuver
4. Six man lift
5. Sitting-up lift
a) 1
b) 2
c) 3
d) 4
e) 5

8. Patients suspected of having sustained a spinal cord injury should be:
1. Placed in the prone position
2. Placed in the supine position
3. Placed in the lateral decubitus position
4. Placed in the sitting position
5. Left in the position in which they were found
a) 1
b) 2
c) 3
d) 4
e) 5

9. Important considerations when planning transportation from the accident scene to the hospital or between hospitals include:
1. Vehicle and personnel resources
2. Patient's cardiopulmonary status
3. Traffic conditions
4. Weather conditions
5. Neurological status
a) 1 and 3
b) 1, 2 and 3
c) 1, 2, 3 and 4

    d) All of the above

    e) None of the above

10. Patients being transferred between hospitals should have:

    1. Oxygen

    2. Nasogastric tube

    3. Spine immobilized

    4. All records (x-rays, laboratory, ER, etc.)

    5. Intravenous line established

    6. Foley catheter inserted

    a) 1 and 3

    b) 2 and 4

    c) 3, 4 and 5

    d) All of the above

    e) None of the above

Answers on page 391.

Emergency Room Management for Neurological Trauma and Disease

Bernard Elser, M.D.

Objectives

1. To understand the role of the emergency department physician in evaluating and treating patients with neurological trauma and disease.
2. To review the mechanisms by which CNS trauma or disease produces neurological lesions and symptoms.
3. To understand the factors which may complicate the primary lesion.
4. To briefly review the emergency room diagnosis and treatment of these disorders.

The emergency room physician is usually the first doctor to see a patient with an obvious or occult neurological or neurosurgical problem. Even though this is also true for most other emergencies, in few other conditions are the initial clinical observations and therapeutic responses to them as critical in preventing transient deficits from progressing to permanent damage.

The birth of emergency medicine as a specialty was brought about by many factors, including the increased utilization by patient and physician alike of the emergency room with its diverse and extensive facilities for all types of real or imagined emergencies. As a result, the emergency room physician has developed expertise which cuts across classical specialty lines in order to be able to stabilize, diagnose and treat the myriad problems which may at any time present to the emergency room.

Bernard Elser, M.D., Associate Professor of Medicine, University of Miami School of Medicine; Medical Director, Emergency Room, Jackson Memorial Hospital, Miami, Fla.

Neurological and neurosurgical emergencies have frequently been a difficult problem for the nonspecialist. The complexity of the nervous system in association with its dominant position in determining the quality of life is probably the major factor in the sense of urgency which is experienced by most emergency room physicians when treating patients with these disorders and is probably also the major reason for the errors, both in commission as well as in omission, which occur in the treatment of these patients. Nevertheless, the large number of elderly patients in our society and the growing complexity of our way of life are rapidly increasing the number of patients who present to emergency rooms with neurological and/or neurosurgical problems. Therefore, emergency room physicians have been forced to develop a growing expertise in assessing, stabilizing and providing for the initial treatment of these patients.

What follows is an attempt to describe the role of the emergency physician and some of the clinical considerations in caring for patients with neurological and neurosurgical problems. The specialist provides the definitive diagnosis and ultimate treatment of these disorders. The initial evaluation, stabilization and disposition of these patients is the function of the emergency room physician.

Rather than review all the well-described classical disorders, their diagnosis and treatment, I thought it would be more appropriate in this setting to select several important concepts within this large area for review and special comment.

Diagnosis

A common presenting problem to the emergency room is the patient in coma, with or without focal neurological signs. The history and physical examination, combined with routine laboratory and radiological studies, are often sufficient to establish a working diagnosis. Another important diagnostic modality is the progression of clinical findings. For example, change in mental state with time is a very important clinical sign. However, the use of poorly defined terms in describing alterations of mental status such as obtunded, stuporous and even coma blunts this important diagnostic tool. These subjective words often prevent accurate description of the progression of a lesion and as a result interfere with the precise determination of the natural history of a disease entity and the results of therapy. A major improvement has been the recent development of the Glasgow Coma Scale (Table 1) which uses a few easily measured parameters of nervous system function to obtain an objective definition of the clinical state of a patient at a single point in time. As a result it is possible to achieve more precise determination of the progression of the disorder and the results of therapy. To be most effective, this evaluation must be initiated as early as possible, in the emergency room, or at the scene of the event.

Understanding the mechanism of brain injury in head trauma is often helpful in estimating the type and anatomical location of a resulting lesion. Additionally, this knowledge permits an understanding of some of the clinical manifestations in circumstances where there is progression of a lesion. To this end, it is useful to classify the head into four compartments: the brain, the extracellular space, the cerebrospinal fluid and the vascular space.

As a result of rapid accelerative and decelerative forces which may occur even in the absence of direct trauma, the brain invariably shifts around inside the head, rocking from side to side and back and forth while the inferior surface slides over the

Table 1. Glasgow Coma Scale

A. *Eyes open*	Spontaneous	4
	To sound	3
	To pain	2
	Never	1
B. *Best verbal response*	Oriented	5
	Confused conversation	4
	Inappropriate words	3
	Incomprehensive sounds	2
	None	1
C. *Best motor response*	Obeys commands	6
	Localized pain	5
	Flexion (withdrawal)	4
	Flexion (abnormal)	3
	Extension	2
	None	1
		3 – 15

G. Teasdale and B. Jennett, *Acta Neurochirurgica* 32:45-55, 1976.

rough orbital surfaces of the base of the skull. As a result one may see contusive injuries, particularly to the frontal and temporal lobes, while the occipital and parietal lobes, surrounded by relatively smooth skull, are less commonly affected by this mechanism. Another important consequence of this motion of the brain within the skull is the torsion and tugging on anchored structures such as the brain stem and superficial blood vessels. These forces may tear veins which bridge the cortex as well as the superior sagittal sinus and may lead to a subdural hemorrhage. Alternately, or concomitantly, there may be compression and dysfunction of the reticular activating system of the brain stem leading to alterations of the mental state.

The brain, encased in a rigid skull, will suffer when any one of the compartments of the brain is increased, either as a result of a hematoma or edema, and impinges upon or displaces another compartment. Initially there are compensatory forces which tend to minimize these effects. For example, a small amount of spinal fluid, blood or extracellular fluid can be squeezed out of the brain and intracranial vault and reduce the intracranial volume when one of the other compartments has increased. Finally, however, as the lesion progresses, compression of brain substance with its displacement into an area of lesser resistance (herniation) may occur. The resulting pressure and ischemic effects on structures such as the third nerve herald this ominous and progressive development. These may occur at variable times following the initial injury and lead to focal or systemic physical signs which, at least initially, may be reversible with adequate therapy.

The often quoted remark "a CT scan of the head is worth more than a roomful of neurologists," while acknowledging the great usefulness of this test in assessing neurological and neurosurgical disorders, minimizes the importance, speed and availability of the more classical methods for diagnosing these clinical problems. The pupils, their size and reaction to light, the level of consciousness, vital signs, activity of cranial nerves, normal and abnormal reflexes and the position and response of the extremities are very valuable in assessing function of the nervous system. Changes in any one of these parameters over a period of time are as important in evaluating progression of disease and effect of therapy as they are in diagnosing and localizing the disorder.

It is easy to direct all one's attention to the obvious injuries and miss less apparent, potentially more critical and urgent ones. Therefore, a rapid, but thorough systematic neurological examination must be completed together with a comprehensive systemic physical examination on all patients.

The level of consciousness, described objectively as noted above, should be frequently evaluated and may provide valuable information about the progression of the lesion.

Various patterns of abnormal vital signs, including blood pressure, pulse, respirations and temperature, may suggest a focal or diffuse neurological injury or give information about a systemic injury. A head injury, for example, may be associated with any one of several abnormal respiratory patterns. As intracranial pressure rises initial slowing of the respiratory rate may be noted, but as the pressure continues to rise, the rate may become rapid. On the other hand, a rapid respiratory rate may reflect a primary respiratory problem such as difficulty with oxygenation and/or ventilation or possibly draw attention to a metabolic disorder as the initiating or secondary event. Arterial blood gases and/or a set of electrolytes may differentiate those disorders; central nervous system causes of abnormal breathing patterns usually show "normal" blood gases assuming there is no associated primary respiratory injury, while metabolic causes of abnormal breathing patterns show abnormal blood gases in the form of hypoxemia, hypercarbia or electrolyte changes consistent with a metabolic acidosis.

The pulse rate is also an important physical sign, not only as an indication of extracranial injuries, i.e., hemorrhage or hypoxemia, but also as a result of its occasional inverse association with increased intracranial pressure producing bradycardia. As intracranial pressure continues to rise, or when associated with other extracranial injuries, the bradycardia will change to tachycardia and is frequently an ominous sign.

An elevated blood pressure may also indicate elevated intracranial pressure although it might reflect nothing more than anxiety or pain.

Evaluation of the function of the cranial nerves should be rapidly completed and assists in localizing lesions based on abnormalities or asymmetry of function. Stretch reflexes and the presence of abnormal reflexes or abnormal movements such as decerebrate or decorticate posturing should be noted. Pathological reflexes or other "unusual" actions such as yawning or hiccuping also suggest increasing intracranial pressure.

Assessing extremity function, both from the point of view of motor responses as well as sensory function, is helpful in noting paralysis or hemiplegia and, as a result, assists in localizing injuries within the brain or spinal cord.

The oculocephalic and oculovestibular reflexes provide valuable information about the function of the brain stem.

While these functions are important initially in assessing severity of injury and location, they may change at any time and indicate progression of the lesion or the effects of any therapy which might have been employed.

One of the more confusing situations, unfortunately all too frequent, is the patient who is brought into the emergency room comatose, unresponsive to verbal or painful stimuli and in whom there are signs — sometimes subtle, otherwise overt — of trauma. Determining whether this clinical state is the result of major trauma to the central nervous system (epidural hematoma, subdural hematoma, cerebral contusion, intracerebral hematoma) or a consequence of medically induced cause of coma (drug or alcohol overdose, postictal state, hypoglycemia, hypoxia, ischemia) is a confusing but critical determination. It is important to remember that up to 75% of all cases of coma admitted with an unknown etiology are the result of a metabolic or diffuse cerebral disorder rather than a structural lesion. Although there are few if any easily performed tests available within the emergency room which readily permit differentiation of these disorders, the pupils are a rapid and valuable guide. Because the pupillary pathways are relatively resistant to metabolic insult, the bilateral presence of the pupillary light reflex in the patient with coma is a very important sign which suggests a metabolic cause of the coma. In addition, because the areas in the brain stem controlling consciousness are contiguous to those controlling the pupillary light reflex, changes in the size and reactivity of the pupils are an important guide to the presence and location of brain stem lesions causing coma.

Even a unilaterally dilating pupil suggestive of herniation secondary to an expanding lesion, if still reactive to light, indicates potential reversibility of the lesion while demanding immediate attention and action.

As with all other physical signs, pupillary changes must be evaluated in conjunction with other neurological and systemic signs. An isolated pupillary finding may be due to direct trauma to the eye or may unknowingly have been present for a long period of time and may be far less significant.

While primary insult to the central nervous system may often be severe, secondary pathophysiological factors may at times accelerate the progression of the primary lesion. Hypoxemia, for example, is almost invariably present after most cerebral injuries and is a frequent cause of death. It results from a combination of factors including upper airway obstruction, injury to the central nervous system causing depression of ventilation, associated chest injuries and/or aspiration of secretions, blood or vomitus because of loss of gag reflex. As a result of these mechanisms, severe hypoxemia may occur, itself lead to cerebrovascular dilatation with edema and congestion of the vascular and extracellular spaces of the brain and further complicate or exacerbate the primary lesion.

Similar mechanisms cause hypercarbia and the resulting elevation of CO_2 is likewise a potent cerebral vasodilator and may worsen intracranial bleeding and pressure.

Acidosis, either respiratory in origin secondary to inadequate ventilation or metabolic as a result of systemic hypotension and the accumulation of lactate, also leads to vasodilatation of cerebral vessels and aggravation of any existing cerebral edema or bleeding.

Ventilation, oxygenation and tissue perfusion must therefore be stabilized and maintained as rapidly as possible in order to prevent any worsening of the original insult. Stabilization of vital functions and the assessment of the location and extent of any injuries are the most important functions of the emergency room physician when presented with a patient with signs or symptoms of a neurological or neurosurgical disorder.

The patient who has been the victim of a neurological or neurosurgical catastrophe frequently dies or suffers additional damage as a result of complications of factors outside the central nervous system. Hypoxia, for example, is probably one of the most common causes of death in patients with central nervous system disease or injury and may be the result of coma with inability to protect the airway, aspiration, associated chest injuries and/or loss of central control of respiration. As a result, the establishment of a secure airway with provision of adequate ventilation and oxygenation is probably the first and most urgent function of the emergency room physician in dealing with these patients.

The assessment and maintenance of adequate cardiovascular function is an equally urgent responsibility. Many patients who present with catastrophic neurological events or those with simultaneous chest injuries often have associated cardiovascular disease and the stabilization of this function is important in preventing additional insult or worsening of the initial disorder.

Signs of associated trauma, whether as a result of an initial medical problem (falling down after having suffered a syncopal episode or CVA) or when an injury is the initiating event, are not always readily apparent. A search for blood loss, occult trauma and other signs or causes of volume depletion should be rapidly undertaken. A patient with an isolated head injury generally does not present in shock and, when present, should initiate a thorough search for other associated injuries.

At times, even the most obvious head injury may in fact be of secondary urgency. The emergency room physician must search for and assess the extent and urgency of all the injuries in determining treatment priorities. A rapidly expanding epidural hematoma or major injuries to the cardiovascular system are examples of lesions which must be treated rapidly. It is the responsibility of the emergency room physician to determine treatment priorities and coordinate the efforts of the specialists and/or subspecialists in treating the entire patient.

The rapid and extensive growth of both laboratory and radiological means of assessing organs and systems has improved our accuracy in diagnosing various traumatic and medical disorders. Recent examples include Computerized Axial Tomography and its newer cousin, Positron-Emission Tomography. These methods permit reasonably accurate, noninvasive means of assessing many different disorders in areas heretofore inaccessible with the classical techniques. Unfortunately, all these methods require sophisticated devices and extensive time for completion. Nevertheless, they have revolutionalized the diagnosis of neurological and neurosurgical disorders and should be used to diagnose and more accurately localize lesions. Their greatest danger lies in the speed that is sometimes exercised to use these tests before appropriate stabilization of vital functions and a rapid physical assessment of the entire patient is completed.

Self-Evaluation Quiz

1. In any group of unselected patients who present to an emergency room in coma, trauma is the most common cause.
   a) True
   b) False
2. Factors which may complicate a neurological lesion include:
   a) Hypoxemia
   b) Hypercarbia
   c) Respiratory acidosis
   d) Metabolic acidosis
   e) All of the above
3. All of the following are true about neurological trauma *except*:
   a) Occasionally, associated trauma to other organs or systems may demand a higher treatment priority than damage to the central nervous system
   b) The most common cause of death is hypoxemia secondary to respiratory failure
   c) The brain, encased in a rigid skull, cannot adapt to increasing pressure or an enlarging hematoma
   d) The pupils are often helpful in distinguishing between traumatic and metabolic causes of coma
   e) The CT scan of the brain should precede the complete neurological physical examination
4. Vital signs, including blood pressure, pulse and respirations, rarely give information about the severity of a lesion in the central nervous system.
   a) True
   b) False

Answers on page 391.

Intensive Care Evaluation of the Comatose Patient

Joseph R. Berger, M.D. and
Robert B. Daroff, M.D.

Objectives

Coma is a frequent and major concern in the intensive care unit. The paper presents a detailed bedside examination of the comatose individual with an emphasis on possible etiologies. The pathophysiology and prognosis of coma are addressed briefly.

Introduction

Although there are subtle differences in various definitions of "coma," we have elected to use that proposed by Plum and Posner of an "unarousable unresponsiveness" [1]. "Stupor" is defined as an "unresponsiveness from which the subject can be aroused only by vigorous and repeated stimuli" [1].

Coma results from either a physiologic failure of both cerebral hemispheres or of the reticular activating formation of the brain stem; the latter projects to the cortex and serves to maintain consciousness. There are essentially four general pathophysiological causes of coma [2]; (1) supratentorial mass lesions, (2) infratentorial mass or destructive lesions, (3) metabolic encephalopathy and diffuse cerebral disturbances and (4) psychogenic "coma." The first two produce coma by altering the brain stem reticular formation. Supratentorial mass lesions affect the brain stem in one of two fashions, "uncal" or "central" herniation [1]. In the former, lateral displacement of

Joseph R. Berger, M.D., Department of Neurology, University of Miami School of Medicine, Fla. and Robert B. Daroff, M.D., Professor and Chairman, Department of Neurology, Case Western Reserve University School of Medicine, Cleveland, Ohio.

the temporal lobe over the tentorial edge compresses the midbrain. Initially, there is a third nerve palsy on the side of the lesion with ptosis and pupillary dilatation preceding ophthalmoplegia. Alteration of consciousness then follows and either contralateral hemiplegia or ipsilateral hemiplegia (from compression of the contralateral midbrain against the tentorial edge) appears. Decerebrate rigidity ultimately occurs and the respiratory pattern deteriorates in a rostral-caudal manner. Central herniation results from downward displacement of the diencephalon and adjacent midbrain. Stupor is an early manifestation followed by Cheyne-Stokes respiration. Both pupils are small. Contralateral hemiplegia precedes the decorticate and decerebrate rigidity that develop as coma deepens. Metabolic encephalopathy produces coma by interfering with metabolism of both brain stem and cortical neurons.

In a series of 386 patients seen by a neurologist for "coma of unknown etiology," there were 261 with metabolic and diffuse cerebral disorders, 69 with supratentorial mass lesions, 52 with subtentorial lesions and 4 with psychiatric disorders [1].

Akinetic Mutism and the "Locked-in" Syndrome

There are a variety of conditions resembling but differing from true coma for which there is no general agreement as to nomenclature [3-5]. These are akinetic mutism, persistent vegetative state, apallic state, coma vigil and coma depasse.

The "locked-in" syndrome or the de-efferented state is a specific condition occurring when an individual is incapable of communicating by word or movement, but retains consciousness. While this picture may evolve in such conditions as severe polyneuritis or myasthenia gravis, it typically refers to individuals with destructive lesions of the base of the pons with an intact tegmentum [1]. In this instance, the patient has both quadriplegia and bulbar paralysis with normal consciousness. The ability to blink and to move the eyes in a vertical plane is usually retained. These are circumstances in which no voluntary movement is possible and only a "normal" EEG can distinguish this condition from coma.

General Examination

A brief general examination of the unconscious patient is frequently very rewarding. Inspection of the head may disclose evidence of trauma, such as periorbital ecchymosis ("racoon eyes") or Battle's sign. Battle's sign is the mastoid swelling and hematoma that develop when a fracture extends into the mastoid portion of the temporal bone. It is most apparent two to three days after the traumatic event [6]. Palpation of the scalp may reveal a visually unsuspected bogginess over sites of trauma or even a palpable skull fracture. Otoscopic examination may demonstrate hemotympanum denoting underlying skull fracture, as may the presence of otorrhea or rhinorrhea.

When trauma has been eliminated as an etiologic possibility, passive neck flexion may be performed. Resistance to this maneuver is suggestive of meningeal irritation from infection or blood. Head retraction may be apparent when meningeal irritation is severe. Variants of passive neck flexion include Kernig's and Brudzinski's signs. Kernig's sign is the resistance encountered to extension of the knee when the lower extremity is flexed at the hip; Brudzinski's neck sign consists of flexion of both thighs and legs following passive flexion of the head on the chest [7]. These signs may be misleadingly absent in deep coma [8].

The integument may bear witness to systemic diseases, such as the myxedematous changes of hypothyroidism, uremic frost, the stigmata of cirrhosis, the sallow complexion of Addison's disease and the cherry red complexion of carbon monoxide poisoning. The skin should be inspected for the characteristic antecubital needle tracks of the IV drug abuser. Bullous skin lesions suggest the possibility of drug-induced coma [9]. Although these lesions have been most frequently reported with barbiturate overdose [10], imipramine, meprobamate, glutethimide, carbon monoxide and phenothiazine have been implicated as well. Rashes characteristic of viral, bacterial or rickettsial disease may be apparent. The state of hydration as gauged by skin turgor and sweating may be a helpful diagnostic aid.

When alcohol, uremia, hepatic failure or diabetic ketoacidosis play a role in the comatose patient, it may be detected by careful attention to breath odor. Intoxication by certain commercial and pharmacological agents also gives rise to characteristic breath odors [11].

The nature of the vital signs (pulse, blood pressure, temperature and respiration) is, of course, essential. Abnormalities of pulse and blood pressure may reflect a primary cardiac event as the etiology of the patient's disorder. On the other hand, it is well established that central nervous system pathology, particularly subarachnoid hemorrhages, may result in cardiac arrhythmias [12]. Hypertension may be a reflection of the pressure effect of rising intracranial pressure, the Kocher-Cushing reflex. It is frequently accompanied by bradycardia, but the latter can occur independently of blood pressure elevation [13]. The presence or absence of the Kocher-Cushing reflex may be as dependent upon the nature and location of the intracranial lesion as the level of intracranial pressure [14].

Hypothermia and hyperthermia result from various disorders affecting the CNS. Additionally, these two conditions have primary effects upon cerebral metabolism. Hypothermia may occur with Wernicke's encephalopathy [15], other hypothalamic lesions, myxedema, hypopituitarism, exposure and a variety of drug overdoses, including alcohol, phenobarbital and phenothiazines. Apart from the rather rare hypothalamic lesions, hypothermia almost always implies metabolic depression of the CNS [16]. Altered consciousness [17] and isoelectric electroencephalographs (EEG) [18] may occur in the presence of hypothermia. Unlike hypothermia, hyperthermia generally does not alter consciousness except when it accompanies heat stroke [1]. In this disorder, disturbance of consciousness is the presenting sign [19]. In addition to heat stroke, hyperthermia may complicate infections, tumor necrosis, delerium tremens, drug toxicity and thyroid storm.

The respiratory pattern can be an important localizing sign [16]. The examiner must also be aware of the possible influence on respiration of a metabolic disorder that coexists with a structural CNS lesion. Listed in Table 1 are the neuropathological correlates of breathing abnormalities.

Cheyne-Stokes respiration is a pattern of periodic breathing in which hyperpnea regularly alternates with apnea, the transition being made in a smooth crescendo-decrescendo

Table 1. Neuropathological Correlates of Respiration [1]

Forebrain damage
  Epileptic respiratory inhibition
  Apraxia for deep breathing or breath-holding
  Pseudobulbar laughing or crying
  Posthyperventilation apnea
  Cheyne-Stokes respiration (CSR)

Midbrain-rostral pons tegmentum
  Central neurogenic hyperventilation

Pontine base
  Pseudobulbar paralysis of voluntary control

Lower pontine tegmentum
  Apneustic breathing
  Cluster breathing
  Short-cycle anoxic-hypercapneic CSR
  Ataxic breathing

Medullary
  Ataxic breathing
  Slow regular breathing
  Loss of automatic breathing with preserved voluntary control

fashion. The period of hyperpnea most often exceeds that of apnea. This breathing pattern implies bilateral neurological disturbance, usually deep in the cerebral hemispheres or diencephalon [1]. While anoxia or prolonged circulation time may augment this respiratory periodicity, the neurologic lesion is necessary for its appearance [20].

Central neurogenic hyperventilation is a rapid, regular, deep respiratory pattern that reflects disease in the brain stem tegmentum between the low midbrain and middle pons [21]. Hyperpnea cannot be ascribed to a central etiology when the arterial pO_2 is less than 70 to 80 mm Hg or the arterial pCO_2 is greater than 40 mm Hg [22].

A prolonged pause after full inspiration occurs with apneustic breathing. It generally reflects a disturbance at the mid or caudal pontine level, usually an infarction [1]. Ataxic breathing is a grossly irregular pattern of rate and depth of respiration that is seen with medullary disease [1].

Apnea is the *complete* cessation of respiration and is an invariable criterion of brain death. Occasionally, in the initial ten seconds after a patient is detached from a respirator, a few brief shallow breaths attributable to diastolic cardiac movement may be detected and should not be confused with spontaneous respiration [23]. The diagnosis of absolute apnea requires the absence of spontaneous respiration at a carbon dioxide tension (pCO_2) of at least 60 mm Hg [24]. This level of pCO_2 can be safely obtained by the technique of apneic oxygenation in which 100% oxygen is delivered endotracheally for a ten-minute period [24]. Blood gases should be performed to confirm the pCO_2.

Ocular Examination

Pupil size and reactivity are essential to the evaluation. Pupil size is dependent upon ambient light, dual sympathetic and parasympathetic innervation and the sense of nearness. The latter is eliminated as a factor in the comatose patient. The sizes and regularity of the two pupils in dim illumination should be made. Then, reactivity is determined with a bright flashlight. Any degree of pupillary constriction indicates reactivity. A common cause of a widely dilated, fixed pupil is the instillation of mydriatics by a previous examiner. Since the effects of the mydriatics may wear off at unequal rates (the rate of metabolism is faster in an injured eye), pupillary asymmetry may be noted. There are myriad causes of anisocoria [25].

Symmetrically small and reactive pupils may reflect a diencephalic disturbance of either a structural or metabolic nature. Midposition or slightly widened pupils that are unreactive to light, but spontaneously fluctuate in size, result from midbrain damage in the pretectal or dorsal tectal region. When pupils are midposition, fixed to light, slightly irregular and often unequal, a nuclear midbrain lesion is implicated. A unilateral widely dilated, fixed pupil indicates oculomotor nerve compression such as that associated with uncal herniation where the dilatation may herald the event. When the parasympathetic pathway functions unopposed, as may occur with pontine tegmental lesions that interrupt the descending sympathetic pathway, small, pinpoint pupils result. Careful examination with a magnifying glass will verify the presence of the pupillary light reflex [26].

A variety of metabolic disturbances and pharmacological agents affect pupil size and function. The ingestion of atropine and other parasympathetic blocking agents may result in widely dilated and fixed pupils. Opiates generally produce pinpoint pupils. Glutethimide, massive barbiturate overdose and hypothermia may fix the pupils. Pupillary dilatation may follow circulatory arrest, although it is not an invariable accompaniment of irreversible coma [27].

Other helpful ocular signs include eye closure, doll's eyelid phenomenon, evoked blinking and the corneal reflex. In general, comatose patients have complete or near complete eyelid closure. The tone of the closed lids varies inversely with depth of coma, as does the length of time the lids remain open after arousal [8]. The gradual closure of an eyelid after its passive elevation cannot be duplicated by the hysteric. The doll's eyelid phenomenon is the reflex opening of the eyes when the neck is flexed. It is present in light or moderate coma, particularly in subarachnoid hemorrhage, and allows assessment of levator palpebrae function [8].

Blinking can be evoked by bright light, loud sound or threat. Its presence with bright light indicates that optic tract, lateral geniculate bodies, upper and mid brainstem and facial nerves are intact. It does not necessarily imply intact geniculocalcarine connections. When elicited by loud sound, auditory nerve function is established. To evoke blinking by threat, the eye should be approached from the side so air currents do not result in a corneal reflex. Its presence denotes the functional integrity of the visual pathways and facial nerve.

A strong stimulus may be required to obtain the corneal reflex in the comatose patient. A midbrain lesion at the level of the oculomotor nucleus with intact lower brainstem is indicated by bilaterally brisk corneal reflexes and dilated fixed pupils [8].

Ocular motility should be examined in their resting position after the patient has been aroused maximally since dysconjugate eye positions may normally occur during sleep [28]. Slight horizontal dysconjugacy is not uncommon in the comatose patient. Conjugate deviation laterally or vertically may be noted. Forced deviation of the eyes downward and medially usually denotes a thalamic lesion and increased intracranial pressure [29]. Conjugate lateral deviation reflects ipsilateral hemispheric or contralateral brain stem disease. On occasion, a large thalamic-basal ganglionic hemorrhage whose caudal extension is limited to the midbrain may result in conjugate ocular deviation contralaterally [30].

Nystagmus superimposed on conjugate ocular deviation is suggestive that a seizure disorder is the cause of the altered level of consciousness. An EEG is the best diagnostic test.

Skew deviation (vertical ocular dysconjugacy) generally indicates brain stem disease and in 66% of the cases the lesion is on the side of the hypotropia [31]. Ocular bobbing, a fast downward deviation of the eyes with a slow return to midposition, generally signifies an extensive pontine disorder, but extrapontine compression, obstructive hydrocephalus or metabolic encephalopathy may be responsible [32].

Not infrequently, the comatose individual with intact brain stem will exhibit roving eye movements. These slow eye movements, which may be conjugate or dysconjugate, are of no localizing value except to indicate integrity of brain stem structures responsible for the eye movements in that particular direction.

The oculocephalic reflex (doll's head maneuver) is elicited by turning the head in either vertical or lateral planes; the eyes turn an equal amount in the opposite direction. This reflex involves both labyrinthine and, to a lesser degree, tonic neck receptors. Evidence of oculomotor, trochlear and abducens nerve damage, as well as an internuclear ophthalmoplegia, may become apparent during oculocephalics. The presence of full horizontal excursions of the eyes generally excludes a supra-medullary brain stem lesion as the cause of coma [33].

Cold caloric testing is typically performed by instilling up to 50 cc of ice water in the ear canal via syringe with the head at a 30° elevation from horizontal. It is a stronger vestibular stimulus than oculocephalics. This procedure should only be performed after otoscopic examination has ruled out a ruptured tympanic membrane. Stimulation of the semicircular canals by thermal conduction results in nystagmus, with the fast phase directed away from the ear irrigated with cold water. Nathanson has devised a useful classification of response to cold calorics (Table 2) [34]. A sedative-hypnotic drug overdose should be suspected when calories induce forced downward ocular deviation of one or both eyes [35].

Papilledema may develop within hours of a subarachnoid or intracerebral hemorrhage [36]. The presence of retinal hemor-

Table 2. Nathanson Classification of Response to Cold Calorics [34]

Stage 1

Cold calorics produce arousal with normal ocular responses as seen in wakefulness; that is, quick and slow phase nystagmus, most apparent on gaze opposite to the side stimulated, somewhat less on direct forward gaze and least on gaze to side stimulated.

Stage 2

Cold calorics produce tonic conjugate deviation to side of stimulus with fine nystagmus.

Stage 3

Cold calorics produce tonic conjugate deviation of eyes to side of stimulus without nystagmus.

Stage 4

Cold calorics produce no ocular response, the eyes remaining in or near midposition.

---

rhages bespeaks a sudden, severe increase in intracranial pressure that most commonly occurs following rupture of an aneurysm, but also in trauma [37]. Occasionally, with these dramatic intracranial pressure elevations, vitreous, conjunctival and orbital hemorrhages occur.

Motor Examination

One should look for the presence or absence of spontaneous limb movement which may be asymmetrical and indicative of a focal lesion. Pinching or deep pressure is appropriate noxious stimulus. Lateral abduction at the shoulder is the only movement that is always purposeful. Other movements, such as forward flexion, may represent an unconscious reflex.

Resistance to passive movement is than determined. Paratonic rigidity or gegenhalten is a plastic rigidity that is present to equal degrees during flexion and extension. The more rapidly the limb is moved, the greater the resistance. It generally reflects diffuse forebrain disease, either metabolic or structural. Spasticity has a predilection for certain muscle groups (flexors of the arms and extensors of the legs).

Various postures, either resting or stimulus-induced, may be helpful diagnostically. Decorticate rigidity is recognized by adduction of the upper extremities with flexion at elbows, wrists and fingers and extension and internal rotation of the lower limbs with plantar flexion. It usually indicates diffuse bihemispheric lesions [1]. Decerebrate rigidity, in extreme form, is an opisthotonic posturing with extension, adduction and pronation of the arms and extension of the lower limbs with the feet plantar flexed. Its presence implies brain stem damage caudal to the red nucleus and rostral to vestibular nuclei [38]. In addition to structural lesions where decerebrate rigidity may even be unilateral, it may also result from severe metabolic disorders. Lesions of the pons at the level of the trigeminal nerve may result in a decerebrate posturing of the upper extremities and flaccidity or weak flexor responses of the lower extremities [1]. Alternatively, large pontine lesions may cause flaccid upper and spastic lower limbs.

Hysterical Unresponsiveness

On occasion the physician is faced with an unresponsive patient who has no organic pathology. This hysterical "coma" seldom lasts more than a few minutes and is rare, accounting for only 1% of a large series of comatose patients collected by Plum and Posner [1]. Most frequently, these patients lie quietly with jaws shut and eyes closed. The respiratory pattern is eupneic. Muscle tone and deep tendon reflexes are normal. Pupils are symmetric and reactive. There is a resistance to passive eyelid raising during which the globes deviate outward and upward (Bell's phenomenon), unexpected in the truly comatose. Roving eye movements are never present. Calorics show a normal response and also invariably "awaken" the patient when more conventional noxious stimuli have failed.

In contrast to hysterical "coma," catatonic unresponsiveness may last for days. The muscle tone is increased and limbs tend to maintain their posture after passive movement.

Ancillary Studies

Routine laboratory studies in the comatose individual should include glucose, sodium, potassium, chloride, bicarbonate, calcium, blood urea nitrogen, liver function tests and urinalysis. When respiration is irregular or acid-base imbalance is suspected, arterial blood gases should be obtained. Additionally, toxicology screen of serum, urine and gastric contents should be performed in patients without a readily apparent etiology.

In the absence of head trauma, skull x-ray is rarely rewarding. When trauma is apparent, cervical spine as well as skull x-rays may be helpful. Computerized axial tomography (CAT) of the brain is invaluable. It is normal in metabolic coma and is often normal in meningitis and subarachnoid hemorrhage. Cerebral infarction may not be apparent by CAT very early after the insult [39] and subdural hematomas may be missed [40].

Once a mass lesion has been ruled out by CAT and no evidence of retinal hemorrhage or papilledema exist, a lumbar puncture may be performed to determine evidence of infection or bleeding. Opening pressure should be recorded and all appropriate cerebrospinal fluid studies performed.

The EEG may reveal unsuspected seizure activity. A nonlocalizing EEG suggests a diffuse process, such as a metabolic disturbance or involvement of subcortical brain stem structures [41]. A normal study is incompatible with organic coma and should raise suspicions of locked-in syndrome or psychogenic coma.

Predicting Prognosis in Coma

Numerous attempts have been made to find predictors of prognosis for comatose patients. Some of the commonly used parameters are (1) age, (2) duration and depth of coma, (3) the nature of the intracranial lesion, (4) associated extracranial lesions and (5) electroencephalographic findings [42].

Scales based on clinical assessment, such as the Glasgow [43] and Munich [44] Coma Scales, have been devised to gauge depth of coma. The Glasgow investigators define coma as simply an inability to obey commands, to speak or to open the eyes [43, 45]. Their scale, based on these easily assessed features, is displayed in Table 3. Numerical values have been assigned to different responses. When the sum of these parameters was less than or equal to 7, the patient was comatose; when the sum was 9 or more, he was not. Pupil reaction and eye movements correlated reasonably well with level of responsiveness [45]. The predictive value of this combination of simple observations has been demonstrated [46]. While developed for the evaluation of post-

Table 3. Glasgow Coma Scale [45]

Eye opening	E	
Spontaneous		4
To speech		3
To pain		2
Nil		1
Best motor response	M	
Obeys		6
Localizes		5
Withdraws		4
Abnormal flexion		3
Extends		2
Nil		1
Verbal response	V	
Orientated		5
Confused conversation		4
Inappropriate words		3
Incomprehensible		2
Nil		1

traumatic coma, the scale has been applied to nontraumatic coma as have the guides to brain stem function enumerated by Plum and Posner [47]. We feel these scales are most helpful for nurses and nonneurological physicians.

Coma complicating a medical illness generally portends a grave prognosis. Seventy percent of patients in coma from medical illness remained comatose or in a vegetative state at one month [48]. Only 16% had a moderate to good recovery. When any of the following signs were exhibited during the first 24 hours, the chance of recovery doubled: any verbal response, eye following, calorics, motor responses to command or stimulus or normal skeletal muscle tone. On the other hand, the chance of even a moderate recovery dropped to less than 8% if any of the following were absent after six hours of coma: pupillary reactions, oculovestibular reflexes, corneal reflexes, motor responses to stimulation or deep tendon reflexes [48].

The prognosis for recovery of neurological function following cardiac arrest is dependent upon depth and duration of postarrest coma [49]. Patients who are awake within two days of hospital admission have a much improved chance of neurological recovery [50]. Provided these patients survive subsequent cardiac arrest and other medical complications, they have an 80% probability of good neurological function several years later [51].

While not absolute in their predictive capacities, these scales and clinical parameters do provide a reasonable means by which to assess the effects of therapy and gauge eventual prognosis. Further studies, no doubt, will improve upon them.

References

1. Plum, F. and Posner, J.B.: Diagnosis of Stupor and Coma. Philadelphia:F. A. Davis Company, 1972, pp. 1-286.
2. Posner, J.B.: The comatose patient. JAMA 233:1313-1314, 1975.
3. Jennett, B. and Plum, F.: Persistent vegetative state after brain damage. Lancet 1:734-737, 1972.
4. Ingvar, D.H. and Brun, A.: Das komplette appalische syndrom. Arch. Psychiatr. Nervenkr. 215:219-239, 1972.
5. Pagni, C.A., Giovanelli, M., Tomei, G. et al: Long term results in 62 cases of posttraumatic complete apallic syndrome. Acta Neurochir. 36:37-45, 1977.
6. Boles, R.: Facial, auditory and vestibular nerve injuries associated with basilar skull fractures. *In* Youmans, J.R. (ed.): Neurological Surgery. Philadelphia:W. B. Saunders Company, 1973, vol. 2, pp. 1013-1014.
7. Wartenburg, R.: The signs of Brudzinski and of Kernig. J. Pediatr. 37:679-684, 1950.
8. Fisher, C.M.: The neurological examination of the comatose patient. Acta Neurol. Scand. 45 (Suppl. 36):1-56, 1969.
9. Pinkus, N.B.: Skin eruptions in drug induced coma. Med. J. Aust. 2:886-888, 1971.
10. Gröschel, D., Gerstein, A.R. and Rosenbaum, J.M.: Skin lesions as a diagnostic aid in barbiturate poisoning. N. Engl. J. Med. 283:409-410, 1970.
11. DeGowin, E.L. and DeGowin, R.L.: Bedside Diagnostic Examination. New York:The MacMillan Company, 1969, pp. 142.
12. Vidal, B.E., Dergal, E.B., Cesarman, E. et al: Cardiac arrhythmias associated with subarachnoid hemorrhage: Prospective study. Neurosurgery 5:675-680, 1979.
13. Edholm, O.G.: The relationship of heart rate to intracranial pressure. J. Physiol. 98:442-445, 1940.
14. Weinstein, J.D., Langfitt, T.W. and Kassel, N.F.: Vasopressor response to increased intracranial pressure. Neurology 14:1118-1131, 1964.
15. Koeppen, A.H., Daniels, J.C. and Barron, K.D.: Subnormal body temperatures in Wernickes encephalopathy. Arch. Neurol. 21:493-498, 1969.
16. Plum, F.: Examination of the unconscious patient. Br. Med. J. 1:49, 1972.

17. Rosin, A.J. and Exton-Smith, A.N.: Clinical features of accidental hypothermia, with some observations on thyroid function. Br. Med. J. 1:16-19, 1964.

18. Bennett, D.R., Hughes, J.R., Korein, J. et al: Atlas of Electroencephalography in Coma and Cerebral Death. New York:Raven Press, 1976, p. 3.

19. Shibolet, S., Coll, R., Gilat, T. et al: Heatstroke: Its clinical picture and mechanism in 36 cases. Q. J. Med. 36:525-548, 1967.

20. Brown, H.W. and Plum, F.: The neurologic basis of Cheynes-Stokes respiration. Am. J. Med. 30:849-860, 1961.

21. Plum, F. and Swanson, A.G.: Central neurogenic hyperventilation in man. Arch. Neurol. Psychiatry 81:535-549, 1959.

22. Plum, F.: Hyperpnea, hyperventilation and brain dysfunction. Ann. Intern. Med. 76:328, 1972.

23. Finklestein, S. and Ropper, A.: The diagnosis of coma: Its pitfalls and limitations. Heart Lung 8:1059-1064, 1979.

24. Schafer, J.A. and Caronna, J.J.: Duration of apnea needed to confirm brain death. Neurology 28:661-666, 1978.

25. Thompson, H.S. and Pilley, S.F.J.: Unequal pupils. A flow chart for sorting out the anisocorias. Surv. Ophthalmol. 21:45-48, 1976.

26. Fisher, C.M.: Some neuro-ophthalmological observations. J. Neurol. Neurosurg. Psychiatry 30:383-392, 1967.

27. Schwartz, B.A. and Vendrely, E.: One of the problems posed by the diagnosis of irreversible coma: The flat EEG and pupil diameter. Electroenceph. Clin. Neurophysiol. 28:648, 1970.

28. Fluur, E. and Eriksson, L.: Nystagmographic recording of vertical eye movements. Acta Otolaryngol. 53:486-492, 1961.

29. Gilner, L.I. and Avin, B.: A reversible ocular manifestation of thalamic hemorrhage. Arch. Neurol. 34:715-716, 1977.

30. Keane, J.R.: Contralateral gaze deviation with supratentorial hemorrhage. Arch. Neurol. 32:119-122, 1975.

31. Keane, J.R.: Ocular skew deviation. Arch. Neurol. 32:185-190, 1975.

32. Susac, J.O., Hoyt, W.F., Daroff, R.B. et al: Clinical spectrum of ocular bobbing. J. Neurol. Neurosurg. Psychiatry 33:771-775, 1970.

33. Daroff, R.B. and Troost, B.T.: Supranuclear disorders of eye movements. In Glaser, J.S. (ed.): Neuro-ophthalmology. Hagerstown: Harper & Row Publishers, 1978, pp. 201-218.

34. Nathanson, M.: In Bender, M.B. (ed.): The Oculomotor System. New York:Harper & Row Publishers, 1964, pp. 484-488.

35. Simon, R.P.: Forced downward ocular deviation. Arch. Neurol. 35:456-458, 1978.

36. Pagan, L.F.: The rapid appearance of papilledema. J. Neurosurg. 30:247-249, 1969.

37. Keane, J.R.: Retinal hemorrhages. Arch. Neurol. 36:691-694, 1979.

38. Fog, M. and Hein-Sorenson, O.: Mesencephalic syndromes. In Vinken, P.J. and Bruyn, G.W. (eds.): Handbook of Clinical Neurology. Amsterdam:North Holland Publishing Company, 1969, pp. 281-283.

39. Davis, K.R., Taveras, J.M., New, P.F.J. et al: Cerebral infarction

diagnosis by computerized tomography. Am. J. Roentgenol. 124:643-660, 1975.

40. Forbes, G.S., Sheedy, P.F., Piepgras, D.G. et al: Computed tomography in the evaluation of subdural hematoma. Radiology 126:143-148, 1978.
41. Silverman, D.: Retrospective study of the EEG in coma. Electroencephalogr. Clin. Neurophysiol. 15:486-503, 1963.
42. Pazzaglia, P., Frank, G., Frank, F. et al: Clinical course and prognosis of acute post-traumatic coma. J. Neurol. Neurosurg. Psychiatry 38:149-154, 1975.
43. Teasdale, G. and Jennett, B.: Assessment of coma and impaired consciousness. Lancet 2:81-83, 1974.
44. Brickmann, R., Von Gramon, D. and Schulz, H.: The Munich coma scale. J. Neurol. Neurosurg. Psychiatry 39:788-793, 1976.
45. Jennett, B. and Teasdale, G.: Aspects of coma after severe head injury. Lancet 1:878-881, 1977.
46. Jennett, B., Teasdale, G., Galbraith, S. et al: Severe head injury in three countries. J. Neurol. Neurosurg. Psychiatry 40:291-297, 1977.
47. Caronna, J., Leigh, J., Shaw, D. et al: The outcome of medical coma: Prediction by bedside assessment of physical signs. Trans. Am. Neurol. Assoc. 1975, pp. 25-29.
48. Plum, F. and Levy, D.: Predicting prognosis in coma. Am. J. Med. 65:224-226, 1978.
49. Snyder, B.D., Ramirez-Lassepas, M. and Lippert, D.M.: Neurologic status and prognosis after cardiopulmonary arrest. Neurology 27:807-811, 1977.
50. Yarnell, P.R.: Neurologic outcome of prolonged coma survivors of out-of-hospital cardiac arrest. Stroke 7:279-282, 1976.
51. Earnest, M.P., Yarnell, P.R., Knapp, G. et al: Long term survival and neurologic status following resuscitation from out-of-hospital cardiac arrest. Neurology 30:443, 1980.

Self-Evaluation Quiz

1. Uncal herniation is characterized by:
   a) A dilated pupil on the side opposite the herniation
   b) Hemiplegia that may be either ipsilateral or contralateral to the site of herniation
2. The most common cause of "coma of unknown etiology" is supratentorial mass lesions.
   a) True
   b) False
3. The "locked-in syndrome" is most often the result of destructive lesions of the base of the pons with intact tegmentum.
   a) True
   b) False

4. Signs of meningeal irritation are invariably present with meningitis.
    a) True
    b) False
5. Isoelectric EEGs may occur with:
    a) Barbiturate intoxication
    b) Dilantin intoxication
    c) Bilateral subdural hematomas
    d) Hypothermia
6. Pupil size is dependent upon:
    a) Ambient light
    b) Autonomic innervation
    c) Level of consciousness
    d) Sense of nearness
7. The Kocher-Cushing reflex is an invariable accompaniment of rising intracranial pressure and always associated with bradycardia.
    a) True
    b) False
8. Bullous skin lesions in the comatose individual suggest overdose by which of the following:
    a) Barbiturate
    b) Imipramine
    c) Dilantin
    d) Aspirin
9. Slow eye movements in the comatose individual are of localizing significance.
    a) True
    b) False
10. Which of the following suggests a skull fracture following trauma:
    a) Raccoon's eyes
    b) Battle's sign
    c) Hemotympanum
    d) CSF rhinorrhea
    e) All of the above

Answers on page 391.

Panel Discussion

Moderator: Dr. Marshall

Panelists: Drs. Daroff, Elser and Green

Moderator: Dr. Daroff, since Dr. John Ward is here from Richmond, maybe we should begin with the issue of decerebration. Richard Greenberg, in an article in the August 1977 *Journal of Neurosurgery*, demonstrated quite nicely that decerebration is not a function of brainstem disturbance, but rather is demonstrable of diffuse hemispheric disturbance. Probably, although from a prognostic viewpoint I certainly would agree with what you have said, it indicates a much more ominous prognosis than does decortication. However, in terms of localization, it is not terribly useful. Would you comment on that?

Dr. Daroff: I think one can hold a symposium on decerebration and decortication and still not answer all the questions. If you tell me that one can have decerebration with an intact brainstem but diffuse bihemispheric disease, I shall accept that, provided the thalamus is involved.

Moderator: Dr. Green, is there a difference between neurogenic and spinal shock?

Dr. Green: There is a difference between neurogenic and spinal shock. When one talks about neurogenic shock, one is referring to a sympathectomy from injury to the brainstem or the spinal cord down to about the T-4 level. This is classically what is termed neurogenic shock. It is a triad of hypotension, hypothermia and bradycardia due to an interruption of the sympathetics and takeover by the parasympathetics (vagus). The important thing about this type of shock is that the primary problem is not with volume, because these patients are not volume-depleted. Therefore, the treatment should not be large volume replacement, but rather should be redistribution of volume with use of the MAST suit and the Trendelenburg

47

position. If the pulse drops below 60, you should give atropine 0.4 mgm IV to start with. We have found with the Swan-Ganz catheter that these patients do not have an adequate cardiac output. Spinal shock is the acute loss of motor, sensory and reflex functions below the level of injury. It is a physiological transection of the spinal cord, not necessarily an anatomical one; actually the majority of these patients do not have a physical transection. In spinal shock, for some reason, at 6 to 12 weeks and sometimes as long as 16 weeks following injury, the patient will convert from a flaccid lower motor preparation into an upper motor neuron preparation with hypertonia and hyperreflexia. This transformation heralds the end of spinal shock. Some authors report that one cannot tell when a person is incomplete or complete until he is out of spinal shock, which is not true. I think that many of the terms we formerly used, such as spinal shock, when talking about prognosis are completely useless.

Moderator: Drs. Elser and Daroff, this question is directed to you, and Dr. Green may wish to comment: How do you get the emergency room physician to call a neurologist or neurosurgeon promptly? Dr. Elser, please start.

Dr. Elser: Stabilization of the patient, including the checking for dysfunction of other systems, or evaluating the patient with multisystem trauma is the first priority. Resuscitation and maintenance of vital signs, especially the airway, breathing and ventilation, are also critically urgent. I don't believe there is any reluctance to call the neurologist or neurosurgeon; we just seek to make a rapid assessment and stabilize the patient before calling the specialist. Very rarely, the need for a neurologist or neurosurgeon may not be immediately evident.

Dr. Daroff: I would like to pass on that question because my residents are in the audience and they know I have not been in an emergency room for six years.

Moderator: Dr. Daroff, I have a question for you, and then we will come back to the spinal cord, which seems to be a major focus of interest. In general, comment about the prognosis for patients who are locked in. Have you ever seen a patient who has been locked in who has completely recovered?

Dr. Daroff: Yes, I know of a case of a college student whose roommate decided to commit suicide and turned on the oven gas. The girl died but the innocent student, my subsequent patient, became locked in and ultimately recovered, but she was cortically blind. You do not have to have fixed structural disease to be paralyzed. A person can be temporarily locked in.

Moderator: Dr. Green, I shall combine some questions in the interest of saving time. How do you keep the number of spine boards that are required in south Florida from proliferating at a rapid rate, since emergency rooms tend to steal them and keep them? How do you make them available? Do you have a program of interchange between emergency rooms and between emergency medical services?

Dr. Green: In Illinois a state grant purchased under contract several thousand boards and they were distributed throughout the state. They were free to all of the fire rescue departments. When boards arrived at a hospital, they would be left and the emergency personnel would take another one.

Dr. Elser: It is a problem and the way in which they have solved the problem here is this: They have painted a color on the edge of it so you can identify it rapidly. It is really the ambulance personnel who cause the problem, because they steal from the fire rescue, and vice versa. So they painted the edges of them so they can be identified better.

Moderator: Dr. Green, why is system care less expensive than patients who receive care in a nonsystem kind of environment? Specifically, you showed a slide of spinal cord injuries showing that the average cost of patient care in a system — that is, in an organized, comprehensive approach to spinal cord injuries — was significantly less expensive. Would you comment on the reason for that?

Dr. Green: Patient cost is related to the severity of the injuries as well as to the number of complications and length of hospitalization. An organized system that is established to handle each stage of the patient's care and to expedite passage through these phases of care with a multidisciplinary team that is committed to treating this relatively rare but complicated patient results in shortened hospitalization. It is not a matter of one physician performing a better operation than another or possessing better medicine. Rather, it is staffing with a team with volume experience must result in a better care program than a place which gets one patient per year. I think the answer lies in those two phrases: committed multidisciplinary team and volume experience.

Moderator: That is very appropriate. I think that has been the experience throughout the country, that the cost of care, when it is well organized, just tends to be less expensive. I think that is the experience in San Diego with thoracic injuries. The patients are usually operated upon earlier and stabilized earlier. Also, the cost of transporting patients from one hospital to another is not as significant because laboratory tests tend to be repeated.

Dr. Green, when you take a patient off the board, do you transfer him following the myelogram or diagnostic procedure to a Rotor-Rest bed, to a hospital bed or to a Stryker frame? If you choose one of these three listed, please explain briefly your preference for one over any other for a patient with a spinal cord injury.

Dr. Green: Without belaboring the point I shall simply say that it is our opinion at this center that the Rotor-Rest is the only available equipment that effectively immobilizes spinal cord injuries. There are many papers in the literature that have reported that the Stryker and the circle electric bed are actually dangerous to patients because they do not immobilize the spine adequately. We use just the Rotor-Rest bed.

Moderator: Do you believe that patients with head injuries — and I do not agree with what you have said, by the way, about head injuries — and spinal cord injury should always be transported in the Trendelenburg position, as you stated in your presentation?

Dr. Green: Yes, I do.

Moderator: Let me rephrase the question. In the patient who has already had an Esophageal Obturator Airway placed, the standard method of management, certainly, in our region of the country for patients with injuries involving respiration, that is, head, spine or chest, is to transport them head up. What advantage is gained in a patient in whom the blood pressure is being constantly monitored or relatively constantly monitored in transporting the patient in such a way that one may endanger the intracranial space, when you can adequately measure the blood pressure and you have already adequately protected the airway?

Dr. Green: There is no advantage. I agree with you, if you have done that, if the patient is intubated and he is not shocky, then I do not think this is necessary but these measures cannot be counted on in most cases even in San Diego, so I still prefer the general use of the Trendelenburg position in all neurological injuries in the pre-hospital phase.

Moderator: Are soft cervical collars of any use in transporting a traumatized patient? Dr. Green, I think you can answer that, and I think we can expand the question in this way: Is the soft collar of any value in the emergency room? Dr. Elser, please also answer the question.

Dr. Green: I think I have already expressed my answer to that. I think collars are contraindicated in the pre-hospital phase. I think they are very good for sprained necks. Without them, where would our attorney friends be? We do use them for soft tissue sprains, but not for immobilization.

Moderator: Dr. Elser, in the emergency room, are they of any value?

Dr. Elser: I basically agree with what Dr. Green has said. I would like to comment on the previous question, if I may, about transporting a patient in the Trendelenburg position. If any of you have ever had the opportunity to ride in a fire rescue truck and be a part of the fire rescue team, you will realize that constant monitoring is really something you can only write about. It is very difficult to take a blood pressure and monitor anything that is going on except visually, as long as you are not turning a corner and trying to stay on the seat yourself. These things are nice to write about but they actually do not occur very often. For that reason, I support what Dr. Green originally said.

The Multiple Injury Patient

George H. Rodman, Jr., M.D.

Objectives

To delineate priorities of multiple system trauma into life-threatening, urgent and delayed priorities. Early treatment of hemorrhagic shock will be discussed. The reader will learn the appropriate use of the military anti-shock trouser. Specific chest-related injuries will be discussed.

Management of the multisystem trauma patient principally involves priority of activities. Despite the divergent interests between the neurosurgeon, general surgeon, orthopedic surgeon and the emergency room physician, all must agree upon initial priorities in patient management and what specific life-saving techniques must be undertaken. Other diagnostic and therapeutic endeavors must be staged in order of descending importance.

Life-threatening injuries include those which affect the respiratory system. Central nervous system injuries must be recognized immediately and require urgent type of therapy. Other urgent, not clearly life-threatening complications include abdominal or thoracic visceral injuries and some central nervous system injuries.

Delayed priorities are primarily orthopedic in nature. Few fractures require immediate reduction. Those that do are associated with neurovascular compromise, such as humoral or supracondylar fractures. A fractured femur with ischemia distal to the fracture site because of acute vascular injury also falls into this category.

The entire approach to therapy must prevent the delayed sequelae that have been advertised as occurring secondary to

George H. Rodman, Jr., M.D., Assistant Professor of Surgery and Anesthesiology, University of Miami School of Medicine, Fla.

hypovolemic shock. These primarily occur within the cardio-vascular and respiratory systems.

Resuscitation of the multisystem trauma patient still evokes the time-honored approach of the ABCs to therapy. Life depends upon the adequate flow of oxygenated blood and requires the cooperation of both the heart and respiratory system. Maintenance of an airway includes removal of foreign bodies, dentures, debris and other assorted materials.

Very few patients require invasive attempts, such as a tracheostomy, to establish an artificial airway. In almost all instances, emergency airway support can be provided with endotracheal intubation. Some care must be taken with this technique, especially with an associated neck injury. Otherwise the injury may be worsened by further neck manipulation. Facial fractures are associated with a significant degree of swelling during the first several hours after the injury. If during that time the patient is going to be moved throughout the hospital for various diagnostic procedures, airway compromise may occur. Early intubation may be reasonable while circum-stances are still controlled.

Shock easily resuscitated is most likely due to mild volume loss. However, the hemorrhage may still be occurring. As the patient becomes hypotensive there is obviously going to be less blood loss. With resuscitation and restoration of more normal blood pressure, significant hemorrhage may recur. Large-bore 14 or 16 gauge intercaths permit multiple intravenous infusions at rapid rates. The central venous catheter is not required during the early resuscitation period. With a combative patient cannulation of a central vein is associated with a much higher incidence of pneumothorax or inadvertent arterial puncture.

Any resuscitation can be adequately carried out with the use of balanced electrolyte solutions such as normal saline or Ringer's lactate. Not only do these replace the intracellular but also the extracellular fluid losses which are occurring. Blood is unnecessary during the early resuscitation period. Patients with adequate volume replacement can withstand a hematocrit of 15% to 18% without any ill effects.

Obvious, frank bleeding must be controlled. Extensive cranial-facial bleeding, secondary to mid-face fractures, can be controlled with the use of Foley catheters inserted into the external nares. Extensive blood loss from massive scalp lacerations can be controlled with pressure applications, tourniquets are only used on extremity bleeding when complete or near complete amputation has occurred. With the advent of reimplantation of limbs, even this practice has fallen into question.

The MAST (Military Anti-Shock Trouser) has been particularly useful controlling intra-abdominal hemorrhage. Having three compartments, each leg or the abdominal portion can be blown up separately or together. The "G" suit has been used at the scene of the accident by the emergency medical technicians. The MAST suit can be inflated up to a maximum pressure of 105 mm Hg. At lower pressures, usually about 40 mm Hg, some 500 to 750 ml of blood can be transferred from the lower extremities back into the central circulation. The effect of this autotransfusion is oftentimes a marked improvement in blood pressure and probably cardiac output. With high MAST pressures, sometimes higher than arterial pressure, blood flow may be redirected from the lower extremities to more vital organs including the lungs, liver and brain. The indication for the "G" suit in trauma patients is shock at the scene of the accident. Some precautions must be taken when the patient arrives in the emergency room with the MAST suit inflated.

The MAST suit must not be removed to complete a physical examination. Sudden decompression may result in severe hypotension resulting in cardiac arrest. Resuscitation can be extremely difficult under these circumstances. The MAST suit should not be deflated until those responsible for patient care are ready to take immediate, direct intervention such as an abdominal laparotomy. The MAST suit is not deflated until the subject is in the operating room and is ready for immediate surgical intervention.

Advantages of the MAST suit include limitation of duration of shock and minimization of hemorrhage. Less blood loss results in fewer transfusions and patients are less likely to develop problems such as dilutional coagulopathies or infectious hepatitis.

What is recurrent shock? What is happening to the patient who continually develops shock after resuscitation is apparently successful? It may be due to blood loss or may involve another problem, such as cardiac tamponade. Tension pneumothorax may also have the same presentation. Another cause of recurrent shock includes direct myocardial contusion with inability to maintain adequate stroke volume.

Myocardial contusion is a rather difficult diagnosis to make. First, one needs to have a high index of suspicion, which is usually fostered by an adequate history. Other signs include any bony abnormality of the anterior chest or any sign of disruption of the bony thorax, as might occur in deceleration injuries during automobile accidents. The most useful screening test is the electrocardiogram, which would demonstrate any arrhythmias or ischemia.

Blunt chest trauma with development of underlying pulmonary contusion also has diagnostic signs. Fractures of the scapula and upper ribs may hint at more significant injuries. In the patient with a flail chest or sternum, one must suspect that the force required to fracture the sternum has also been transmitted to the heart directly below. Therefore, it is quite reasonable in those circumstances to expect cardiac contusion due to those circumstances. More importantly, it may suggest a very severe, abrupt deceleration, the kind associated with aortic injury.

The routine electrocardiogram analysis can detect subtle arrhythmias not normally diagnosed by palpation of the pulse or auscultation. They may be the only diagnostic clue to cardiac contusion.

The cardiac tamponade with the accumulation of blood in the pericardial space presents with a decreased stroke volume and narrowed pulse pressure. There may be distention of neck veins and a marked increase in central venous pressure. In these circumstances pericardiocentesis can be life-saving. The easiest approach is the subxyphoid route. The needle is directed toward the left shoulder with an alligator clip placed on the needle to monitor the electrocardiographic injury pattern when the epicardium is contacted.

The aorta is a relatively fixed structure at the diaphragmatic hiatus and the ligamentum arteriosum, just distal to the takeoff of the subclavian artery. With sudden deceleration, more mobile portions of the aorta swing forward inducing a tear. Although most times this is a lethal injury, a significant number arrive alive at the hospital. These are usually much smaller tears.

Radiographic findings include a widened mediastinum and loss of the aortic notch. There may be a density in the left upper thorax. Arteriography confirms the diagnosis.

All multisystem trauma patients who develop pneumothorax, or hemopneumothorax, require chest tube placement. Continued massive hemorrhage after placement of the chest tube usually represents significant arterial injury, either an intercostal artery that may have been injured as a result of rib fracture or inadvertently occurring during placement of the chest tube. Internal mammary arteries and aortic injuries can also be associated with massive outpouring of blood from chest tubes. Most times the hemothorax due to a significant pulmonary injury will stop once the blood is evacuated and the lungs are reexpanded.

An adequate abdominal examination is extremely difficult to perform in the multisystem trauma patient. Other injuries and pain make cooperation extremely difficult. Peritoneal lavage is most often recommended in these situations. Before beginning peritoneal lavage both the bladder and the stomach must be emptied. This is carried out with the insertion of a nasal gastric tube and a Foley catheter.

For lavage a dialysis catheter is introduced into the lower portion of the peritoneal cavity, usually the cul-de-sac. A volume of fluid is instilled and the fluid is then returned for a sampling of blood loss. Commercial peritoneal dialysis kits are available to do this. The abdomen is entered in the midline about one third of the distance between the umbilicus and sympathis pubis. After skin infiltration a small stab wound is made, and through this an 18 gauge 2½" needle is inserted into the peritoneal cavity. A guide wire is then introduced through the needle. With the guide wire in place the needle is then removed and the blunt-nosed catheter with multiple perforations in the tip is inserted over the guard wire and down into the pelvis. The diagnosis may in some instances be confirmed by a small quantity of blood which is already collected in the cul-de-sac. Otherwise, an infusion of 1000 ml of balanced electrolyte solution through the catheter begins. After simple side-to-side agitation the now empty infused bottle is placed on the floor and the siphon effect allows the return of some of that fluid. Colormetric analysis helps determine the amount of blood loss and whether or not this corresponds to any abdominal hemorrhage. Any bile in the lavage fluid or any bacteria on gram stain are indicative of a hollow viscus injury. Amylase of the fluid is compared to serum amylase.

After initial evaluation in the emergency department and initial resuscitation, decisions have to be made as to what next happens to the patient. Does he need further diagnostic studies, does he require operative intervention, or does he need placement in the intensive care unit? The stable patient may then be able to receive further diagnostic studies including multiple x-ray examinations. Other patients who are more unstable may require immediate surgical intervention.

The unstable patient is a different problem altogether. A minimal number of interventions and diagnostic procedures are carried out and only those which are of definite help in understanding the complete diagnosis.

In summary, the initial management of the multiple injured patient must follow the ABCs of resuscitative efforts. Shock must be recognized and treated thoroughly. It is only our ability to limit the depth and duration of shock that can be associated with an increase in survival after a significant injury.

Self-Evaluation Quiz

1. Fractured neck is:
   a) A life-threatening injury
   b) An urgent injury
   c) Delayed priority
   d) a and b
   e) b and c

2. Early resuscitation and maintenance of the airway during multiple system trauma includes establishment of a tracheostomy.
   a) True
   b) False

3. All soft tissue injuries about the face require establishment of an artificial airway.
   a) True
   b) False

4. Central venous catheter:
   a) Should be established during resuscitation for hypo-volemic shock
   b) Should always be placed via the subclavian route
   c) Should never be placed in the antecubital approach
   d) Is not required during hemorrhagic shock
5. Select the most appropriate fluid for replacement during hemorrhagic shock.
   a) O negative blood
   b) Typed specific blood
   c) Balanced electrolyte-containing solution
   d) Colloid-containing solution
   e) Low molecular weight dextran
6. Recurrent shock may develop:
   a) After the initial resuscitation
   b) As a result of tension pneumothorax
   c) As a result of cardiac tamponade
   d) All of the above
7. Diagnosis of myocardial contusion includes all of the following *except*:
   a) A high index of suspicion
   b) Chest wall abnormality
   c) Myocardial ischemia
   d) Arrhythmias
   e) Atrial fibrillation
8. Cardiac tamponade is diagnosed by all of the following *except*:
   a) Narrow pulse pressure
   b) Decreased stroke volume
   c) Elevation of central venous pressure
   d) Neck vein distention
   e) Bradycardia

Answers on page 391.

Fluids, Salts and Blood

T. J. Gallagher, M.D.

Objectives

To define fluid lossess occurring during hemorrhagic shock. The reader will learn the appropriate types of fluid to be used during resuscitation and the pros and cons of each. Differences between balanced electrolyte and albumin-containing solutions will be discussed. Complications after transfusion therapy will be described as well as appropriate therapy. Appropriateness of micropore blood filters during massive transfusion therapy will also be discussed.

One cannot separate neurological disease from total system involvement. Intravascular volume is a major consideration in multiple system trauma. Today, most of our concepts of fluid resuscitation are based upon the work done by Shirers and his colleagues. In summary, their work using dogs as a hemorrhagic shock model demonstrated that resuscitation carried out with only blood, or blood in conjunction with colloid-containing solutions, was associated with a high mortality approximating 70%. Only with the addition of balanced electrolyte-containing solutions, such as Ringer's lactate solution, was mortality reduced to about 20% to 30%. Volume loss is recognized as a major defect during shock. Hypovolemia induces interstitial fluid movements into the intravascular compartment at the expense of interstitial volume. This form of autotransfusion is the body's attempt to maintain normal circulating volume. During resuscitation, if the interstitial volume is also not replaced, then therapy is inadequate and the previously observed mortality returns. Therefore, electrolyte-containing solu-

T.J. Gallagher, M.D., Associate Professor of Surgery and Anesthesiology, University of Florida College of Medicine, Gainesville, Florida.

61

tions not only restore and maintain intravascular volume, but also replace the interstitial deficits.

This autotransfusion occurs within the first 30 minutes of hypovolemic shock. This means that the head-injured patient arriving in the emergency room in hemorrhagic shock cannot be resuscitated just with the amount of blood lost. Replacement of interstitial fluid loss is required; therefore, resuscitation will consist of both blood and balanced electrolyte-containing solutions.

Fluid resuscitation becomes more complicated in the patient with head injury or neurosurgical intervention. Intravascular volume must be adequate to insure perfusion of all vital organs including the heart, lung, kidneys and liver; but at the same time, fluid resuscitation must not be so overzealous that cerebral edema is exacerbated. The multisystem trauma patient may require large volume infusions in order to maintain intravascular volume. The period of equilibration may occur well into the postoperative period. In order to have a precise understanding of fluid administration invasive monitoring with a pulmonary artery catheter is generally required.

Fluid replacement in the operating room varies depending upon operative site. During intrathoracic or intra-abdominal procedures patients usually lose body fluids at the rate of 7 ml/kg/hr and require at least that infusion rate to maintain homeostasis. On the other hand, minimal fluid replacement is required during neurosurgery.

How is fluid replacement monitored? Generally we follow such signs as blood pressure, urine output and pulse rate. However, as stated in other papers, blood pressure may respond to other stimuli besides intravascular volume. It is at best a poor indicator of tissue perfusion. It is affected by pain, and some patients may develop a hypertensive response in the operative period. Tachycardia can be considered a sign of inadequate intravascular volume replacement. However, patients on propranolol may not be able to mount a tachycardia in response to hypovolemia. Urine output may be increased in high output renal failure because of glucosuria or osmotic agents such as Lasix or mannitol. In all these circumstances urine certainly is not a true indicator of organ perfusion. Trauma-induced diabetes insipidus can also increase urine output. Those patients requiring close monitoring of volume may require interventions such as a balloon-tipped, flow-directed thermodilution pulmonary artery catheter.

Which is the most appropriate type of fluid? There is still a controversy between the use of crystalloid or colloid containing solutions. Colloids are primarily albumin which exerts an osmotic effect. Some investigators have felt that the hydrophylic properties make it an ideal agent to use with increased lung water, such as during respiratory failure or interstitial pulmonary edema. The osmotic effect would draw fluid from the interstitial space back into the intravascular compartment for eventual renal excretion. On the other hand, balanced electrolyte solutions may tend to dilute the amount of albumin present and fluid would then tend to move in the opposite direction, from the intravascular to the interstitial compartment. The result would be an increased lung water and the possible development of respiratory distress syndrome.

Conversely, albumin could also lead to the development of failure and pulmonary edema. Since it is such a powerful osmotic agent, it may tend to markedly overexpand the intravascular compartment as it pulls water from other areas. As a result congestive heart failure and pulmonary edema may develop. Clinically, it is difficult to regulate albumin infusion and maintain adequate intravascular volume, while not overloading the patient.

Various laboratory investigations have indicated that albumin may be a poor fluid choice in patients with generalized sepsis and increased capillary permeability. Under those circumstances, albumin infused may leak out through the capillary and into the interstitial space and exert an osmotic effect. As a result, water can accumulate in areas with already increased interstitial fluid. In addition, during hypo-albuminemia serum albumin levels cannot be increased with infusions of the same product. Albumin will transiently rise and return to baseline.

Which is the best fluid for resuscitation — balanced electrolytes or albumin? This question has been studied by several different investigators. In one series the resuscitation fluid consisted of balanced electrolyte-containing solutions and washed red blood cells. They did not receive one drop of albumin. The second group, in addition to the resuscitation fluid used in group one, also received 150 gm of albumin in each 24-hour period. Physiologic endpoints, blood pressure, urine output and central venous or pulmonary artery occlusion pressure were the same in both groups. Both groups had the same types of injuries, penetrating and blunt trauma. Each had the same number of injuries, approximately 1.4 systems per patient; and the same number of patients were in shock at the time of admission to hospital, approximately 20% in both groups. Eighty-eight were in the group not receiving colloid, while 55 did receive albumin. Over the next five days there was no difference in any parameter in either group. This included intrapulmonary shunt, arterial venous oxygen content difference, mixed venous PO_2, pulmonary compliance, oxygen gradients and cardiac output. In summary, both groups were adequately resuscitated and there were no statistically significant differences in any of the usual physiological parameters messured in the postoperative period. Therefore, it would seem that albumin had no demonstrable benefit. Since it is much more expensive than balanced electrolyte solutions, on a routine basis it may be contraindicated.

How much blood can a patient safely lose and what volume of electrolyte solution should be used for replacement? Most authorities recommend maintaining a hematocrit greater than 30%. Below that value, oxygen delivery to peripheral tissues can be compromised, especially with a low cardiac output state. Various formulas have been described to predict the fluid volume to replace blood loss. From data derived in animal experiments most recommend approximately 3 ml of Ringer's lactate for every milliliter of blood lost. As blood is removed, a continuous infusion of Ringer's lactate maintains blood pressure. At the end of the study the amount of blood loss was calculated as well as the amount of Ringer's lactate given. The ratio originally calculated was 3 ml of Ringer's lactate for every one of blood lost. However, after the Ringer's lactate infusions were begun, the blood loss from the animals was not simply red cells and plasma but also the infused Ringer's lactate. Therefore, the "blood" lost was really blood and Ringer's lactate not containing nearly as many red cells as previously thought. The ratios were recalculated and actually 9 ml of crystalloid was given for every milliliter of blood lost.

Most blood banks now utilize component therapy. Not every patient needs all the products found in a unit of whole blood. However, under certain circumstances such as massive hemorrhage, whole blood simplifies adequate resuscitation. Massive transfusion therapy implies a complete exchange transfusion. In a normal 70-kg patient blood volume is 7% to 8% of body weight or about 5 liters.

Massive transfusion therapy results in some predictable complications. Major blood group incompatibilities can occur during massive transfusion therapy. When patients receive 30 to 40 units of blood, blood typing mistakes can occur. Under general anesthesia transfusion reaction is difficult to diagnose; back pain, fever and chills are absent. The first sign of a transfusion incompatibility may be blood or hemoglobin in the urine. Acidosis and hypotension may occur during severe reactions. A transfusion reaction requires discontinuation of the blood, correction of acidosis and hypotension and institution of massive diuresis to prevent hemoglobin precipitation in the renal tubules. Antihistamine therapy has no role during massive transfusion reactions.

Stored, banked blood is deficient of platelets, factor V and factor VIII and coagulopathies can develop after massive transfusion therapy. These dilutional coagulopathies are most often due to thrombocytopenia. Platelets lose their function within six hours of collection and the process is accelerated by refrigeration. Although Factors V and VIII are also diminished, it is unusual for coagulopathies to develop. In fact, those factors can be reduced as much as 40% and bleeding will still not occur. During massive transfusion therapy if bleeding time is prolonged or oozing is uncontrolled, platelet infusions may be reasonable. Each platelet pack contains about 10,000 platelets.

Factors V and VIII are found in fresh frozen plasma. However, most times a reduction of these factors does not cause any active bleeding.

Cold blood infused at a rapid rate may precipitate cardiac arrhythmias. This is especially true if infusion is through a central venous line. The ensuing hypothermia can lead to massive vasoconstriction and increased myocardial work. Blood should be warmed prior to infusion and can be accomplished with the use of microwave ovens, infrared therapy, or warming coils.

Is there any evidence that would indicate the need for micropore blood filters during transfusion therapy? After the first five days stored blood begins to accumulate particulate materials such as fibrin and cellular debris. Micropore filters adequately filter this debris. However, there has been little evidence whether that was of any clinical significance. We have studied this problem in trauma patients who have developed respiratory failure. Patients with multiple system trauma who required more than 7 units of blood and then developed respiratory failure were randomly divided into two groups. One group received all of their blood via a standard 170 micron filter. The second group received all transfusions through a 40 micron Pall ® filter. Respiratory function was then compared. Each group received approximately 16 units of blood between 9 and 11 days old. There was no difference in either group in the level of positive end-expiratory pressure (PEEP) required to restore intrapulmonary shunt to 15% in both groups. Likewise, there were no differences in the time PEEP therapy was required or the length of mechanical ventilatory support. We concluded that patients with respiratory failure after multiple system trauma and massive transfusion therapy with a standard 170 micron filter had no difference in pulmonary function compared to a similar group receiving blood through a 40 micron filter. The use of micropore filters did not appear to alleviate the level of respiratory dysfunction developed.

In summary, various types of transfusion fluids are available to maintain intravascular homeostasis; all are effective. There are indications for particular fluids which may vary with circumstances, but in general the overall goal remains adequate circulating volume.

Bibliography

Cooper, J.D., Maeda, M. and Lowenstein, E.: Lung water accumulation with acute hemodilution in dogs. J. Thorac. Cardiovasc. Surg. 62:957-965, 1975.

Lowe, R.J., Moss, G.S., Jilek, J. and Levine, H.D.: Crystallid versus colloid in the etiology of pulmonary failure after trauma: A randomized trial in man. Surgery 81:676, 683, 1977.

Shires, G.L., Carrico, C.J. and Canizaro, P.C.: Shock. Philadelphia:W. B. Saunders, 1973.

Skillman, J.J., Restall, D.S. and Salzman, E.W.: Randomized trial of albumin vs. electrolyte solutions during abdominal aortic operations. Surgery 78:291-303, 1975.

Virgilio, R.W., Smith, D.E., Rice, C.L. et al: Effect of colloid osmotic pressure and pulmonary capillary wedge pressure on intrapulmonary shunt. Surg. Forum 27:168-170, 1976.

Self-Evaluation Quiz

1. Increased survival after hemorrhagic shock is due to:
   a) Replacement of lost blood
   b) Infusion of albumin
   c) Replacement of interstitial fluid losses
   d) Vasopressor therapy
2. Fluid replacement therapy is best monitored with a central venous pressure catheter.
   a) True
   b) False
3. Balanced electrolyte-containing solutions include:
   a) Low molecular weight dextran
   b) Ringer's lactate
   c) Normal saline
   d) Hartmann's solution
   e) Hypotonic saline
4. Effects of albumin therapy include all *except*:
   a) Congestive heart failure
   b) Expansion of intravascular volume
   c) Decreased interstitial fluid volume
   d) Prevention of respiratory failure
5. End-points in fluid resuscitation include all of the following *except*:
   a) Blood pressure
   b) Urine output
   c) Pulmonary artery occlusion pressure
   d) Central venous pressure
   e) Pulse pressure
6. Blood replacement with balanced electrolyte solutions should be done at the ratio of 4 ml of balanced electrolyte for every 1 ml of blood loss.
   a) True
   b) False

7. Transfusion coagulopathies are related to all of the following *except*:
   a) Thrombocytopenia
   b) Decreased factor V
   c) Decreased factor VIII
   d) DIC
   e) Decreased factor X

8. Micropore blood filters should be used with the infusion of fresh whole blood.
   a) True
   b) False

Answers on page 391.

Metabolic Considerations

George H. Rodman, Jr., M.D.

Objectives

To discuss various metabolic parameters including hypothermia and alkalosis. Specific complications discussed include low ionized calcium, hypoglycemia and fluid resequestration. Appropriate fluid in salt replacement will be discussed. Appropriate nutritional therapy will also be reviewed. The reader will learn appropriate replacement of protein sources with amino acid therapy.

The initial resuscitation involves various metabolic stages or phases. The stress period with high circulating catecholamine levels usually lasts for 48 to 72 hours after the initial insult. Once intravascular volume has been restored, the deresuscitation can be effectively begun. Positive fluid balance is no longer necessary and diuresis ensues. During the next five to seven days when oral caloric intake is limited, the tremendous waste of the nutritional reserve begins. This is accelerated in the patient already malnourished prior to the onset of his illness.

The immediate post-resuscitative period requires adequate oxygen delivery. This means maintenance and correction of ventilatory abnormalities. This proceeds in concert with aggressive cardiovascular support. Oxygen delivery is maximized by increased cardiac output and maximized hemoglobin levels.

It is almost inevitable that after major surgical interventions some degree of hypothermia develops in the immediate perioperative period. This is related to the major body cavities being exposed to ambient temperature for extended periods.

George H. Rodman, Jr., M.D., Assistant Professor of Surgery and Anesthesiology, University of Miami School of Medicine, Fla.

69

The infusion of room temperature fluids and the unheated anesthetic all contribute to temperature loss. During the rewarming phase shivering may occur. This may be readily apparent although many times it can be difficult to observe clinically. The major problem is that shivering markedly increases oxygen consumption. Although we would prefer patients to begin to breathe spontaneously during this period, one may have to balance this against the exaggerated oxygen consumption because of the shivering required to generate and conserve body heat. Therefore, at least during the rewarming process, paralysis may have an important role in reducing patient metabolic demands.

In a head injured patient, it is usually considered reasonable to maintain lowered intracranial pressure by hyperventilation. The reduction of PCO_2 to 25 to 30 mm range is associated with a marked decrease in cerebral blood flow and accompanying decrease in intracranial pressure. The induced respiratory alkalosis is associated with an increase in oxygen consumption, a shift of the oxyhemoglobin dissociation curve to the left, with a resultant decrease in oxygen availability for peripheral tissues. Also, cardiac arrhythmias are more prevalent during respiratory alkalosis. In addition, hyperventilation with an increased mechanical rate and tidal volume can cause myocardial depression by impeding venous return.

Usual electrolyte abnormalities are related to both potassium and calcium. Specific calcium problems relate not to total but, in fact, ionized calcium levels. These are now able to be measured clinically. Ionized calcium is important for appropriate cardiovascular function. There does not appear to be any direct relationship between ionized and total serum calcium levels. It is not uncommon in trauma patients to be hypocalcemic in the post-resuscitative period requiring up to 2 gm of ionized calcium chloride to improve cardiovascular performance.

Hypoglycemia is another common complication after trauma. This may be related to increased level of circulating catecholamines. Epinephrine has well-known anti-insulin effects. Problems with induced diuresis have been alluded to in another paper. When blood sugar is greater than 250 mg%, insulin is used in small dosages preventing both the hyperosmotic effects as well as inappropriate diuresis.

Salt therapy may be important in the resuscitation of the multiple trauma patient with head injuries. Salt intake is limited in patients with chronic congestive heart failure or cirrhosis. This does not mean that this cannot be a useful form of therapy during acute illnesses in even this group of patients; however, these patients already have a salt water overload. If they are then resuscitated with hypotonic or salt-poor solutions, homeostasis may be further compromised. By the ADH effect, water excretion is minimized to maintain intravascular volume. If free water is added, serum osmolarity is further diluted and the kidney cannot excrete its free water load, because now it labors under the influence of the stress aspects of the ADH excretion. It is not difficult to monitor intravascular status using a pulmonary artery catheter.

Fluid sequestration is not uncommon in the postoperative period. This can occur in the wall of the intestine in the peritoneal space and the like. There may also be a functional loss of fluid due to the inability of fluid to move back and forth between the interstitial and intravascular compartments. The sodium-potassium pump at the cellular membranes is an energy-dependent system. In the stress state the body attempts to generate its own energy from combustion of endogenous sources.

What other parameters need to be measured? The well-resuscitated patient will most likely be hypocalcemic after massive transfusion therapy; pH and other blood gas parameters including PO_2 and PCO_2 are monitored. GI losses in terms of both volume and electrode composition are monitored. In the complicated patient, such as one with an anastomotic leak or who has developed sepsis, one must pay particular attention to all fluid therapy. Every fluid loss must be assessed for both volume and electrolyte composition. This includes chest, abdominal and nasogastric and bladder drainage. Improved types of nasogastric catheters result in an increase in GI losses. Primarily stomach fluid contains hydrochloric acid. Hypochloremia and increased biocarbonate losses lead to a relative metabolic alkalosis. Hypokalemia develops not from gastric losses, but with the development of metabolic alkalosis potassium levels are driven into the cellular compartment. In addition because of the hypochloremia bicarbonate becomes a reabsorbable anion in the renal distal tubules and for every bicarbonate reabsorbed one hydrogen ion is lost.

Potent loop diuretics such as Lasix and ethacrynic acid operate by blocking chloride reabsorption in the loop of Henley. They then perpetuate this problem of hypochloremia and metabolic alkalosis. The preservative in blood, citrate, is also converted to bicarbonate and metabolic alkalosis can develop after massive transfusion therapy.

Therapy includes replacing chloride. This increases chloride levels permitting normal anionic and cationic changes to occur in the kidney and eventual normalization of the acid base properties. With severe forms of alkalosis and massive gastric fluid loss hydrochloric acid infusions may be necessary to restore normal parameters. Hydrochloric acid is infused through a central vein in order to avoid thrombosis. Eight milliliters of a 12 molar solution is dissolved in 1000 liters of D5W with a resultant concentration of .8 mEq of acid per milliliter fluid. The replacement dosage is based upon the same calculations used for bicarbonate.

Since the alkalosis is also due to chloride, one must replace great amounts of chloride anions. The volume distribution of chloride is some 30% of total body weight. The difference between the actual serum chloride concentration and the desired serum chloride concentration multiplied by the volume distribution equals the total chloride ion deficit. This can then be replaced over the next 24 to 72 hours by infusions of appropriate chloride-containing solutions.

Nutritional response after major surgery or trauma goes through several phases. During the first phase, organ system function is maintained by generation of increased energy. In the absence of exogenous nutritional resources protein stores are mobilized. At this stage exogenous nutritional support has no active role. However, as the stress period begins to wane, the onset of nutritional therapy can begin to interrupt and reverse the destruction of body proteins. With protein synthesis wound healing can begin and the lost protein regenerated.

There are three obvious sources of energy: carbohydrates, proteins and fats. Each individual requires some 1800 kcal per day. Energy developed comes from adenosine triphosphate, ATP. Carbohydrates are principally stored in the liver in the form of glycogen with some available in the skeletal muscle. These glycogen stores are usually depleted within 24 to 36 hours after the onset of stress. Although fat supplies twice as much calories per kilogram (9 cal/kg) than do proteins or carbohydrates, it cannot be utilized at times of stress. This is especially true of the brain. Other systems unable to function with fat metabolism include leukocytes and fibroblasts. Therefore, the most abundant and useful energy source is protein. Breakdown of protein sources provides amino acids for energy substrate utilization.

It is not unusual to excrete at least 10 gm of nitrogen per day. This is done at the expense of about 60 gm of protein. This works out to a loss of lean body mass of one half pound per day. In order to prevent these detrimental effects, exogenous sources of energy substrates must be available. The preferred route is the GI system. However, in the early stages of illness, most patients have minimal gut function and this route is not always available. Therefore, carbohydrates and proteins are combined in the form of intravenous hyperalimentation therapy. Patients require nitrogen in the amount equal to that which is being presently utilized. Also, patients require various cofactors in terms of vitamins and trace elements. Some fat is also required. Other intracellular components need to be added in significant quantities, particularly potassium. Acidosis secondary to the amino acid load is not an uncommon complication and may require correction.

Another major complication of intravenous hyperalimentation therapy is hyperglycemia. A critically ill patient may react like a diabetic simply because of the major injuries and stress, making hyperglycemia always a constant threat. Sliding insulin scales or continuous infusions are used to maintain normal glucose levels. Patients also require some fat infusions. Ten to twenty percent solutions are now commercially available. These are isotonic and can be given through peripheral veins.

Nutritional therapy begins after the initial stress period of 24 to 48 hours during which patients are unable to tolerate high glucose infusions. Dextrose in 5% to 10% solutions plus some amino acids can then be started. Total nutritional support involves higher concentrations of glucose: providing

2,000 to 3,000 calories per 24-hour period of time. As GI function improves, the patient can then be switched to interval therapy. In summary, then, this type of patient requires precise and close monitoring of all electrolyte, metabolic and nutritional components. By paying particular attention to these areas, one can minimize or prevent complications developed in the postoperative period.

Self-Evaluation Quiz

1. After multiple system trauma, hyperalimentation therapy should be gotten immediately.
   a) True
   b) False
2. Hypothermia always decreases oxygen consumption.
   a) True
   b) False
3. Complications of alkalosis include all of the following *except*:
   a) Decreased oxygen availability
   b) Cardiac arrhythmias
   c) Increased oxygen consumption
   d) Hyperkalemia
4. If serum calcium is normal, further calcium therapy is not indicated.
   a) True
   b) False
5. Hyperalimentation therapy consists of replacement of all of the following *except*:
   a) Carbohydrates
   b) Proteins
   c) Trace elements
   d) Fats
   e) Calcium
6. Nitrogen loss usually exceeds 10 gm in a 24-hour period.
   a) True
   b) False
7. Complications of hyperalimentation therapy include all of the following *except*:
   a) Hyperglycemia
   b) Hypoglycemia

   c) Hyperosmotic state

   d) Renal diuresis

   e) Metabolic alkalosis

8. The multiple trauma patient usually requires in excess of 3500 calories for a 24-hr period.

   a) True

   b) False

Answers on page 391.

Renal Function Syndromes

David J. Jaffe, M.D.

Objectives

To discuss three clinically encountered syndromes of fluid and osmolar imbalance from a pathophysiological, clinical and therapeutic standpoint.

There are several syndromes encountered in contemporary neurological and neurosurgical practice the pathogenesis of which intimately involves renal function. I shall discuss three of these syndromes: hyperosmolar states; diabetes insipidus; and antidiuretic hormone excess syndrome, particularly the syndrome of inappropriate ADH (SIADH).

Body fluid balance is normally regulated by an osmostat (osmotic receptor) located in the brain in the region of the hypothalamus. This very sensitive receptor detects changes in osmolarity or blood plasma particle content relative to plasma water. The physiologic adaptations occurring in an individual are determined by the intactness of the osmostat and the direction of osmotic changes taking place.

Osmolarity can be determined or estimated by several methods. One can collect a specimen of blood and submit it to the laboratory where osmotic content will be determined by measuring changes in the freezing point of water. Solutions of higher osmolarity lower the temperature to which water must be cooled before it will freeze. The value reported is referred to as the measured plasma osmolarity. The second commonly used method estimates plasma osmolarity utilizing values obtained from the profile-6 (electrolytes, glucose, plasma urea (BUN)) according to the following formula:

David J. Jaffe, M.D., Assistant Professor of Nephrology, University of Miami School of Medicine; Clinical Assistant Professor of Nephrology, Jackson Memorial Hospital, Miami Veterans Administration Hospital, Fla.

$$pOsm = 2(Na^+) + \frac{glucose}{18} + \frac{BUN}{3} + (X)$$

$(X) =$ unmeasured osmotically active particles

For mathematic simplicity glucose can be divided by 20 and BUN can be divided by 3. The factor (X) refers to substances which are usually unmeasured by the laboratory which can be osmotically active and contribute to the overall osmotic pressure (e.g., mannitol and ethanol). As an example, if the serum sodium of an individual is 136 mEq/liter, the glucose = 100 mg/dl and the BUN = 18 mg/dl with no unmeasured osmotic particles present the calculated osmolarity will be 283 mOsm/liter.

$$pOsm = 2(136) + \frac{100}{20} + \frac{18}{3}$$

$$= 283 \text{ mOsm/liter}$$

The brain osmostat is "set" at an osmolarity of 284 ± 5 mOsm/liter. Slight increases above this level will stimulate the osmostat and result in ADH production in the hypothalamus, transport to and release from the posterior pituitary. ADH will then exert its physiological effect on the kidney causing an increase in fluid reabsorption and ultimately plasma osmolarity will normalize. Decreases in osmolarity will conversely suppress ADH production and release, less fluid will be reabsorbed by the kidney and this will result in normalization of plasma osmolarity.

In addition to the above ADH effect, increases in plasma osmolarity will stimulate the hypothalamic thirst center(s) leading to an increase in fluid intake by normal individuals. A neurologically impaired or postoperative patient may have the thirst mechanism transiently or permanently impaired. These individuals may not sense the need for increased fluid intake or may be incapable of drinking and may require fluids by IV route.

Some individuals may be encountered who have developed a hyperosmolar state, a state of increased plasma osmolarity (with pOsm values often approaching or greater than 350 mOsm/liter) (Table 1). Such states may develop in patients who have had glucose administered pre-, intra- and postoperatively or in those

Table 1. Hyperosmolar States: Occurrence

A. Mannitol and glucose administration
B. Diabetes (especially the elderly)
C. Dialysis
D. Hyperalimentation
E. Burns
F. Drugs (diuretics, steroids, alcohol)

infused with mannitol. In contemporary neurological/neurosurgical practice mannitol is administered in an attempt to prevent or treat cerebral edema. In other specialties, e.g., cardiovascular surgery, mannitol has been infused to prevent development of renal insufficiency. Both substances are osmotically active and can increase plasma osmolarity if administered to any patient in excess of that patient's ability to metabolize them. Glucose is a measured osmotic substance while mannitol is not commonly measured by the clinical laboratory (X factor in calculation).

Other patients who have not received exogenous glucose or mannitol may spontaneously develop hyperosmolar states. Elderly diabetic patients in addition to developing diabetic ketoacidosis are particularly prone to the development of hyperosmolarity. This propensity must be considered carefully whenever such patients require surgical intervention. Individuals undergoing dialysis (hemodialysis or peritoneal) have developed the state when certain glucose-containing infusate solutions were used and more fluid removed. The administration of parenteral alimentation solutions in the hospital setting has precipitated hyperosmolar states including coma. Use of various drugs, particularly alcohol, steroids and diuretics can result in the clinical picture with these patients appearing to be "presensitized." Osmolarity should be monitored closely in any of these patients especially if surgery is contemplated. It has been clearly demonstrated that the *majority* of patients developing hyperosmolar states either for the first time or recurrently have mild to moderate *underlying* renal insufficiency.

The hyperosmolar state has several major characteristics (Table 2). First, hyperosmolarity is present with plasma osmolarity equal to or greater than 350 mOsm/liter. Second,

Table 2. Hyperosmolar States: Characteristics

A. Hyperglycemia (often ≥ 1000 mg/dl)
B. Plasma hyperosmolarity (≥ 350 mOsm)
C. *Absence* of ketoacidosis
D. Depressed sensorium
*E. Profound dehydration The mean water loss is 9.1 liters or 25% of body weight

*Most significant characteristic.

hyperglycemia is usually seen, often with plasma glucose values greater than 1,000 mg/dl. This may represent decreased insulin secretion or decreased effect. Diabetic patients with the hyperosmolar state must be differentiated from those with ketoacidosis. The hyperosmolar patient will not usually have detectable ketoacids (lab or Ketostix) and the rapid Kussmaul respiration/acetone odor of breath seen in ketoacidosis. Depressed sensorium, the third main characteristic, results from changes in osmolarity, fluid shifts into or out of cells or from hyperglycemia. Finally, hyperosmolar patients have been shown to be profoundly fluid depleted with an average water loss of 9.1 liters or approximately 25% of their body weight in kilograms. *Fluid depletion is the key characteristic* of the syndrome — water is lost in excess of the loss of osmotic particles.

Two pathophysiologic mechanisms have been proposed for the production of the hyperosmolar state. The first occurs in the presence of substances which are freely permeable between extracellular and intracellular spaces, most commonly urea and ethanol. Far advanced renal insufficiency with extremely high BUN values constitutes the only clinical situation currently where hyperosmolarity is due to urea. This is very infrequently encountered today because intervention in the form of dialysis is instituted earlier in the course of renal failure than in previous times. More commonly one may encounter the ethanol-intoxicated patient, especially those with head trauma. When ethanol is consumed it enters the vascular space as well as the intracellular space where it is metabolically degraded. This results in a situation in which ethanol levels are greater in plasma than within the cell. The circulating ethanol exerts an osmotic effect raising the plasma osmolarity by 22 mOsm/liter for each 100 mg/dl of ethanol present. This increase in osmolarity draws water from the cell and should stimulate ADH release and lead to increased water reabsorption; however, ethanol directly blocks ADH action on the kidney. Despite the increase in plasma osmolarity an excessive amount of water is lost from the body greater than expected. This brings about an even higher blood ethanol concentration and osmolarity. The concept is illustrated in Figure 1.

Because plasma ethanol concentration is not a routine laboratory determination the pOsm *measured* by freezing point depression will be greater than the pOsm *calculated* from the osmolarity formula. This is illustrated by the following clinical example:

Comatose alcoholic patient who is intoxicated and has a blood alcohol level of 100 mg/dl, Na+ = 136 mEq/l, glucose = 100 mg/dl and a BUN = 18 mg/dl.

Measured pOsm = 305 mOsm/liter

Calculated pOsm = $2(136) + \dfrac{100}{20} + \dfrac{18}{3}$ = 283 mOsm/liter

Measured pOsm > Calculated pOsm

(305 mOsm/L)   (283 mOsm/L)

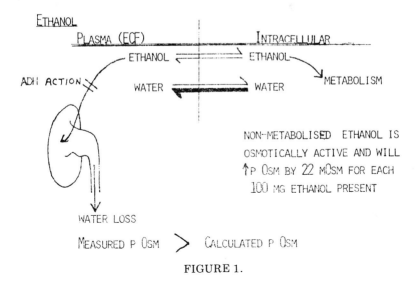

FIGURE 1.

The second pathophysiologic mechanism occurs with glucose or mannitol, substances which are not freely permeable between extracellular and intracellular spaces. In this situation the osmotically active glucose or mannitol remains within the extracellular (intravascular) space. Water is lost from the cells and produces an osmotic diuresis in which one loses more water than osmotic particles. This second mechanism is illustrated in Figure 2.

The following is a typical clinical situation:

Postsurgical patient returns from the OR where he has been administered large quantities of concentrated glucose IV; large urine volumes (=150 ml/hr) are noted. The patient's sensorium remains markedly dulled after the effects of anesthetics should have worn off. Labs reveal serum Na+ = 136 mEq/L, glucose = 1100 mg/dl, BUN = 18 mg/dl.

Measured pOsm = 333 mOsm/liter

$$\text{Calculated pOsm} = 2(136) + \frac{1100}{20} + \frac{18}{3} = 333 \text{ mOsm/liter}$$

Measured pOsm = Calculated pOsm in this instance. (It must be remembered, however, that glucose is measured by the

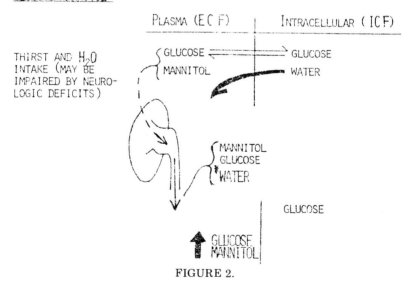

FIGURE 2.

clinical lab while mannitol is not. Were the hyperosmolar state due to mannitol the measured pOsm would be greater than the calculated pOsm.)

Treatment of the hyperosmolar state is trifold. First, fluid deficits should be corrected. Second, hyperglycemia is treated with insulin (ethanol and mannitol, on the other hand, must be metabolized by the body). Third, potassium is supplemented as necessary to prevent hypokalemia. As I have stated previously, the patient manifesting hyperosmolarity is virtually always profoundly fluid-depleted (average 9.1 liters). Fluid should be administered under appropriate hemodynamic and clinical monitoring with two thirds of the deficit administered during the initial 12 hours. The remaining one third of the deficit can then be replaced over the following 12 to 24 hours depending upon the patient's age and cardiovascular status. Normal saline solution has been shown to be the most appropriate replacement solution since it will expand the intravascular space without greatly altering the intracellular milieu. Were one to choose instead half normal saline then the body would be receiving more water than NaCl. This water would then leave the intravascular space and enter the intracellular space. The result would be intravascular volume depletion (even shock) and intracellular edema. When particularly severe, cerebral edema may develop and be devastating.

Hyperglycemia is treated both by the above fluid replacement and by the administration of exogenous insulin which acts to allow glucose to reenter the cell. Only a mild insulin resistance is usually encountered with the average patient requiring small doses of insulin. Indeed, blood glucose levels in the range of 1,000 mg/dl may be normalized by as little as 5 to 10 units of insulin. The administration of larger doses of insulin to these patients has occasionally resulted in profound hypoglycemia.

Potassium deficits resulting from diuresis and K+ shifts facilitated by insulin are replaced according to commonly accepted protocols. Blood potassium levels should be obtained in all patients and serially monitored as therapy is instituted.

The second abnormality of water and osmotic balance to be discussed is diabetes insipidus (DI). There are two forms of DI: neurogenic and nephrogenic. The medical literature sometimes refers to neurogenic DI as central or ADH-sensitive and nephrogenic as ADH-insensitive. I shall not dwell on nephrogenic DI except to state that it is pathophysiologically neither a defect of ADH production nor of its release. Nephrogenic DI represents a defect of the target end-organ, the renal tubule. This defect is characterized by a lack of sensitivity of the tubule to endogenous (and exogenous) ADH. On the other hand, neurogenic DI reflects defective ADH production, transport or release into the circulation.

As discussed earlier the hypothalamic osmoreceptor senses the number of osmotically active particles in blood and the pressure thus generated. When the osmotic pressure of blood increases within or above the normal range (284 ± 5 mOsm/liter) by an increase in number of osmotic particles or water loss from the body, the osmoreceptor is stimulated. This triggers ADH production by the hypothalamus, ADH transport to and release from the posterior pituitary into the circulation. Ultimately ADH is delivered to the kidney where it exerts its effect. Within the kidney the distal tubule and collecting duct, in the presence of ADH, become more permeable to water allowing more water to be reabsorbed. Under conditions of lowered plasma osmolarity (usually water excess) the hypothalamic osmoreceptor is inhibited, less ADH is produced, transported and/or released to the circulation. This ultimately results in less water being reabsorbed by the kidney. Figure 3 depicts the events occurring in normal individuals to maintain normal daily osmotic balance.

In the patient with neurogenic DI, in response to water loss and an increase in osmolarity, less than a normal quantity of ADH is produced and released. Urinary water losses exceed that which should normally occur thus maintaining plasma osmolarity slightly greater than normal. The thirst mechanism can in compensation lead to an increase in water intake and potentially normalize plasma osmolarity when it is intact. The person with a neurological deficit or one who is postoperative may have a functional or structural defect in the thirst mechanism. When adequate fluids cannot be consumed by these individuals, symptomatic hyperosmolarity may result unless IV fluids are provided. Figure 4 depicts the defects occurring in the patient with neurogenic DI as compared with normals.

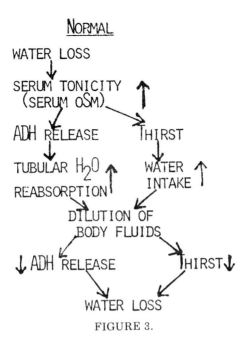

FIGURE 3.

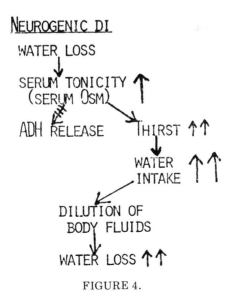

FIGURE 4.

Table 3 summarizes the varied etiologies of neurogenic DI. Functional or structural defects in the osmoreceptor, the ADH-producing area of the hypothalamus, the pituitary stalk or posterior pituitary may produce neurogenic DI. In approximately 40% of cases no anatomic abnormalities can be conclusively demonstrated while 60% occur on the basis of a demonstrable structural defect: posthypophysectomy; posttraumatic; tumors (supra- or intrasellar); intracranial cysts and granulomas; histiocytosis; vascular (including cerebrovascular occlusions); "empty sella" syndrome. One may easily see that the neurologist or neurosurgeon will encounter such patients more commonly than will other physicians.

The clinical manifestations of neurogenic DI are summarized in Table 4. Onset is almost always abrupt and may be triphasic. The first detectable change is the development of polyuria. Urine output increases to reach a peak volume within 24 to 48 hours of onset. Rarely urine volumes greater than 10 liters/24 hours have been reported — urine volumes are *usually* less than this amount. Urine specific gravity is usually 1.001 to 1.005 with corresponding urine osmolarities between 50 and 200 mOsm/liter. This represents nearly maximally dilute urine. Little diurnal variation in urine output can be detected. Plasma osmolarity is usually slightly increased above normal (297 ± 12 versus 284 ± 5 mOsm/liter), representing slight volume depletion. In response the thirst mechanism is stimulated and polydipsia is noted. Some investigators have found that patients with DI have a predilection for consumption of iced drinks.

Table 3. Etiologies of Neurogenic DI (Central)

A. Idiopathic (40%)

B. Neuropathological (60%)
   1. Posthypophysectomy
   2. Posttraumatic
   3. Tumors (supra or intrasellar)
   4. Intracranial cysts
   5. Granulomas
   6. Histiocytosis
   7. Vascular (including CVA)
   8. Other ("empty sella," etc.)

Table 4. Clinical Manifestations of Neurogenic DI

A. Onset *almost always abrupt*

B. May have triphasic pattern
   1. Diabetes insipidus – injury to hypothalamic centers of ADH production
   2. Antidiuresis – release of preformed ADH from necrotic cells
   3. Diabetes insipidus – ADH deficiency

C. Polyurea – urine output usually < 10 L/24 hr
   1. Urine s.g. usually 1.001-1.005
   2. Urine Osm 50-200 mOsmo/L
   3. Usually peaks within 1-2 days
   4. Little diurnal pattern

D. Polydipsia
   1. Preference for iced drinks (±)

E. Slight volume depletion
   1. pOsm ↑ to 297 ± 12 (nl 285 ± 4)

F. May have bladder distention and/or hydronephrosis

This may reflect only a Western cultural bias for iced drinks explaining why this finding is not universally accepted. The neurologically impaired patient with DI and large urine volumes may require IV fluid replacement. Additionally, such patients may have decreased bladder sensation with bladder distention/hydronephrosis becoming a significant clinical problem.

Table 5 summarizes the diagnostic maneuvers which have been utilized to differentiate the patient with DI and clinically similar syndromes (psychogenic water drinkers, IV volume expansion) from the normal patient. The first of these is commonly referred to as the water deprivation test. The patient

Table 5. Diagnostic Maneuvers: Neurogenic DI

A. Water deprivation test:

	Normal	*Neurogenic DI*
urine flow ↓ to < .5 ml/min		*no change* or slight ↓
urine Osm ↑ to ≅ 800 mOsm/l		*slight* ↑ of U Osm

B. Hypertonic saline: dangerous as may result in CHF
   (nl urine flow ↓ to 25% or less of control)

C. Response to exogenous vasopressin:
   1. Normal and neurogenic DI will ↓ urine flow and
      ↑ U Osm appropriately

is fluid-deprived from 12 to 16 hours with urine flow rate and osmotic changes monitored. Individuals who are normal, psychogenic water drinkers or are volume expanded will respond by decreasing urine flow rate to less than 0.5 ml/min and by increasing urinary osmolarity to 700 to 800 mOsm/liter. Those with DI in contrast show no change or only slight decreases in urine flow rate and slight increases of urine osmolarity to 300 to 400 mOsm/liter. The test should never be performed overnight or in circumstances where adequate observation is not possible since the individual with true DI could become significantly volume depleted. If evidence of hemodynamically significant volume depletion occurs at any time, the test should be immediately terminated and fluid deficits replaced. Hypertonic saline administration has a similar effect on urine flow rate and osmolarity as fluid deprivation with the normal patient responding while the patient with DI will not respond. This test is in disfavor because it has led to precipitation or worsening of congestive heart failure in volume-expanded individuals or those with cardiovascular disease. Response to exogenous vasopressin administration can differentiate the normal patient from the patient with DI and can further differentiate neurogenic DI (ADH-sensitive) from nephrogenic DI (ADH-insensitive). The normal patient treated with vasopressin will slightly decrease urine flow rate and slightly increase urine osmolarity. The patient with neurogenic DI will respond to a replacement of hormone deficiency by significantly reducing urine flow rate and increasing urine osmolarity to values approaching those of normally concentrated urine. The patient with nephrogenic DI will show virtually no response to this maneuver.

Therapy for neurogenic DI consists of exogenous ADH administration (Table 6). Aqueous pitressin and longer acting pitressin tannate in oil were used extensively in the past. They have now been relegated to infrequent usage by the successful synthesis and purification of dDAVP (D-amino arginine vasopressin), the active hormone. This preparation has a long duration of action (12 hours) and can be administered intranasally in doses of 5 to 20 μg twice daily to the patient regardless of his mental status.

We will now consider the antidiuretic hormone excess syndromes. Just as there can be situations where ADH is

Table 6. Treatment of Neurogenic DI

A. ADH administration
  *1. dDAVP (d-amino arginine vasopressin)
       intranasally in dose 5-20 μg twice daily
       a. *Long acting*
   2. Pitressin tannate/aqueous pitressin

B. Ancillary measures
   1. Drugs
       a. Chlorpropamide (enhances effect of ADH)
       b. Acetaminophen
       c. Clofibrate
       d. Tegretol (carbamazepine)
       e. Thiazides
            1. Vol. depletion → increased H_2O reabsorption
           †2. Nephrogenic form

*Drug of choice.
†Thiazides have been shown to be of significant benefit in patients with a nephrogenic form of diabetes insipidus.

depleted (DI) other situations can develop where ADH is excessive. When ADH is present in concentrations which are excessive for the underlying clinical situation, the syndrome is termed the syndrome of inappropriate antidiuretic hormone (SIADH).

In review, as the concentration of ADH increases in blood in response to hyperosmolarity or hypovolemia more fluid is reabsorbed by the renal tubule. This brings about a normalization of volume status and suppresses further production and/or release of ADH into the circulation. The patient with an ADH excess syndrome has an excess of endogenous circulating ADH, increased fluid reabsorption, normalized or expanded blood volumes. In this situation further ADH production/release should be suppressed but suppression does not occur.

Antidiuretic hormone excess syndromes are characterized by excessive ADH concentration, increased fluid reabsorption and clinically by (1) serum hyponatremia (Na+ less than 130 mEq/L); (2) plasma hypoosmolarity; (3) low plasma urate levels; (4) low blood urea nitrogen (BUN); (5) relatively concentrated urine with increased urinary osmolarity; and (6) moderate urinary Na+ losses (usually > 20 mEq/L). Serum hyponatremia results from the excess of water intake and reabsorption as well as sodium losses in the urine. Plasma hypoosmolarity occurs with the decrease of serum sodium concentration. A sample osmolarity calculation in a patient with ADH excess follows:

$$\text{Plasma osmolarity} = 2(Na^+) + \frac{\text{glucose}}{20} + \frac{BUN}{3}$$

$$= 2(120) + \frac{100}{20} + \frac{6}{3} = 247 \text{ mOsm/liter}$$

Decreased urate and BUN levels are produced by volume expansion, diuresis and decreased urate and urea reabsorption by the kidney. The association of decreased urate levels with ADH excess syndromes was noted almost 100 years ago and remains clinically relevant. Several recent papers claim that patients suspected of having ADH excess syndromes must have low urate levels or the diagnosis should be questioned. The presence of excess ADH results in increased water reabsorption. Thus, relatively concentrated urine is elaborated with osmolarity usually 100 mOsm/liter greater than plasma osmolarity. Urinary sodium losses result from the natriuresis associated with slight volume expansion. The above characteristics are summarized in Table 7.

The diagnosis of SIADH can be excluded in certain circumstances (i.e., circumstances where changes in ADH levels are appropriate). The patient with SIADH must meet all of the exclusion criteria in Table 8. Individuals with ADH excess are usually clinically euvolemic even though hemodynamic measurements may reveal evidence of mild volume expansion. The presence of volume contraction (i.e., positive tilt test) stimulates ADH appropriately — the volume contracted patient does

Table 7. ADH - Hormone Excess Syndromes: SIADH

	A.	Criteria
		1. Hyponatremia and serum hypoosmolarity
		2. Urine inappropriately concentrated despite hyponatremia (U Osm > pOsm)
		3. Urinary $Na^+ \geq 20$ mEq/l
		4. Depressed [urate] P
		5. Depressed [BUN] P
Definitive		6. Elevated ADH levels
		7. Improvement of hyponatremia after fluid restriction

Table 8. Exclusion Criteria: SIADH

1. "Normovolemia"
2. Normal renal function
3. Normal adrenal function
4. Normal thyroid function
5. "No drugs"

not have SIADH. Thus, if you are evaluating a patient for SIADH check the blood pressure first and make certain that the patient is euvolemic.

Patients with SIADH must have normal renal function. Renal dysfunction can result in an inability of the kidney to respond to ADH, fluid or sodium challenges and produces occasionally a picture clinically similar to SIADH but with normal or depressed ADH levels. The adrenal hormones, cortisone and aldosterone, affect fluid and electrolyte balance. Excess or deficit of these hormones clinically simulate ADH excess syndromes though once again the ADH levels of these patients are normal. It is unnecessary to determine adrenal function by blood tests since clinical evaluation is usually adequate to exclude the cushingoid or addisonian patient. Thyroid function must also be normal since the patient with myxedema cannot excrete water loads adequately; clinical evaluation is usually sufficient. Finally, the patient should not be taking any drugs which might affect release of ADH or potentiate its action. Such drugs include those listed in Table 9.

After excluding the preceding situations the ADH-excess syndromes have developed secondary to a variety of processes. The primary cause is idiopathic hypothalamic dysfunction which accounts for up to 75% of cases. Secondary causes are central nervous system disorders of degenerative, traumatic, infective, malignant or vascular nature and pulmonary path-

Table 9. Drugs ↑ ADH Release or Potentiating ADH Action

1. Oral hypoglycemics: chlorpropamide, tolbutamide
2. Antineoplastics: vincristine, cyclophosphamide
3. Sedatives and analgesics: *barbiturates*
4. Psychotrophics: amitriptyline, phenothiazines
5. Miscellaneous: nicotine, clofibrate, tegretol

ology (tuberculosis and tumors). ADH or ADH-like substances have been eluted from malignant lesions extrinsic to the central nervous system.

Onset is usually insidious though acute onsets have been reported. Symptoms may be confined to the laboratory abnormalities previously elucidated or may be clinically manifested. Most common clinical symptoms are disturbances in neurologic function ranging from subtle personality changes to seizures and coma.

Treatment is directed toward correcting the most potentially serious abnormality, hyponatremia. Severe hyponatremia can be corrected by the administration of hypertonic saline and concomitant use of diuretics. Chronic asymptomatic hyponatremia, on the other hand, is most easily treated by fluid restriction in the cooperative patient. When cooperation is uncertain or impossible, chronic drug therapy has been advocated. Lithium carbonate, which is used clinically to treat manic-depressive psychosis, blocks ADH effect on the kidney resulting in a drug-induced nephrogenic DI-like picture. When administered to the patient with ADH-excess syndromes, hyponatremia usually resolves; however, the toxic effects of this drug have precluded long-term usage. Demeclocycline, a tetracycline derivative, also results in a nephrogenic DI-like picture and has been useful in treating SIADH when one is unable to fluid restrict. Toxic side effects have been described in cirrhotic patients and make its long-term use uncertain. In those patients whose ADH-excess syndrome is tumor-related the appropriate therapy is primary resection of the tumor mass if such is possible.

In conclusion, one should be well aware that each of the syndromes I have discussed can develop in association with neuropathological processes. Each can be devastating if unrecognized but is amenable to medical therapy.

Self-Evaluation Quiz

1. The formula for calculating plasma osmolarity utilizes lab values for:
   a) Sodium
   b) Potassium

    c) Chloride
    d) Glucose
    e) BUN
    f) Unmeasured osmotically active particles
2. Most patients with hyperosmolar states have normal renal function.
    a) True
    b) False
3. The treatment of hyperosmolar states consists of:
    a) Normal saline
    b) Half-normal saline
    c) Insulin, 100 units IV or IM
    d) Insulin, 5-10 units IV
    e) Potassium
4. Patients with diabetes insipidus are usually slightly volume depleted.
    a) True
    b) False
5. Pitressin tannate in oil is the currently accepted treatment for all forms of diabetes insipidus.
    a) True
    b) False
6. Patients with SIADH must have:
    a) Normal renal function
    b) Normal cardiovascular function
    c) Normal adrenal function
    d) Evidence of hypothyroidism
    e) Plasma hyperosmolarity
7. Fluid restriction is the mainstay of treatment of patients with SIADH.
    a) True
    b) False

Answers on page 391.

Panel Discussion

Moderator: Dr. Shapiro

Panelists: Drs. Gallagher, Jaffe and Rodman

Moderator: Dr. Jaffe, if you have a head injured patient who comes to you with very severe hyperosmolality, four or five days posttrauma, who has received large amounts of mannitol and has a serum osmolality of 325 or 330, would you still advocate the use of normal saline for him? How would you resuscitate this patient back to a normal osmolality?

Dr. Jaffe: This patient presents a complex medical problem, i.e., how to appropriately treat hyperosmolarity without impairing neurological or cardiovascular function. It is appropriate to insert a catheter for measurement of central volume status in the patient with multiple injuries and to utilize readings to regulate volume replacement therapy.

Management of the patient in question will depend upon three factors: (1) renal functional status; (2) cardiovascular dynamics and (3) hepatic function. Mannitol is primarily excreted by the kidneys with a small extrarenal component. That fraction not excreted remains within the intravascular space until it can be metabolized in the liver. The patient with normal renal, cardiovascular and hepatic function develops hyperosmolarity secondary to hypermannitolemia as a result of relative excess renal water losses. Adequate fluid replacement should be provided to maintain intravascular volume and normal electrolyte concentrations. In the patient with heart disease or in the patient with decreased renal function who may be unable to excrete water or mannitol ever-vigorous fluid replacement may worsen cerebral edema or precipitate congestive heart failure. These are avoidable complications of aggressive intervention. Such patients require especially close monitoring and may require inotropic agents,

95

diuretic therapy and/or dialytic intervention. Finally, patients with impaired hepatic function might fail to metabolize mannitol resulting in persistent hyperosmolarity and hemodynamic disturbances.

Moderator: Dr. Gallagher, are there any problems connected with the rate at which our medical colleagues might want to do this in the patient I have just described? What other monitoring might you want to do for this patient?

Dr. Gallagher: In this situation, I think one would have a question about volume and about what is going on. The only way to answer these questions would be to accurately measure it, rather than guess at it. But basically I mean the intravascular monitoring of volume status with such things as pulmonary artery catheters to assess what is going on with the cardiovascular function, especially if one is going to go with volume replacement and one is worried about volume overloading the patient.

Moderator: Dr. Rodman, would you also please respond to this question? Is there anything else you might want to monitor in this patient?

Dr. Rodman: If you are talking about monitoring apparatus, no, I cannot think of anything. If you are talking about the aggressive correction of such states, then we have been in this situation often where we have had to do aggressive fluid infusion at the same time we are replacing fluid. We have even done exsanguination forms of therapy, if you will, at the same time we are restoring red cell mass, and even not using sodium chloride, simply because in the excess state you are creating at that time, hypervolemia is a problem. Many times, phlebotomy combined with something that is not quite as isotonic as what is being removed will allow mild, more appropriate shifts of water to occur. But then you begin to have to change back to more standard forms of therapy, such as Dr. Jaffe suggested. Without the ability to do ultrafiltration, i.e., without the ability to squeeze patients correctly, then I have at least on two occasions provided patients with phlebotomy combined with half-normal saline with closely watching their red cell mass.

Moderator: Does anyone watch the central nervous system of the patient during this time? Do you know what I mean, Dr. Gallagher?

Dr. Gallagher: Obviously, one must watch the central nervous system. I mentioned the use of half-normal saline and appropriate amounts of water, and one can intensify cerebral edema in the presence of physical shock in the patient. This must be carefully observed.

Moderator: Why do you not just use plain Ringer's lactate? I think one of the things that can happen, and I have seen this happen, is that we overly aggressively try to reverse what is basically often an iatrogenic problem, that we do it very quickly and very efficiently. The brain is a perfect osmometer if you use an ICP device and monitor the pressure. You will sometimes find that if we want to make trouble fast, we will give just water. The utilization of solutions that are normally constituted can also be dangerous if this is done too fast. The brain can respond very quickly with an elevation of intracranial pressure when you do this, whether it be hemodialysis or whatever technique you use. Monitoring pressure in this particular situation, and I am referring to the head injury patient, is often exceedingly useful in guiding the rate and the choice of the modality that one will use.

I have a number of questions dealing with the controversy over which method one is going to use for volume replacement — a colloid method versus the crystalloid method — when one has a loss of cerebrovascular integrity — blood-brain barrier damage. The questioners are alluding to the fact that was brought up earlier that one can end up with protein in the lung and possibly protein in the brain. Would you comment on that, especially if you have any data that strongly support one technique over another, Dr. Gallagher?

Dr. Gallagher: We do have data involving other organ systems. Dr. Mark Rowe at our institution studied piglets, in which he applied an injury into the bowel. There was increased capillary permeability at the site of injury and he was able to document that in those animals at the site of injury there was an increased accumulation of albumin and protein and an increased amount of edema formation. At the same time, in other areas where there was no injury produced, there was a dehydrating effect, that is, the albumin actually moved fluid from the extracellular fluid compartment back into the intravascular space. I myself am not aware of what goes on or what studies have been done across the blood-brain barrier in terms of moving some molecules, such as albumin.

Dr. Rodman: I will not discuss the blood-brain barrier because of your greater expertise, Dr. Shapiro. In those disease processes, and perhaps it is nothing more than severe injury, where capillary membranes throughout the body are injured, then albumin-loading may in fact not result in the intravascular persistence of albumin. The fact that it gets into the interstitium has been theoretically implied as creating a reverse oncotic effect and dragging water out of the interstitium. Dr. Gallagher and I both agree, based on the data that have been presented in the literature, regarding the measurement of albumin fluxes, exclusive of the brain, that so far no one has been able to suggest there is a bad effect from albumin. Most of the albumin is probably restored in some unknown way through the lymphatic system back into the intravascular compartment. I think everyone has been saying that there does not seem to be any benefit of such therapy in maintaining intravascular volume. In something like the brain, which has a closed, fixed space in which to operate, perhaps it may become more important.

Moderator: Dr. Jaffe, do you medical people have anything to add?

Dr. Jaffe: I am also aware of some of the studies that have been reported. The only information I might add is empiric observations of hemodialysis patients treated with albumin. We have noted some untoward effects. Some patients develop a "pulmonary-edema-like" picture as a result of the oncotic agent entering the pulmonary space. Several studies have been critical of oncotic agents because of their potential for entering third spaces such as lung or abdomen. The central nervous system by being the most confined of body spaces could conceivably be irreversibly harmed by agents entering the space and causing fluid retention or edema.

Dr. Gallagher: It lacks a lymphatic system. What lymphatic function one has in the cerebral spinal fluid becomes progressively attenuated as one gets into pathological situations. Insofar as a carefully controlled laboratory experiment dealing with this question, there are a few dealing with lungs, as far as I am concerned they are nonexistent. In the clinical situation, they are not measurable because there are too many things going on. So I think this is something that will remain unanswered. Possibly someone in the future will deal with this particular issue. Another important issue, as well as the one for which there are no data, is which vasopressor is the appropriate kind to use in a situation where one must use it in conjunction with resuscitation. Is there a vasopressor which will preferentially allow blood to be redistributed toward the brain and the heart? This is what we are looking at. We have some answers with regard to heart and no answers with regard to brain in that particular situation.

Dr. Rodman: While we are talking about ideal fluid therapy, I shall mention that the question of what is an ideal resuscitative medium is one you have heard argued for the past several years. It is based solely on the selection of those solutions containing albumin and those that do not. Now there is a third type. It really provides a twist and it may really have very startling effects in central nervous system function, and that is the hyperosmolar form of intravenous fluid therapy that has been popularized in the burn patient. In burn patients, one of the goals of resuscitation is to prevent edema, simply because it impairs burn wound healing and may indeed enhance the acquisition of burn wound sepsis. In every other kind of patient, so far, it is very difficult to show that acute ankle edema or sacral edema or other interstitial edema either is bad or accumulates to any great degree and just stays there when giving normal, standard quantities and volumes of resuscitation fluids. But if we can reduce that edema throughout the body, then one could assume perhaps that we may have some control over what is going on when fluid resuscitation is given for the brain. The hyperosmolar kinds of resuscitation really have sodium concentrations that are about twice normal. Randomized, prospective studies should be performed and our group is now undertaking such an effort. It is a third type and it may assume more ideal proportions in terms of the fluid than the old argument of colloid versus standard isotonic solution.

Moderator: You have just anticipated a question I was about to ask: Is there a role for early blood replacement as a fourth possible modality?

Dr. Rodman: I think in terms of trying to restore intravascular volume, yes, blood has some ideal characteristics. It probably hangs around a little bit longer than red cell mass does. But the unfortunate aspect of this, as Dr. Gallagher showed in his presentation of shock data from Dr. Shires, is that if one is trying to replace cubic centimeter for cubic centimeter of blood loss (which can be done in experimental situations and can be estimated in clinical conditions) one can match the blood volume, stabilize the hematocrit, and the patient may still be in shock, as defined by low flow states or inadequate oxygen dynamics, when measuring AVO_2 differences. So I think there is an obligatory requirement for giving not just blood cubic centimeter per cubic centimeter after shock. However, if one has a more controlled experiment or a more controlled human condition where the depth and duration of shock have not been severe, then, certainly, blood replacement with equal volume is ideal.

Moderator: Let us do a little philosophizing. How do you decide which specialist has the primary care for a multiple-injury patient? Let us direct this to each panelist.

Dr. Gallagher: I think the primary responsibility for the multiple-injury patient lies with the general surgeon, in terms of when he first arrives at the hospital, he then is familiar enough with all of the systems to make a rapid evaluation of what needs to be done rapidly and where and when. From that point, the patient then enters into the system, and in our institution, the multiple-injury patient ends up in the general surgical intensive care unit, from which time his intensive care course is directed by an intensive care team, which can consist of one person, an anesthesiologist, to an internal medicine person, or whoever, but all are trained in and understand the principles of total system care for the patient who is critically ill.

Dr. Rodman: I agree with that. I would only hedge in this way, by saying that this person who, although here it is designated by specialties, and that is probably true of most institutions, irrespective of his primary orientation has to take the responsibility of total coordination. There is a body of knowledge that is being demonstrated to be peculiar to critical care. I think it is reasonable to expect that person to be geographically based in the critical care area. Whether he has the ability to operate is totally irrelevant, since the coordination sequencing of diagnostic and therapeutic procedures is the key to this whole situation.

Dr. Jaffe: I believe I have an easy answer to that question: not the internist. There is, however, an extremely active role for the internist to play in the management of metabolic, fluid, acid-base and electrolyte problems of the multiply injured patient.

Moderator: This issue could be discussed throughout all eternity. What is the safe maximum daily mannitol dose in head-injury patients, especially with regard to preventing renal impairment in grams per kilogram per day? If there is a renal lesion, could you tell us about it? Let us start with the medicine people.

Dr. Jaffe: To the best of my knowledge no investigator has described a renal lesion associated with the use of mannitol. Since mannitol is an "inert" substance, one would not expect to see a renal lesion. As for maximum "safe" dosages of mannitol there has been no successful quantitation of a universal per kilogram dosage. Dosages utilized have ranged from 0.25 gm/kg/4 hr to 4 gm/kg/4 hr. One can monitor mannitol effects by detection or calculation of changes in serum osmolarity and utilize these values as a basis for fluid therapy. Each patient must have his mannitol dosage titrated to maximize desired effect and minimize complications.

Moderator: Dr. Marshall is not here so I shall attempt to answer for him and for myself. I think the answer is that one must titrate. One must look at what is happening. I think the initial doses of mannitol at 1 or 2 gm/kg q 4 h are gross overdoses. Dr. Marshall and I have done some work looking at that question, in particular looking at lower doses. The high dose of mannitol that is suggested in the literature results from a simple mathematical calculation from the dose of urea that formerly was used before mannitol supplanted it. That particular dose of urea was established in patients who did not have very high intracranial pressure, which means that you must give much more to see any result. So we start with a bias toward overdose. In the study that Dr. Marshall and I did, we found that the use of 0.25 to 0.5 gm/kg was essentially the same in terms of ICP reduction, time of ICP reduction, and the only point where it differed was at the fifth hour. That would tend to indicate that one can use lower doses and not suffer as rapid an electrolyte depletion and dehydration as one might otherwise get with the very high doses and still obtain virtually the same effect as far as ICP is concerned. So we can only help you by saying that a lower dose can be just as effective. It would appear that a 10 mOsm jump each time is about the range one needs. One does not need to go much higher than that in order to see some reduction in ICP.

There is another question here in terms of a better agent than mannitol for ICP reduction, but I think that when one finds one's self at the 48th to the 72nd hour using increasing doses of mannitol in order to be able to maintain the ICP in a desirable range for the clinical condition, then one is beginning to lose the ballgame. One must look toward other modalities to change the outcome, if in fact it can be changed at that point.

Should mannitol be used at all? Are there not better diuretics that often affect intracellular edema and brain swelling? I shall direct this to the panelists but first I would like to say that, to only affect intracellular edema, has no effect on intracranial pressure. One just shifts the water from one place to another. One must shift it and get it out of the head. So that is the basis for this discussion.

What about the loop diuretics as an alternative to other hyperosmolar agents such as glycerol? Dr. Rodman, would you like to answer?

Dr. Rodman: As I recall, there are some data — I think accumulated in the operating room in the craniotomy group of patients — to compare the efficacy of mannitol in one group, and mannitol and Lasix in another group, and a third group with Lasix alone. It seems that the addition of Lasix together with mannitol or alone produced an equal effect as a single dose of mannitol. As a matter of fact, the combination of mannitol and Lasix seemed to create a more marked reduction in intracranial pressure. The adverse properties of giving Lasix that I can think of are the potential for creating further electrolyte abnormalities just because of chloride wasting and adding a potential alkalosis to the situation. That is the extent of my knowledge on that question.

Moderator: I think the paper you are quoting is by Websick from Massachusetts General Hospital. There are additional papers showing the same thing. That is patient material, and there are similar data in animal experiments.

Dr. Gallagher: I agree with Dr. Rodman. I am familiar with that same data, which showed that Lasix is just as good as any other agent. I would only caution about some of the side effects of Lasix therapy, especially the development of hypokalemia and ventricular arrhythmias which may develop as a result of that. I have not been impressed that Lasix has been a very effective agent in reducing peripheral edema. I would guess that its main effect is a decrease in blood volume in terms of decreased intracranial pressure.

Dr. Jaffe: I would agree that in appropriate circumstances one or both agents may be quite effective. There has been a long-standing debate as to whether diuretics or mannitol is more effective therapeutically. Most medical literature has not supported the contention that loop diuretics are effective in preventing postoperative renal failure. Where mannitol has been utilized in patients have elective surgical procedures (especially thoracic surgical procedures), the expected incidence of postoperative renal insufficiency has been shown to be markedly decreased. Several anesthetic agents will produce a state of mild nephrogenic diabetes insipidus in which urinary volume losses will be increased thus further impairing intravascular volume status. Therefore, the rationale for using mannitol infusion to restore volume status also appears to have merit. Diuretic administration in such volume-depleted patients would only lead to further volume depletion and enhance the possibilities for the occurrence of renal insufficiency.

Moderator: I shall tell with prejudice our approach to this particular problem. Dehydration per se will take along with it dehydration in the brain. So we could even use to reduce ICP, if you like, hemodialysis. What we are interested in are mechanisms, and does one of these drugs have any advantage over any other? Furosemide, in terms of its general dehydration effects, will dry a sponge out in the brain. It does not have any special blood-brain barrier activity, such as that which we have when we use osmotic particles in the blood. It does, however, have an effect on cerebrospinal fluid secretion rates. I am sure that the preliminary studies that are now being done will be validated to show that it reduces cerebrospinal fluid secretion rates. But here we are talking about chronic utilization, not acute utilization. In the acute situation, the onset time for mannitol is about 10 to 15 minutes. The onset time for furosemide is considerably longer, in terms of bringing about an ICP reduction. The use of both agents will lead to a more rapid onset and a more profound reduction, perhaps because one bypasses some of the increase in central venous pressure that one sees when one uses mannitol alone. That has to contribute to some extent to the pressure inside the head. The mannitol, though, appears to have some advantage for rapid decompression. There are instances, however, which we all face, that is, the patient who has congestive heart failure or has a potential for that to occur. Since oxygenation of the brain is the critical factor here, then in that situation I would electively choose to go with Lasix and recognize that it is going to take a little bit more time to get to our desired position. With both of these agents, the subject of rebound has at least to enter into one's head. In my practice, and from what I see in the literature, if one does not go about replacing cubic centimeter for cubic centimeter the volume that is lost, rebound will not occur because the patient will remain in a general dehydrated state and one should be replacing about two thirds of the volume that is lost acutely in order to stay away from the problem of rebound. I do not think there is any special advantage to the use of loop diuretics or for hemodialysis for this. I think mannitol does have a special advantage in this situation in terms of rapidity of onset. I caution additionally that when one uses mannitol, as any hyperosmotic agent can be shown to do, if one infuses it in a very rapid fashion, I call that the "macho" administration, that is, as fast as one can push it in, one will cause an increase in intracranial pressure that is not related to the CVP and a drop in peripheral vascular resistance that is due to the hyperosmolar effect and, transiently, one may in fact have a precipitous increase in ICP and a drop in the blood pressure. So the method of administration has merely switched to intravenous drip rather than bolus administration. The drop in blood pressure is well recognized in the anesthetic literature. The problem with the intracranial pressure increase is also recognized but not so well popularized.

Physiologic Basis for Monitoring Cardiovascular Systems

T. J. Gallagher, M.D.

Objectives

To present an explanation of the differences between measurements of central venous and pulmonary capillary wedge pressure. Placement and complications of pulmonary artery catheters will be described. In addition, the reader will learn to analyze cardiovascular function in terms of preload and contractility.

Many patients with neurological disease also have involvement of the cardiovascular and respiratory system. Presently, cardiovascular and respiratory monitoring have reached a significant degree of sophistication.

The primary purpose of the cardiovascular system is to deliver oxygen to peripheral tissues for uptake and utilization. Several different manipulations can accomplish the task. Variations of the oxyhemoglobin dissociation curve can affect oxygen delivery and utilization. A rightward shift of the curve increases the amount of oxygen availability to tissues by decreasing the oxygen affinity to hemoglobin molecules. This commonly occurs in such things as acidosis or an increase in 2-3-DPG. Leftward shifts of the curve have the opposite effect as do such factors as alkalosis and decreases in 2-3-DPG.

A second mechanism to improve oxygen delivery is to increase the oxygen carrying capacity. This is principally accomplished by increasing the hemoglobin concentrations. Both mechanisms are somewhat limited in their scope of

T.J. Gallagher, M.D., Associate Professor of Surgery and Anesthesiology, University of Florida College of Medicine, Gainesville, Florida.

usefulness. Changes in the oxyhemoglobin dissociation curve are only transient in nature and hemoglobin concentration can be increased only to levels of 14 or 15 mg%. Otherwise, viscosity markedly increases resulting in compromise of micro-vascular flow.

Therefore, the major manipulation of the cardiovascular system is enhancement of cardiac output or stroke volume. As a result flow is increased throughout the entire system, increasing the amount of oxygen being delivered to any particular unit.

In the critically ill patient the usual methods of evaluation may not be very helpful or, in fact, may be shaded by other circumstances. Usually tachycardia is taken as an indication of inadequate volume replacement. However, patients with such conditions as sick sinus syndrome may simply be unable to increase their heart rate.

Peripheral perfusion is often assessed in terms of skin temperature and color. However, hypothermia is not an uncommon problem in the postoperative period. This is related to the ambient temperature in the room as well as the cold solutions used for intravenous fluid replacement and having the abdomen or chest opened for a prolonged period. With hypothermia skin perfusion is markedly decreased. Obviously, artificial lighting or skin pigmentation can also interfere with the assessment of peripheral perfusion.

The level of consciousness is often thought to be a function of adequate tissue perfusion. As cardiac output or flow to the brain decreases, patients become more obtunded. However, drugs, anesthetics and direct head injury may also interfere, making assessment extremely difficult.

Blood pressure is not a very reliable indicator of the adequacy of intravascular volume. Patients may be markedly hypovolemic and still be able to maintain a peripheral blood pressure. The usual response is vasoconstriction in an attempt to maintain the required perfusion pressure. It is only in the late stages, as hypovolemia continues uncorrected, that sudden precipitous falls in blood pressure may occur.

Urine output is also not a very adequate indicator of intravascular volume. Commonly, adequate urine output is thought to reflect renal and overall tissue perfusion. However, urine output may be maintained despite inadequate intra-vascular volume with an osmotic diuretic agent such as glucose or mannitol. Therefore, under all these circumstances more specific information is required to better evaluate cardiovascular response.

Specifically, patients at maximum physiologic stress who require an improvement in resting cardiac output to maintain adequate tissue perfusion include those with multiple-system trauma, including brain injury, marked blood loss, chest or abdominal injuries and intra-abdominal sepsis. It is not un-usual for the head-injured patient to have severe multiple-system involvement or overwhelming sepsis, both of which fit into the above categories.

Normally, the well-trained athlete or the young neonate both increase cardiac output by increasing heart rate. The neonate has a stiff ventricle and cannot significantly increase stroke volume while the athlete increases stroke volume but simultaneously increases heart rate. Above 150 to 180 beats per minute, cardiac output may actually begin to decrease primarily due to diminished diastolic filling time. Stroke volume is consequently decreased and cardiac output falls. In patients with preexisting coronary artery disease with limited coronary flow, the increase in cardiac rate occurs at the expense of increased oxygen consumption far out of propor-tion to delivery. Contractility becomes less efficient due to decreased available oxygen.

Impaired myocardial function requires invasive cardio-vascular monitoring and intervention. Compromised function may result from preexisting disease such as coronary artery insufficiency, hypoxia at the time of the initial injury, direct myocardial contusion, or various combinations of the above. These patients cannot maintain an increased cardiac output simply by increasing heart rate. They must resort to increased stroke volume. This is best done by taking advantage of the so-called Starling's Law.

If a myocardial muscle fiber is stretched to any length, the energy of contraction is proportional to the stretch length. The greater the stretch, the greater the energy of contraction and more work is obtained. This is analogous to a slingshot; the further one pulls back on the elastic, the further the pellet or rock is propelled.

In the heart as ventricular volume is increased, left ventricular diastolic pressure is also increased. The greater the volume, the greater the pressure and the further the myocardial muscle fiber is stretched. Increased stretch increases the energy of contraction with resultant enhanced stroke volume.

Since increases in pressure relate to increases in volume, measurement of left ventricular end-diastolic pressure (LVEDP) is directly related to left ventricular end-diastolic volume (LVEDV) which, in turn, is directly related to myocardial muscle fiber length.

What clinical tools do we then have available for these measurements? Since systemic perfusion is of utmost importance, we are primarily interested in left heart function. The balloon-tipped, flow-directed, thermodilution pulmonary artery catheter is well suited for measuring left heart function. When in place the catheter passes through the right atrium, out the right ventricular outflow track and into a small branch of the pulmonary artery. Inflation of the balloon tip with 1.5 cc of air totally occludes flow beyond the catheter. In effect we now have a static column of blood across the pulmonary vascular bed through the pulmonary vein and to the left atrium. This is analogous to a closed pipe filled with fluid and without flow. Then, pressure at one end of the pipe is equal to pressure at the opposite. Similarly, when the pulmonary artery catheter balloon tip is inflated, wedge or occlusion pressure is equal to pressure at the other end of the system, namely, left atrial pressure.

In the absence of mitral valvular disease left atrial pressure is equal to LVEDP. Therefore, pulmonary artery occlusion pressure directly relates to left atrial pressure which is the same as LVEDP.

LVEDP reflects LVEDV which is an estimate of myocardial fiber length. Increased pulmonary artery occlusion pressure secondary to an increase in intravascular volume stretches the myocardial fibers. The increased energy of contraction results in increased stroke volume.

Can central venous pressure measurements substitute for pulmonary capillary wedge pressure in the critically ill patient? Central venous and pulmonary capillary wedge pressure are not directly related. In some patients, when central venous pressure is simultaneously recorded with pulmonary capillary wedge pressure, wedge pressure is much higher than central venous pressure. In others, central venous is much higher than wedge. If the right and left side of the heart functioned in parallel with a common atrium, then right-sided pressures would accurately reflect left-sided heart function. However, the heart is actually in series and there is no reason that right-sided pressures should equal left-side pressure. Interposed between the right and left heart is the entire pulmonary vascular bed. Each ventricular function curve has a different form and slope. In addition, the units of work vary by a factor of 10. The left ventricle pumps against a much greater systemic pressure (70 to 80 mm Hg) than does the right ventricle pumping against a low pressure pulmonary vascular system. Therefore, in the critically ill patient information on left heart function can only be obtained by utilizing a pulmonary artery catheter.

The pulmonary artery catheter is usually inserted percutaneously into the internal jugular, subclavian, femoral or antecubital vein. Cutdown is avoided because of the increased risk of infection. Catheter movement is monitored by electrical transduction coupled to an oscilloscope display. Once in the superior or inferior vena cava the balloon tip is inflated and the catheter is passed into the right atrium, through the right ventricle and out into the pulmonary artery where it finally wedges in a small branch of the artery. When the balloon is deflated, the familiar pulmonary artery tracing with an elevated diastolic pressure reappears.

Complications related directly to the pulmonary artery catheter are quite rare. Those reported with insertion include pneumothorax, ventricular arrhythmias, perforations, right bundle branch block and knotting. The design of the catheter has been changed so that the balloon has a blunt dull surface markedly reducing the incidence of arrhythmias as it passes through the right ventricle. Most arrhythmias are transient in nature and require little or no treatment. Once the catheter passes through the right ventricle they usually subside spontaneously. However, an occasional premature beat may require treatment with intravenous lidocaine. Resuscitation by countershock is extremely rare. Perforations generally are associated with the Seldinger technique in which a wire is placed in the vein. If the wire is advanced too far, there is a risk of perforation, usually the right atrium. Pneumothorax is not related to the catheter itself, but rather to cannulation of the central vein. Appproximately 8% to 10% of the patients develop a transient right bundle branch block after placement of the catheter. This is usually not of any great clinical significance except when there is already a left bundle branch block. In those situations an electrical cardiac pacing wire should be on standby. Knotting or kinking of the catheter usually occurs when the tip fails to pass out of the right ventricle. Continued passage of the catheter leads to coiling in the ventricle with possible development of a knot. In the usual size adult, the catheter should be in place after passage of 50 to 55 cm.

With the modified Seldinger technique a central vein is first cannulated and a central venous pressure type catheter inserted. This extra step insures actual cannulation of the vein. A soft-tipped cardiac wire is then passed through the central venous catheter and on into the central vein. The catheter is then removed leaving only the wire in the vein. Over that wire is introduced a dilator and a 8 Fr. plastic introducer. They both follow the track over the wire and into central vein. The dilator and wire are then removed leaving only the introducer in the vein. The pulmonary artery catheter can then be introduced via the plastic introducer.

Catheter colonization or sepsis is a frequent occurrence and can be related to a cutdown incision. In addition, studies by our group have indicated that at the end of 72 hours, in patients with intra-abdominal sepsis catheter colonization approaches 50%. For that reason, all catheters are removed at the end of three days. If it is determined that the patient still requires invasive monitoring, a new catheter is placed in a new site. These types of devices are prone to infection since they may have to be consistently manipulated to determine wedge pressure; they are disconnected for cardiac output determinations, and blood is continuously removed through the catheter for various laboratory procedures.

Thermodilution cardiac output is quickly determined at the bedside. A thermistor in the catheter tip is directly connected to the cardiac output computer. This thermistor is a Wheatstone bridge mechanism, a series of resistors all balanced so that no electrical flow occurs. Cardiac output is determined by the injection of a known volume of solution at a known temperature into a port some 30 cm back from the thermistor. Blood flowing past is cooled and the temperature change causes a difference in resistor settings and current flows. The current flow is plotted against time and the area under that curve corresponds to the cardiac output. The whole procedure takes some 30 seconds. The reproducibility is within 2% to 3% and is accurate to within 10% of the dye dilution method.

Evaluation of cardiac performance can be divided into preload, contractility or afterload. Preload refers to filling pressures of the left and right heart. Left-sided preload is measured by pulmonary capillary wedge pressure. In general, cardiac output is related to filling pressure, that is, as we increase the pulmonary capillary wedge pressure we should expect a concomitant increase in cardiac output or work. With low filling pressures in a compliant ventricle small increases in pressure effect rather large increases in work. As the heart becomes full, significant increases in filling pressure are necessary to effect much increase in cardiac work. In fact the curve descends if the ventricle is overfilled.

In each instance a particular ventricular function curve is developed for each patient. The goal is to find the maximal cardiac output related to the minimal filling pressure required. Often this will range between 14 and 18 mm Hg. However, each particular case may vary. It is incumbent to find the filling pressure which results in the maximal improvement in cardiac output. This will obviously vary from one patient to the next. It makes no sense to keep the wedge pressure at 18 mm Hg if cardiac output is the same at 10 mm Hg. Patient demands and cardiac performance may vary over time; therefore, inadequate filling pressure at one point may be quite satisfactory at a later date.

Cardiac contractility is the intrinsic quality of myocardial muscle contraction. This is difficult to measure clinically, since strain gauges are not normally placed on the myocardial tissue. If filling pressure has been maximized and cardiac output still judged inadequate, the problem may be one of inadequate contractility. At any particular filling pressure cardiac output may vary. A decrease in cardiac output at the same filling pressure is usually related to an alteration or a decrease in cardiac contractility. This is the same as a shifting of the ventricular function curve down and to the right. Agents which improve cardiac contractility include digitalis, calcium chloride and those given by continuous infusions such as dopamine, epinephrine and dobutamine. With the use of inotropic agents cardiac output can be enhanced at the same filling pressure or in fact maintained at lower pressures.

In summary, accurate and precise measurement of cardiovascular function is afforded with the use of various invasive monitoring devices. Such devices as a pulmonary artery catheter allow accurate surveillance of intravascular volume as well as precise determinations of cardiac performance. By utilizing these methods one is then able to appropriately interact at specific levels of cardiac function and have direct feedback of the response.

Bibliography

Chiariello, M., Gold, H.K., Leinbach, R.C. et al: Comparison between the effects of nitroprusside and nitroglycerin on ischemic injury during acute myocardial infarction. Circulation 54:766-773, 1976.

Civetta, J.M., Gabel, J.C. and Laver, M.B.: Disparate ventricular function in surgical patients. Surg. Forum 22:136-139, 1971.

Civetta, J.M. and Gabel, J.C.: Flow directed-pulmonary artery catheterization in surgical patients: Indications and modifications of technic. Ann. Surg. 176:753-756, 1972.

Cohn, J.N.: Vasodilator therapy for heart failure: The influence of impedance on left ventricular performance. Circulation 48:5, 1973.

Forrester, J.S. and Swan, H.J.C.: Acute myocardial infarction: A physiological basis of therapy. Crit. Care Med. 2:283, 1974.

Langer, G.A.: The mechanism of action of digitalis. Hosp. Pract. 6:49-57, 1970.

Sarnoff, S.J. and Berglund, E.: Ventricular function. I. Starling's law of the heart studies by means of simultaneous right and left ventricular functions curves in the dog. Circulation 10:706, 1954.

Shell, W.E. and Sobel, B.E.: Protection of jeopardized ischemic myocardium by reduction of ventricular afterload. N. Engl. J. Med. 291:481, 1974.

Stanley, T.H., Isern-Amarai, J., Liu, W.S. et al: Peripheral vascular versus direct cardiac effects of calcium. Anesthesiology 45:46-58, 1976.

Swan, H.J., Ganz, W., Forrester, J. et al: Catheterization of the heart in man with use of a flow-directed balloon-tipped catheter. N. Engl. J. Med. 283:447-451, 1970.

Self-Evaluation Quiz

1. Oxygen delivery is affected by all of the following *except*:
   a) Oxyhemoglobin dissociation curve
   b) Hemoglobin concentration
   c) Acidosis
   d) Serum albumin
   e) Cardiac output
2. Hypothermia is always associated with a low cardiac output state.
   a) True
   b) False
3. Blood pressure accurately reflects intravascular volume.
   a) True
   b) False
4. Starling's Law states that the greater the stretch length of the myocardial muscle fiber the greater the velocity of contraction.
   a) True
   b) False
5. The Swan-Ganz catheter helps measure or calculate all of the following *except*:
   a) Preload
   b) Cardiac output
   c) Oxygen consumption
   d) Arterial venous oxygen content difference
   e) Renal vascular resistance
6. Complications in pulmonary artery cathetering include all of the following *except*:
   a) Perforation
   b) Premature ventricular contractions
   c) Pneumothorax
   d) Right bundle branch block
   e) Knotting
7. Distal placement of the catheter tip results in an inordinately high cardiac output.
   a) True
   b) False
8. Cardiac contractility can be directly measured.
   a) True
   b) False

9. Positive inotropic agents include all of the following *except*:
   a) Isoproterenol
   b) Calcium chloride
   c) Dobutamine
   d) Nitroprusside
   e) Nitroglycerin

Answers on page 391.

PEEP and IMV:
Definition and Utilization

Bradley H. Ruben, D.O.

Objectives

1. To present a brief description of the pathophysiology of acute and chronic adult respiratory distress syndrome (ARDS).
2. To relate how PEEP prevents airway closure.
3. To describe the mechanism and advantages of IMV.
4. To list the criteria for use of PEEP and IMV.

This paper will present modes of ventilatory support, namely, PEEP and IMV, in relation to the adult respiratory distress syndrome (ARDS), with implications to the neurologically injured patient.

ARDS is characterized by low PaO_2's, and low $PaCO_2$'s in individuals who had normal pulmonary function prior to the onset of respiratory failure. They are trying to increase their PaO_2's physiologically by increasing their minute ventilation. Consequently, the patient's $PaCO_2$'s are low, and there is an associated respiratory alkalemia.

Another hallmark feature of this disease process is that there are generally no x-ray changes in the early stages. This disease process, acute respiratory failure, is diagnosed on the basis of blood gas exchanged, arterial blood gases.

Late respiratory failure, like acute phase disease, is characterized by low PaO_2's but they are usually less than 50. There is relatively little improvement in oxygenation with increasing

Bradley H. Ruben, D.O., Assistant Professor of Anesthesiology and Neurological Surgery, Medical Director, Neurosurgical Intensive Care Unit; Associate Director, Department of Respiratory Therapy; Associate, Surgical Intensive Care Unit, University of Miami School of Medicine, Fla.

inspired oxygen concentrations even as high as to 100%. These patients are also hypercarbic, despite rapid ventilatory rates.

If pulmonary mechanics are measured, one would find that compliance is reduced. Compliance is the pressure required to deliver a certain volume of gas to the lung. Also in late respiratory failure, there are severe x-ray changes characterized usually by severe bilateral infiltrates, with only small areas where normal gas exchange can occur. There may also be evidence of increased susceptibility of the lung to pulmonary barotrauma, such as pneumothorax and pneumomediastinum. This disease involves patients who had previously normal lungs, i.e., not those who had chronic lung disease, bronchial asthma or restrictive diseases.

In summary, the characteristics of respiratory failure include (a) variable onset 0 to 48 hours after the predisposing event, (b) hypoxemia, (c) the hypoxemia is refractory to oxygen therapy and to intermittent positive pressure ventilation, (d) respiratory alkalemia, secondary to hyperventilation and (e) decreased pulmonary compliance, because of a decreased functional residual capacity (FRC) which is secondary to atelectasis and ventilation perfusion abnormalities.

A most interesting facet of the problem relates to the predisposing factors associated with ARDS especially with regard to neurologically injured patients. In the case of the multiple trauma patient, with chest injury, i.e., multiple fractured ribs, it is not the trauma per se to his chest wall, but the underlying lung contusion that causes respiratory distress.

In the case of fat embolism in the multiple trauma patient with long bone fractures — it is not the fat per se that causes respiratory distress, but rather the release of free fatty acids which affects the alveolar capillary membrane. The resultant increase of interstitial water in the lung causes respiratory failure.

Sepsis, with the release of endotoxins, affects alveolar capillary membranes.

Pancreatitis is a common finding in patients with high cervical spinal cord injury. In this condition, it is the release of enzymes that affects alveolar capillary membranes and destroys surfactant in the lung.

Disseminated intravascular coagulation is probably not a cause per se of respiratory failure, but it can be associated in late stages of severe or late respiratory failure with the appearance of coagulopathies.

Shock is probably not a cause of respiratory failure in the hypovolemic individual, but in the patient with other associated lesions producing shock, such as cardiogenic, septic or neurogenic, respiratory distress is frequently noted.

Aspiration of gastric contents, especially with a pH less than 2.5, can result in respiratory failure associated with a high mortality. Acid stomachs should be treated with antacids to prevent the acid aspirations, although pneumonitis associated with antacid aspiration also causes respiratory failure. The neurologically compromised patient is especially at risk of such aspiration and its associated morbidity and mortality.

Another cause of respiratory failure is fluid overload associated with congestive heart failure. Viral and bacterial pneumonias are also significant predisposing causes of respiratory failure.

Finally, oxygen toxicity, that is, FIO_2's of greater than 50% oxygen, is associated with respiratory failure. It is not really known what the cause and effect relationship to respiratory failure is, but it is thought that the high oxygen concentrations are toxic to enzyme systems within the lung, causing breakdown of the alveolar capillary membrane. Oxygen toxicity is related to the FIO_2 and to the duration of exposure to oxygen. For example, breathing 100% oxygen, one may get respiratory symptoms within six hours, that being a decreased vital capacity or pain in the chest. Breathing 60% oxygen, it may take several days to develop these same symptoms.

The gross appearance of the lung in which severe or late respiratory distress is found would be wet in appearance, beefy-red, liver-like and airless. The contour of the lung would be normal, but the lung weight would be approximately two to three times normal. Under the microscope, it would be noted that there are few areas of atelectasis, but also only few areas where normal gas exchange can take place. The alveoli and interstitium would be occupied by fluid in the form of blood and serum.

In an oversimplified manner, if one considers upper lung alveoli as compared to lower lung alveoli, it is noted that the upper alveoli are larger than the lower alveoli. This is because the weights of the lung and the blood in the lung, which are gravity dependent, are greater in the lower lung. Because of the greater hydrostatic pressure and consequently greater pleural pressure, the lower alveoli are smaller.

With inspiration, the distribution of gases is greater to the lower lung segments. The change in volume of lower lung alveoli is larger than those in the upper lung fields. This is due to the fact that since there is greater pleural pressure in the lower lung segments, there is a lesser pressure differential between lung parenchyma and the alveoli; i.e. the transpulmonary pressure is less. Consequently, gas is going to flow to an area of least resistance or least pressure differential. The lower alveoli are more compliant, i.e., with small pressure changes, there are larger volume changes.

In respiratory distress (ARDS), there are two factors that exhibit abnormal physiology. First, there is a collection of fluid in the interstitium surrounding the alveolus and in the terminal alveolar ducts. This reduces the cross-sectional area of the terminal airway ducts, which causes gases to have an increased resistance to flow. With fluid in the alveolar interstitium, the alveolus decreases in size. The net effect would be a decrease in lung volume, specifically in FRC. The second occurrence is that fluid collects in the alveolus. This impedes diffusion of oxygen across the alveolar capillary membrane and also destroys surfactant. Surfactant is in the alveolus for the purpose of reducing surface tension, thus preventing alveolar collapse. If surfactant is not present, alveoli collapse.

With a decrease in size or volume of the alveoli, or collapse because of lost surfactant, it is found that although the alveolus continues to be perfused, it is not effectively ventilated. Because of not being ventilated, consequently, blood perfusing this alveolus is not adequately oxygenated. This poorly oxygenated blood mixes with blood from other areas of the lung which has been adequately oxygenated, with the result that the PO_2 of arterial blood is lowered. We can measure this tendency to lower the PaO_2 as venous admixture or shunt. Intrapulmonary shunt is the percentage of blood which is going through the lung which is not being exposed to alveolar oxygenation. A 20% shunt would mean that 20% of the blood or 20% of the cardiac output has not been exposed to alveolar oxygenation.

FRC of the lung is that volume of gas remaining in the lung at the end of tidal expiration. Within the FRC is what is referred to as the closing volume. The closing volume is simply that volume needed in the lung to prevent alveolar collapse. If FRC is decreased, the closing volume would increase and there would be a tendency for alveolar collapse. This is found normally in the aged, in heavy smokers, the obese, in lying supine and in respiratory insufficiency. In ARDS, then, there is a decreased FRC, the closing volume is increased, such that alveolar collapse takes place during tidal breathing with the production of a shunt and, consequently, the tendency toward hypoxemia.

Physiologically then, a person with ARDS breathes rapidly. This attempt serves two purposes: to try and increase intra-thoracic pressure to open alveoli, which they are unable to do, and to increase oxygenation by increasing minute ventilation, which has only a minimal efect because only the remaining alveoli are ventilated, with no new alveoli recruited.

With intermittent positive pressure breathing (IPPB), enough intrathoracic pressure can be developed to overcome closed alveoli. But when the ventilator cycles off, the alveoli collapse. Put in another perspective, when the ventilator fires during inspiration, airway pressure rises. At some point in time, a critical opening pressure is achieved and the alveoli open, while the ventilator continues to fire and airway pressure rises. When the ventilator cycles off, airway pressure falls, and at some point in time, the critical closing pressure of the alveolus occurs, and the alveolus collapses. If the alveolus open time is plotted against total inspiration time, it would be noted that the duration of alveolar inflation would be approximately half that of the total inspiratory time with IPPB. The net effect is that there is little or no improvement in oxygenation.

With the addition of positive end expiratory pressure (PEEP), there is an increase in FRC. Consequently, the closing volume is now below tidal ventilation. Mechanical ventilation is used to recruit collapsed airways and PEEP is used to prevent their collapse at end expiration. PEEP improves arterial oxygenation by preventing alveolar collapse and maintaining alveolar patency through the inspiratory cycle. Now the alveolus is open, ventilation to the alveolus occurs, with restoration of the normal ventilation-perfusion relationship with the consequent improvement in the shunt.

PEEP is increased in increments of 3 to 5 cm of water, until as an end-point a 15% shunt is achieved. In some individuals, small changes in PEEP will lead to large changes in arterial oxygenation, while in others, it will take greater amounts of PEEP to achieve the same effect. There are several ways to utilize PEEP (by saturation, best compliance), but on our service a shunt of 15% is used. If calculations are made, it would be noted that the symptoms of respiratory failure (tachypnea, alkalemia) would occur at a shunt of approximately 15%. So this seems like a logical therapeutic goal.

In order to calculate a shunt, a pulmonary artery catheter must be in place so that a mixed venous blood sample can be obtained. By application of the shunt formula, a shunt value can be obtained.

But, a catheter to monitor cardiac output with the effects of PEEP is not generally needed until 15 cm water of PEEP is used. If less PEEP than this is used, it can be titrated incrementally using the shunt of 15% or the PaO_2/FIO_2 ratio greater than 300. Again, this ratio is used when a pulmonary catheter is not being utilized. For example, if a patient is on 30% oxygen and he has a PaO_2 of 90, his PaO_2/FIO_2 would be 300, and we could surmise that his shunt is 15% or less. This would be in comparison to a patient who may have a PaO_2 of 60 on 30% oxygen. His PaO_2/FIO_2 ratio would then be 200, and we could thus surmise that his shunt would be greater than 15%.

Some of the effects of PEEP include the following: with PEEP applied to the airway it can be transmitted across lung parenchyma, affecting the great vessels in the chest. By so doing, venous return to the heart may be reduced, and consequently cardiac output may be reduced. Also, since venous return is impeded, intracranial pressure may increase. But two aspects must be remembered. Generally, with ARDS, pulmonary compliance is reduced, and consequently the effects of PEEP are not transmitted as readily across the lung. Generally, if PEEP of greater than 15 cm of water is used, a pulmonary catheter is used to monitor cardiac output. Also, at these levels an intracranial monitoring device would be indicated in the patient susceptible to increased intracranial pressure.

With an intermittent mandatory ventilation (IMV) ventilator, a preset volume of gas can be delivered to the patient at a
preset time. Between ventilator breaths, there is a flow cartridge
affixed to the ventilator that delivers a continuous flow of gas.
Consequently, a patient can have a continuous flow of fresh gas
between ventilator breaths. This is opposed to a conventional
ventilator that delivers a preset volume at a preset time, but
does not have a continuous flow of fresh gases between
ventilator breaths. Consequently, if the patient is breathing on
his own, he would be inspiring against resistance and may
inspire carbon dioxide from the expiratory limb of the
ventilator. This would cause the patient to be agitated and
"fight the ventilator," thus necessitating either paralysis or
heavy sedation of the patient. With IMV, since the patient has
no resistance to breathing and a fresh volume of gas from which
to inspire, there is no agitation and the need for paralysis or
sedation is decreased. Also, with controlled ventilation, a
greater positive minute airway pressure is applied to the airway,
thus cardiac output may be impaired. With IMV, spontaneous
breaths between IMV rates would decrease minute positive
airway pressure, thus tending to improve cardiac output as
compared to controlled ventilation.

IMV is added when the $PaCO_2$ is greater than 45, when the
pH is less than 7.35 and the spontaneous respiratory rate is
greater than 30. How, then, does one wean from IMV? As will
be seen, the patient dictates this: if his pH is 7.35 or better, a
normal $PaCO_2$, and his respiratory rate is less than 30. This is
opposed to weaning from conventional ventilation, in which at
some point in time the patient is taken off the ventilator,
observed and then placed back on. Each time he is taken off the
ventilator for longer periods of time until he reaches a point
where he is completely off the ventilator.

IMV combined with PEEP is used in the following manner:
IMV is used to normalize the $PaCO_2$ and the pH, while PEEP is
used to recruit and maintain patent alveoli and thus improve
oxygenation. Normal ventilatory patterns are reinforced; the
patient is able to ventilate between IMV breaths. There is
improved cardiovascular performance and thus oxygen transport. There is not the increased airway pressures and consequently increased intrathoracic pressures that are found with

controlled positive pressure ventilation. It is much easier to wean a patient from IMV, because he dictates when to wean. There would be no need to sedate or paralyze a patient on IMV, which is an advantage if the ventilator becomes disconnected. It is also noteworthy to point out that the incidence of pulmonary barotrauma (pneumothorax, subcutaneous emphysema, mediastinal emphysema, pneumoperitoneum and gastric distention) is no greater with PEEP and IMV when compared to controlled positive pressure ventilation.

In conclusion, in dealing with respiratory failure, we have three important therapeutic tools to consider: the use of titrated PEEP, IMV and cardiovascular monitoring — not one more important than the other. It must be stressed that cardiovascular monitoring, although mentioned here briefly, is just as important as the others, but is discussed elsewhere in this volume.

Self-Evaluation Quiz

1. ARDS is acutely diagnosed on the basis of chest x-ray.
   a) True
   b) False
2. Along with hypoxemia, carbon dioxide retention accompanies late ARDS.
   a) True
   b) False
3. PEEP is used to recruit collapsed airways.
   a) True
   b) False
4. Higher IMV rates (greater than 6/min) are associated with a decreased cardiac output, especially when PEEP is being utilized.
   a) True
   b) False
5. If cardiac output has been optimized, the PaO_2 then determines if PEEP is indicated.
   a) True
   b) False

Answers on page 391.

Surgical Intensive Care Unit Computerized Data Management System

Jeffrey S. Augenstein, M.D., Ph.D.

Objectives

1. To describe the intensive care unit in terms of a data management problem.
2. To describe the reasons why automated data processing technology has previously not worked in intensive care.
3. To describe why computers and other forms of data processing technology should work at this time in intensive care.

Intensive Care Automation

Intensive care has provided some of the greatest advancements in medicine over the last decade. For example, in the late 1960s the mortality from respiratory failure after trauma was over 50%. In most ICUs in the United States the mortality for the same clinical problem is less than 10%. However, this form of medicine is extremely expensive in terms of dollars and labor. The ICU generates the most data per patient, per unit of time, with the most significant implications of any hospital care facility. Managing information is the most time-consuming and costly aspect of care. The costs of manually handling data are increasing steadily. These are basically personnel costs, i.e., nurses, clerks. On the other hand, automated data processing has increased in capability and decreased in cost each year. Furthermore, the performance and reliability of this equipment,

Jeffrey S. Augenstein, M.D., Ph.D., Assistant Professor of Surgery and Anesthesiology, Department of Surgery, University of Miami School of Medicine, Fla.

particularly computers, have improved sufficiently to provide not only affordable but reliable, highly functional data management systems at this time. Not only are the human resources that manage information increasing in cost, but they are becoming scarcer. There is a nationwide shortage of the most active ICU data management personnel — nurses. Many of the present "intelligent" computer applications, e.g., automated arrhythmia monitoring, are as clinically accurate as that of nurses and physicians. On a regular basis, greater demands are being made not only for increased information availability by clinicians, but also for legible, well-documented records and variable reports by medicolegal factions and third party payers, such as Medicare. Computers have advantages over manual recordkeeping in many situations.

Computers have been used for more than 15 years to provide (1) more automated monitoring and therapy and (2) recordkeeping.

The former applications include (1) arrhythmia monitoring; (2) respiratory function monitoring, e.g. pulmonary mechanics; (3) brain function evaluation, e.g., evoked potential monitoring; (4) delivery and measurement of drug and fluid infusions; and (5) output measurements. Many of these applications provide continuous surveillance which is more than 80% as accurate as that of a clinician. Moreover, this monitoring is never interrupted for coffee breaks or inattention.

Few systems exist which manage all or even most of the information which comprises the total ICU clinical record or data base. The record includes at least medications; notes; orders; vital signs; calculations; fluid input and output; laboratory reports; special procedure results; billing data; history; physical exam; and operative reports. Many commercial and university based computer systems can handle parts of this total mass of data. Certain advantages are available to owners of these systems, e.g., production of legible lists of information or instantaneous calculations. Yet many of these systems encumber the user with diffusing the data. Some data are present in the traditional chart and other data exist on the computer's display. In some installations, data must be doubly entered into the computer and the standard chart to satisfy requirements. None of these systems have been shown to be cost-effective or capable of increasing clinical power.

The times are appropriate for the development of computer-based systems which will truly improve the delivery of critical care. There are a number of developments which contribute to this position. First, many programming tools for providing flexible data organization schemes, e.g., data base management protocols, presently exist. Some are already existent in medical applications, but many more exist in other environments such as the airline passenger information systems. Second, critical care in many institutions has evolved to a well-orchestrated and often protocol-based science. These approaches lend themselves to "computerization." Third, other hospital computer installations provide good data organization and data transmission, e.g., laboratory computer systems. This can reduce the manual entry requirements, both increasing efficiency and decreasing error.

The dedicated monitoring and control applications, e.g., arrhythmia monitoring, require only limited development and cost reduction to become price-effective. However, the data management approaches need some major improvements to become truly useful and cost-effective. The primary requirements are described as "interface" demands. The interface or interaction capabilities between the clinical user and the ICU computer as well as the ICU computer and other hospital computers are typically limited. To provide for appropriate user interaction some extensive human factors analysis must be performed. This would generate the blueprint for the design of human factors-efficient facilities. Standardized vocabularies (e.g., for notes) and mechanisms of communication (e.g., special function keyboards and video displays) need to be developed. Communication protocols between computers, e.g., between the laboratory and ICU computer, must be provided. Presently, few computers can communicate with other computers primarily because of proprietary concerns of individual manufacturers.

A needed approach at this time is the analysis of the information processing requirement in intensive care with the development of prototype equipment to meet the user and interface needs. The prototype design should take into account cost considerations, growth potential as well as user needs. A period of evaluation must follow, determining if in fact the user's demands are being met and that the design provides reasonable cost-effectiveness. As the ratio of computer power to costs continues to increase, it is likely that within the next few years literally any capability can be provided at an acceptable cost. Unfortunately, the very critical evaluation, design, development, assessment and development program has not been followed in intensive care data automation to an appropriate degree. Nor were many of the existing systems designed with the present low-cost high-power computers. Thus, while numerous intensive care computer systems exist, none provide the necessary capability or cost-effectiveness. The tremendous demands for adequate information handling in intensive care require that this approach be taken immediately.

The University of Miami School of Medicine Department of Surgery Information Systems Laboratory has taken an aggressive approach in analyzing the information requirements in the Surgical Intensive Care Unit and in designing prototypic equipment to meet these needs. The analysis led to a design which maintained the basic information management at the bedside utilizing a color cathode ray tube display to allow for input and display of all information. The system design provides for data management simultaneously on 16 beds. The plans at this time are to do additional development and evaluation in a mock-up laboratory setting. The evaluation and development program will continue in the Surgical Intensive Care Unit in 1981. Initially a single bed will be utilized progressing to 16 beds over an 18-month period. Detailed examinations will be made to determine if the system is meeting its design requirements of reducing data management costs, increasing care flexibility and increasing clinician's efficiency. The approach provides for analysis, planning, prototyping, evaluation and commitment to final computer and program configuration. This strategy has been shown to be the most productive and cost-efficient in other industries where data processing has been automated.

Self-Evaluation Quiz

1. How accurate is computer based monitoring in some applications, e.g., arrhythmia monitoring?

a) 20% is accurate as a clinician
b) 40% is accurate as a clinician
c) 60% is accurate as a clinician
d) >80% is accurate as a clinician

2. The primary problem in providing computer based intensive care data management is:
   a) Interface demands
   b) Hardware reliability
   c) Computer availability
   d) Interested users

Answers on page 391.

Panel Discussion

Moderator: Dr. Gallagher

Panelists: Drs. Augenstein and Ruben

Moderator: If we really have computers at such a point that we can direct complex airplane traffic around cities and send men to the moon, why is it that medicine really has not taken advantage of this, Dr. Augenstein? We seem to be a stepchild, as it were, in terms of the utilization of what is available in terms of computers.

Dr. Augenstein: I think it probably relates to a difference in philosophy that permeated medicine versus some of the other areas. Medicine is partially an art and the discipline required by computers is somewhat incompatible. We are now maturing to another level of medicine, one where we realize that very accurate organization of data is critical. Part of that maturation for all of medicine really grew out of critical care. So I think medicine really did not articulate its interest in computers in the same way that traffic control did. Therefore, it has been late in utilizing the potential.

Moderator: Dr. Ruben, please explain what the shunt fraction is and how it is utilized. Just exactly what information is needed to be able to calculate the shunt fraction, what does it tell us and why do we need to use it?

Dr. Ruben: The determinants of the shunt fraction are the pulmonary capillary content at the alveolus, which is determined by the alveolar gas, the content of oxygen in arterial blood, and the determinant of oxygen in the mixed venous blood. Consequently, we need to use the Swan-Ganz catheter to be able to obtain the mixed venous blood sample.

Moderator: If we simply look at PO_2's that can be influenced by cardiac output. A low cardiac output will also show a low PO_2. By shunt fraction or venous admixture, that is an estimation of the amount of blood going to the lungs that is

131

not completely oxygenated and really relates only the pulmonary function. Therefore, in critically ill patients with multiple system failure, if one can delineate what the cause of the low PO_2 is, for instance, with a low PO_2, one would not want to increase PEEP, which may depress cardiac output, if indeed the problem was due to a low output and not due to respiratory dysfunction. That is how we can delineate the differences between those two.

Dr. Ruben, what is the average PO_2 that is maintained in your patients with multiple trauma? Is there any advantage for a patient to be kept at PO_2's of greater than 125 mm Hg?

Dr. Ruben: We do not treat PO_2's per se. We treat a shunt to 15%. So consequently, we are not looking at PO_2's; we are looking at the shunt, and the shunt is derived from the shunt equation. Certainly, if cardiac output has been maximized and the shunt is 15% and the PO_2's are high, that is, 150 or greater, perhaps we would tend to lower the FIO_2's.

Moderator: Does everyone need to be treated to a 15% shunt? Where does the number 15 come from?

Dr. Ruben: I alluded to this in my presentation. If one reviews the literature, one would find that probably the onset of respiratory distress or the symptoms of respiratory distress would occur at about a shunt of 15%. So it would seem reasonable, then, to treat to this level.

Moderator: That is what we have used at Jackson Memorial Hospital, although it is fair to point out that there are different end-points. Others may give only enough PEEP to insure that the patient is not hypoxic and still breathing less than toxic concentrations of oxygen, that the PO_2 is at 70 or less than 50% FIO_2, is also certainly a safe range. Other people treat to the best compliance.

Dr. Ruben, how exactly do you measure compliance? What is the difference between static and dynamic compliance?

Dr. Ruben: One has in essence a manometer on the ventilator, and one would note the pressure at peak inspiration delivered from the ventilator. At this point in time we would get an assumption of compliance and that would be static compliance. In order to obtain static compliance, one would have to hold inspiration momentarily at peak inspiration to get that figure. It is an approximate way of noting if the patient's respiratory status, i.e., his compliance, is decreasing. For example, if one was requiring higher pressures to deliver the same tidal volume, then one would probably assume that his compliance is probably decreasing.

Moderator: Dr. Ruben, how do you decide in your unit with the neurosurgical patient just what level of mechanical ventilation is supplied? Is it how long you need to hyperventilate patients? Is hyperventilation prolonged for several days? Is it very reduced intracranial pressure? How do you approach that problem in the brain-injured patient?

Dr. Ruben: Certainly, initially, and within the first 36 to 48 hours, hyperventilation is beneficial until some point in time at which the cerebrospinal fluid pH returns to normal. Probably then cerebral perfusion reestablishes itself to the same levels it had before quite readily. Frequently, one will find a patient with a PCO_2 of 25 and after a few days his intracranial pressure begins to rise again. We have to rehyperventilate that patient.

Moderator: Is it effective at that stage?

Dr. Ruben: Yes, it is effective at that stage.

Moderator: Is it effective in all cases?

Dr. Ruben: Yes, in a majority of cases.

Moderator: So if intracranial pressure went back up, you would continue hyperventilation?

Dr. Ruben: Yes, I would.

Moderator: Provided that you were monitoring intracranial pressure?

Dr. Ruben: Yes, of course, it would have to be monitored.

Moderator: Dr. Augenstein, this question relates more to the surgical intensive care unit. Do you allow the nurses in the unit to remove Swan-Ganz catheters? Is there any reason why they should or should not do this?

Dr. Augenstein: I am not sure we have any definite policy on this question. I think in general the resident physicians are doing that. But the danger that one must be concerned about is minimal. One first makes the decision of whether to monitor the patient with a Swan-Ganz catheter based on some criteria. Equally important criteria need to be applied in deciding when to discontinue this level of monitoring. At that decision point the question is one of the technique of removing the catheter. It is the same kind of problem as removing a central venous catheter. If the patient's head is elevated when one is removing it, one could conceivably have an aspiration of air into the venous system. One must increase the venous pressure at the time that one is removing it. The possibility of arrhythmia exists. As Dr. Gallagher has pointed out, the incidence today of arrhythmias with the Swan-Ganz catheter being inserted is very low. I am not aware of the incidence of arrhythmias on removing catheters. The point is that care must be rendered in removing the catheter. It is just a question of being careful.

Moderator: No, we do not have a policy. We let our nurses pull those out. We have never had a problem with which I am familiar. I think the worst thing that happened was a mistake I made one time when I inserted a catheter. This was when I was a Fellow. It did not go in the right place, it went into the left chest. Unfortunately, there also was some blood in there at the same time and we could aspirate blood back, and we could also get a tracing that looked like a wedge pressure. We thought we were okay, but things just did not seem right. The chest x-ray showed where it was. The mistake was made to remove the catheter at that time. So the patient had a very bad bleed for a short period of time. Fortunately, we were able to stop the bleeding. But I think if one is in the wrong spot and one has gone through the vein, then I would be very careful about who removes it and when, and think it through very carefully.

I have been asked in terms of the Swan-Ganz catheter placement, what do I do in the patient who needs a pulmonary artery catheter, but who has a complete left bundle branch block. As far as I know, the incidence, from data done at the VA Hospital in Miami and in other places, is that right bundle branch block does occur on the order of 10% to 15% with Swan-Ganz catheter placement and is a transitory type of thing. However, obviously, if someone has a left bundle branch and develops a right bundle branch, too, then one is going to be in big trouble. Therefore, we advocate inserting a pacemaker first in those patients with that particular problem who are also going to need a pulmonary artery catheter. The Edwards Corporation, who first developed the Swan-Ganz catheter, has currently developed in limited production a catheter which has incorporated pacing wires into it. There are a series of bands wrapped around it that will allow sequential atrial and ventricular pacing at the same time. So, theoretically, in a situation where a pacer is needed, then one could insert this particular catheter in place of inserting a temporary pacemaker first. Obviously, one runs the risk of, after having put the temporary pacemaker in, then inserting the Swan-Ganz catheter and dislodging the pacemaker while getting the Swan-Ganz catheter in place. Then one will get into big problems. Unfortunately, with the new catheter, I talked about the fact that one can normally place it simply by monitoring the transducer. However, with this catheter, you need fluoroscopy to get it into place. One difficulty we have noticed is that, as the catheter curves through the heart, with patients who are on mechanical ventilators, it does not lodge in the trabecula as the normal pacemaker wire would. As the ventilator cycles on and delivers a breath to the patient, what can happen in many instances is a transient increase in pulmonary artery pressure, the pressure delivered to the lungs which gets transmitted across all the intrathoracic structures. So the transient increase in pulmonary artery pressure which causes then a dilatation of the right side of the heart and as it dilates up the catheter then loses contact with the heart wall and you lose the pace during the time the ventilator cycle is on. So there are still some inherent problems with the use of that particular catheter. We have not solved all of these problems yet.

Dr. Augenstein, regarding evoked potentials, you alluded to the use of those, are they currently clinically helpful? Is there any information we can derive or base interventions on the use of evoked potentials? What information do you have on that?

Dr. Augenstein: I think the people who are using it clinically in San Diego are saying that it is an early warning system for intracranial disaster which is earlier than pressure changes. Interventions designed to deal with mass effects would be appropriate here. It is a technology which is very exciting. There is some basic research literature that is even more exciting about its ability to differentiate between a barbiturate-induced cerebral dysfunction and brain death which, as you know, from an EEG or functional point of view is very difficult to evaluate. I think you will see in the literature in the near future that this will be a clinically useful technique in intensive care.

Moderator: What about such things as power spectrum analysis of the electroencephalogram? Is that helpful at all in taking care of the injured in the operating room?

Dr. Augenstein: You are still taking the same gross signal and trying to just process it. The problem with the EEG is that it is very nonspecific. Whereas, if you tie in stimulus and response, as in evoked potential, function can be more precisely defined. If one takes the gross EEG and filters it or does power analyses or any of the spectrum analysis, one is still dealing with a signal that is nonspecific.

Moderator: Dr. Ruben, basically this question relates to the problem of increased intracranial pressure with the use of positive end-expiratory pressure (PEEP). How do you balance the problem of hypoxia versus increased intracranial pressure and their detrimental effects upon cerebral or brain function? Is PEEP contraindicated in these circumstances?

Dr. Ruben: After reviewing the literature I could not find that PEEP up to 20 cm of water had any effect upon intracranial pressure, whether intracranial pressure was increased or normal. If in ventilatory support we do find a detrimental increase in intracranial pressure, I would want to probably maintain cerebral function. I would probably then want to go to other modes, for example, increasing FIO_2's realizing, of course, the deterrents for using increased FIO_2's.

Moderator: Since not every patient who has brain injury still gets some type of intracranial pressure monitoring, what do you do if during mechanical ventilatory therapy or with PEEP therapy you see a rise in central venous pressure? Does that affect your therapy at all?

Dr. Ruben: No, it does not, not at this point. We are very aggressive in intracranial pressure monitorings. If there are problems in our ICU, we will monitor. For that reason, this is what I am following, and I think this is the best we have right now.

Moderator: I would like to make a point. In the patient who really has pulmonary disease, who has respiratory failure, because of alterations in decreased compliance, most of these pressures that you then apply to the airway really are not transmitted across. In effect, if I saw a patient who had an elevation in central venous pressure as a result of these modalities being used, I would infer that there is a relatively good chance that the patient has too much positive pressure, that we have reexpanded the lung and so improved compliance and now these pressures are being transmitted across. In that case, I might want to back off. Unfortunately, in the surgical unit, we probably do not have as much intracranial pressure monitoring as we would like to have, as compared to the neurosurgical unit.

This is an interesting question, but I am not sure that I fully understand it: Dr. Augenstein, why cannot voice synthesizers be used in medicine?

Dr. Augenstein: There are two ways one could use a voice synthesizer. One is to replace voice in people who do not have voice. Texas Instruments recently marketed a talking translator. If you type in the English word, it will write the French word in the little calculator-like thing and it will pronounce it for you. Conceivably, these kinds of packages could be made available to voiceless people to articulate the basic kinds of things they need in order to get around. Considerable work is being done in this area right now. The other area of voice synthesis is in communication from a machine back to a user. Conceivably, like when one dials the wrong number on the telephone and a voice answers and says, "Dial this number," you could call into a computer system and ask for the blood pressure of the patient and you could have a voice synthesizer give you that information. That technology is here and it is here now. There is nothing terribly unique about that. It just has not really fit into medicine yet.

Moderator: This question is asked of me: Patients with spinal cord injury that have been monitored by cardiac outputs, where have the observations been with regard to the cardiac output in that group of patients?

That is a very difficult question to answer from the standpoint that most of these are young patients to begin with that we normally see who come to our unit. They usually have other associated injuries. As a result, one would expect them to have a hyperdynamic state and an increase in cardiac output. Obviously, when one measures them, because of the sympathectomy that has occurred, such things as systemic vascular resistance is markedly decreased. On the whole, they do seem to have a hyperdynamic state. I am not sure that we have enough data available to be able to differentiate whether or not it is due to the sympathectomy and decreased peripheral resistance or whether it is simply due to all of the other associated injuries which have occurred.

Dr. Ruben and Dr. Augenstein, since both of you take care of patients, you may both answer this question: This is a theoretical patient with multiple trauma with two or more system involvement, 19 to 26 years of age group and no history of cardiac disease. I would presume that he may have had a head injury in addition to that. Dr. Augenstein, would you place a Swan-Ganz catheter in this patient when he comes into your ICU?

Dr. Augenstein: It depends upon the clinical setting. I think one has to utilize the monitoring available and adapt them to the needs of the patient. A patient who has everything functioning normally, even though he has had multiple trauma, is much like the elective surgery patient. For every cholecystectomy, we do not put in a Swan-Ganz catheter. Therefore, one must be somewhat selective. What are our criteria? If a patient is not responding to fluids and we add the problem of a head injury to that, the indications would probably be a little bit more liberal for catheterization. One might want to keep this patient drier and one might want more sensitivity to his overall cardiopulmonary adequacy, rather than just gross urine output. By contrast, the postoperative patient out of the operating room without the head injury who is really in pretty good shape, who is doing everything normally, we would not insert the Swan-Ganz catheter. But if his urine output did not respond to fluids, if his ventilatory status was such that he was going to require aggressive ventilatory therapy, if he is acidotic — if any of the things that indicate an abnormal reaction, he would definitely get a Swan-Ganz catheter inserted very early.

Moderator: Dr. Ruben, what would you do?

Dr. Ruben: I feel my thoughts are similar to Dr. Augenstein's. I may just add that, again, the patient dictates to us what we need to do as far as the lines. Again, what is the nature of the trauma? Does he have a chest injury? Does he have possible underlying myocardial contusion? What are his gases? Are his gases not responding? Are his gases low? You ask yourself the question: Why is his PO_2 low? Is it due to a pulmonary contusion? Is it due to a low cardiac output state? I think these are some of the things one has to ask one's self.

Again, what is his heart rate? What is his urinary output? If one wants to fine-tune this patient and these questions cannot be answered, then I think the Swan-Ganz catheter insertion is indicated.

Moderator: Dr. Augenstein, how permanent are the data recorded from a computer?

Dr. Augenstein: It can be as permanent as one would like it to be. The problem with most computer systems is that they have limited storage capabilities. Therefore, after 24 hours or so, in order to get new data into the computer, they have to purge the data that they already have, which typically means that instead of having immediate access on the CRT, they print it out much the way you would have written it out on paper. That is not a very good way. One of the breakthroughs in technology over the recent past has been in increasing storage capabilities at very low cost. So I do not think in the future we are going to be limited by our ability to store as much information. Once we store it, we can put it into any of a number of technologies that can make it as permanent as we want it to be.

Moderator: Is there any commercial system being marketed that is worth purchasing at this time? From what you have said, I gather that there are problems with all of them.

Dr. Augenstein: I think if you are going to do arrhythmia monitoring, there are a number of systems that are adequate, provided you accept about an 85% accuracy. If you want to do information management, and your goal is to set up a system wherein at the patient's bedside all the information would be available and flexible, that does not exist. The most sophisticated development to date is the Hewlett-Packard offering. It is the most popular right now.

The Pre- and Postoperative Patient: Intracranial Considerations

Harvey Shapiro, M.D.

Objectives

1. To review basic physiologic and pathologic mechanisms involved in cerebral and intracranial pressure dynamics.
2. To explain current concepts in the pharmacologic management of these problems.

Until recently the neurointensive care field generated little interest because, except for the most knowledgeable neurologists and neurosurgeons, most intensivists essentially had little information regarding intracranial dynamics.

Two factors led to the development of modern neuroanesthesia and modern neurointensive care: the utilization of the ICP measuring devices now provides the dynamic details of intracranial pressure events and ICU nurses can now recognize ICP changes. This continuous ICP information dramatically changes the time course of our responses to impending neurologic catastrophes. Intensive care dictates that we respond quickly and not sit and wait for 24 hours for bad things to happen. Getting this on-line information has made the whole area much more exciting. In addition, along with continuous ICP measurements, we have the development of cerebral blood flow methodology.

These two monitoring improvements enabled us to develop a rational approach and arrive at some understanding of events occurring in the intracranial space. I shall discuss the results of CBF studies and the results of ICP studies and how the

Harvey Shapiro, M.D., Professor of Anesthesiology and Neurosurgery, University of California School of Medicine at San Diego; Veterans Administration Hospital, San Diego, Calif.

coalescence of these factors has helped us formulate a modern basis for neurologic supportive care.

All of us recognize that the intracranial contents of tissue, blood and CSF are enclosed in a rather tight box and that volumes here could have reciprocal kinds of changes in them. Major volume buffering is via CSF displacement.

If one increases the blood volume and CSF cannot shift extracranially, then tissue displacement follows. That equates with herniation syndromes. In the maximally decompensated intracranial volume state distortion of tissue and compression of vasculature occur in some areas. This vascular compression causes ischemia. In other areas dilation of cerebral vasculature results in an augmented blood volume compartment. The intravascular compartment now adds mass effect of the already swollen brain. When this happens, the normal pathways down through the spinal subarachnoid space for volume compensation are obliterated, as well as the CSF absorptive pathways.

An ICP of greater than 15 torr in a supine position is abnormal. In terms of intensive care, I think it is very important to always have a zero reference point for the ICP transducer established when the patient is horizontal, and then be very careful about positioning. For instance, if the patient stands up, we get almost negative pressures in the intracranial space, so it makes the interpretation of what is occurring very important to keep in mind that gravity has great effects upon the CSF system.

If we look at the effect of gradually adding volume to the closed box intracranial compartment we go back to some rather simple principles, most recently enunciated by Langfitt and his group [1]. Intracranial pressure: intracranial volume relationships are such that, in this semiclosed system, the gradual introduction of a volume will lead to no pressure change until compensation, that is, what is provided by the CSF, is exhausted, and then an accelerating, exponential increase in ICP ensues. This means that a single ICP measurement that is within normal limits has a poor predictive value in terms of subsequent ICP changes, i.e., one really does not know where one is in terms of the potential for rapid change in pressure with a volume change. It also means that if one is at the point of spatial decompensation, a small addition of a volume can lead to a very precipitous increase in pressure.

This is what we call the concept of intracranial compliance. In some institutions, they actually will test this compliance to find out where the patient is on the curve. Compliance testing is not without its dangers.

Obviously, the result of being on the high end of that curve is intracranial hypertension. In terms of neurointensive care, that is one of the major areas about which we are concerned. I shall discuss some of the problems attendant to that in a pathological sense.

But first, let us examine how often increased ICP can occur in clinical practice. Here one will think about clinical situations that are relatively common: in tumor, head injury, hydrocephalus, osmolar imbalance syndromes, pseudotumor, dialysis complications, metabolic encephalopathy, infectious encephalopathy and large strokes. So one can see that the final wastebasket of ICP is much more than that just associated with the typical mass-occurring problems that we deal with in neurosurgery. Many of these disorders require pharmacologic and nonsurgical management. The treatment principles I shall discuss for mass lesions also apply to some of the other processes that result in an increase in ICP.

Let us consider the rates of volume changes in these various compartments we have talked about. Brain tissue volume changes very slowly, unless one is going to squeeze it out of the head through a burr hole or down through one of the foramina. When we see reductions in brain volume, we think of compression atrophy. There are experimental circumstances, where one has blood-brain barrier damage and deranged cerebrovascular autoregulation, where one can force water into the brain very acutely and very rapidly (minutes). Reversing this process with osmotic diuretics can require an hour or more.

Cerebrospinal fluid changes at moderate to very fast rates following a cough or sneeze instigate volume-pressure buffering changes in the CSF which occur almost instantaneously.

The blood volume compartment is the one that we manipulate in the operating room most frequently. It is very dependent upon oxygen and carbon dioxide tension changes. That compartment can change very quickly, and I shall discuss some of the factors that affect that blood compartment momentarily.

Obviously, the end result of a decompensated state is a displacement of tissue. I do not think this was especially appreciated until Lassen's recent CBF studies revealed that one can have a mass lesion in one place and have relative ischemia and hyperemia in other places within the brain. Lassen has shown that if one then increases the blood pressure, in the presence of an intracranial mass lesion, the brain will suddenly swell because it has altered CBF autoregulation. As the blood pressure increases in the ICU, and I think one can imagine many instances in which the blood pressure increases, such as with suctioning and other kinds of noxious stimulation, then one can then convert one of these areas with poor autoregulation into expansile masses. Those of us who have worked in ICUs have recognized how often the potential for herniation can be very much enhanced by having a blood pressure increase.

One of the consequences of an ICP increase is a reduction on the cortical surface of the brain. Remember that when the brain becomes acidotic, either for exogenous or endogenous reasons, carbon dioxide sensitivity as well as autoregulation will be very much blunted.

In an experimental circumstance, where the blood pressure does not change and the ICP rises, the cerebral perfusion pressure (which is the blood pressure minus the ICP) must be reduced. The initial response to a mass increasing inside the head is one of cerebral vasodilation, as witnessed by an increase in the cerebral blood volume. With autoregulation, the same thing would happen if we just dropped the blood pressure, but in the presence of a mass lesion, autoregulation compensation itself is actually adding to the intracranial volume. This happens because vascular resistance decreases in an effort to keep flow constant. At some critical point, this whole process becomes a vicious circle and the ICP becomes so high that CBF declines along with the metabolic rate for oxygen. The basis for this is the increased cortical tissue or brain tissue hydrogen ion concentration as previously discussed.

With this information at hand, we can go back to some of the first recordings that were made by Risberg and Lundberg in the early 1960s. Keep in mind that we discussed how cerebral blood volume increases with an increase in ICP. We did not say which came first necessarily, but in this situation reported by

Risberg spontaneous ICP waves occur (plateau waves) to over 80 torr. Their study found increases in cerebral blood volume in various areas of the brain accompanying the ICP plateau waves. So there is a very close association between ICP and cerebral blood volume when intracranial compliance is low. All of what we have been talking about fits together very nicely in Risberg's clinical demonstration of the relationship between blood volume and ICP.

This brings us to a discussion of CBF. We deal with ICP in the ICU; we do not measure CBF. I hope I can show you that CBF is important. I think we can establish a very exquisite relationship between CBF, drugs and their potency for increasing ICP. I want to point out that large changes in CBF and cerebral blood volume take place in a normally reactive brain between a $PaCO_2$ of 20 torr to 80 torr. In this CO_2 range cerebral blood volume goes from about 2 ml/100 gm of tissue up to about 5 ml/100 gm. If one multiplies that times the weight of the brain, there is a volume change of between 35 and 40 cc. That is considerable volume. Those who have worked in ICUs realize that if one were to take a syringe with 20 cc of volume and inject that into one of the ventricles, one would see some rather dramatic changes in the patient's intracranial status, especially if a mass lesion was already present.

We arrive at a very simple, possibly oversimplistic rule: techniques and drugs which elevate CBF can also increase ICP.

There is no study in the literature that deals only with an intracranial measurement that can tell you everything about the potency of a particular drug to change ICP because those measurements are performed usually in clinical circumstances at very different places on the compliance curve. So when one wants to get a number concerning relative ICP potency, one must start at the CBF end of the equation, not at the ICP end. That end will tell you that the drug has the ability to raise ICP but when one wants a potency number down, i.e., is this drug more potent than another, then one must go back through the equation to CBF data. The CBF measurements, although we do not do them commonly in the ICUs, are very important in terms of rational drugs used in acute neurologic disease.

There is a basic need to understand the effects of changes in carbon dioxide, blood pressure, brain function and autoregulation. The latter is the ability of the brain's vasculature to adjust itself to a change in perfusion pressure so that CBF remains constant.

If one can imagine a schematic representation, then at a high BP one would have very tiny constricted vessels and at a low BP have very widely opened vessels. A cerebral blood volume change occurs across the spectrum of autoregulation. When autoregulation fails at a low BP, ischemia occurs. Failure at a high BP results in hypertensive encephalopathy. Oxygen has minimal effects until one reaches into the pathologically low ranges. Then one gets a CBF increase. At very high PaO_2 ranges of one atmosphere there is about a 10% to 15% decrease in CBF.

$PaCO_2$ has extreme effects through the ranges with which we normally deal, and as we drop below a $PaCO_2$ of 25 torr, there is progressive attenuation of CBF, carbon dioxide sensitivity and, according to some investigators, signs that flow *that low* actually leads to the development of tissue hypoperfusion. Squat down and hyperventilate for a few minutes, then stand up quickly. You will have stressed autoregulation at a point where flow is very critically reduced, and I think you will feel some symptomatology that you can relate to cerebral ischemia.

Finally, not very often recognized in intensive care is the patient's anxiety level. There is a very good relationship between function and flow and, therefore, blood volume. When brain function increases, metabolism and flow will increase. Another way to do this is with noxious stimulation. I believe that some of the older and more barbaric techniques for examining patients by applying noxious stimulation may, in fact, lead to great difficulties in controlling ICP. I think we should reevaluate some of the overzealous stimulation techniques in the light of recent knowledge about the relationship between function, flow and intracranial blood volume.

As I mentioned earlier, the central tonic factor in maintaining cerebrovascular tone is the hydrogen ion concentration. There are other modifying factors involved in acute changes. Brain metabolism, obviously, results in a change here. We now understand that the blood gases have their effect, with carbon dioxide getting across the blood-brain barrier quickly, with oxygen actually causing an increase in hydrogen ion concentration via its relationship to metabolism. Suffice it to say that there are neurogenic influences which modulate cerebrovascular tone, usually under extreme stress rates, not commonly appreciated. There are intrinsic vascular responses that also modify the response to various challenges, usually over a small blood pressure range and usually they can be thought of as a rapidly reacting system.

When autoregulation is lost, either through tissue acidosis, brain pathology or through hypercapnia, the blood pressure determines the CBF. Let us now consider drugs. We will focus upon the potent anesthetic agents and the various sedative drugs. A drug which alters CNS function must alter cerebral metabolic rate and CBF. Some drugs do this in a coupled fashion, such as the barbiturates. Some drugs uncouple the CBF-CMR relationship, such as the volatile anesthetic agents.

The anesthetic barbiturate, thiopental, results in a paired reduction in flow and metabolism. This paired reduction is associated with a maintained couple of function, a maintained couple of metabolism and flow. As I shall show you subsequently, volatile agents have the ability to uncouple this relationship and to greatly alter autoregulation and carbon dioxide sensitivity. Nitrous oxide increases ICP. Its potency is less than that associated with halothane. Ketamine is really not a good drug to use for a minor orthopedic procedure in a patient who has a head injury. It is not a safe drug. It leads to very brisk, intense increases in ICP associated with EEG activation.

Then there are the drugs that have a minor effect in reducing ICP and maintain coupling. They are the narcotics and the sedative type of drugs that we use in ICUs.

When one has a situation such as a brain tumor patient undergoing the induction of anesthesia, all these principles are at work. The patient receives oxygen by mask, and we are looking at the ICP and the blood pressure. Then laryngoscopy is performed in a patient who is very lightly anesthetized. An increase in blood pressure occurs and is associated with an ICP increase up to 50 torr. Then barbiturate is given again and the ICP falls. The introduction of halothane, which is a cerebrovasodilator, increases the ICP and, more importantly, decreases the blood pressure at the same time. At this point CSF removal is attempted but after that happened there is still a very high ICP, because one can take the CSF out, but if a very strong stimulus for vasodilation exists, then the head just refills with blood. The treatment here is not CSF removal, but rather some maneuver which increases cerebrovascular resistance, such as hyperventilation or, in this case, the addition of pentothal.

Thirty minutes later and in the presence of a potent and stable level of anesthesia a profound stimulation occurs. The head prongs are inserted and the ICP goes up again. Studies which I shall discuss show that part of that ICP is due to a noxious stimulation and resultant cerebral vasodilation. When one administers a volatile anesthetic, a progressive dose-dependent vasoparalysis and loss of autoregulation occur. This means that volatile anesthetic agents can obliterate autoregulation and also potentially decrease the brain's ability locally to redistribute blood flow. There are different metabolic rates throughout the brain and this loss of autoregulation could lead to local metabolic-flow mismatching.

A study was recently reported by Kuramoto which demonstrates the cerebral effects of noxious stimuli in anesthetized dogs [2]. As the halothane concentration increases, the CBF response to pain also increases and without much change in metabolic rate. This kind of phenomenon may be partly responsible for laryngoscopy-associated ICP increases that have been previously described by us. The same pain-related CBF increase occurs during morphine anesthesia which we know does not cause pronounced cerebral vasodilation. This is the icing on the cake in terms of proving that this stimulation is appreciated in the brain despite anesthesia.

All of us use vasoactive agents. We use these agents in the operating room and in ICUs to support peripheral blood pressure. Suffice it to say that the brain is not cardiac output-dependent, as long as the perfusion pressure does not change. The emergency use of a vasopressor makes sense in terms of preserving brain perfusion. If the brain vasculature reacted in the same way that the peripheral vessels react, then one would *not* have a preferential redistribution, but one would have an extraordinarily high blood pressure with no blood really going any place preferentially. Whether a drug has an effect on CBF depends upon its ability to cross the blood-brain barrier.

As I shall discuss, vasodilators do cross the blood-brain barrier, while commonly used vasopressors do not.

Drugs which cross the blood-brain barrier then have access to the affector mechanism in the vascular smooth muscles. Drugs which do not will not change cerebrovascular resistance. For instance, if you were to administer sodium nitroprusside, you would see a reduction in blood pressure and an increase in ICP when an intracranial space occupying lesion is present.

Some investigators feel that this ICP increase does not happen with nitroglycerin. We have seen ICP increases to 50 torr with the administration of nitroglycerin. That should not be too surprising since we are all familiar with patients reporting pounding headaches when they take nitroglycerin. So this drug offers a lower toxicity in terms of cyanide toxicity, but it certainly does not get the patient out of the woods in terms of cerebral vasodilation.

Turner studied induced hypotension in clinical patients [3]. He contrasted nitroprusside with trimethaphan under two states, a normocapnic state and a hypocapnic state. He found that with nitroprusside there is such a strong vasodilation that one sees essentially no change in its ability to increase ICP as the blood pressure falls to 70% of control. With trimethaphan, there is no increase in ICP. That means that this drug might be preferable to control blood pressure in a situation where ICP is already high.

If, on the other hand, one is speaking of elective hypotension, in the absence of increased ICP, I would choose nitroprusside because that drug will be associated with better brain perfusion and trimethaphan, if the ICP is high, simply because it restricts the ICP increase further as it lowers the blood pressure. If the ICP is not high, and one is going to go to very low levels of blood pressure, select this agent, which also causes cerebrovasodilation. Of course, trimethaphan is a very different drug. It is a ganglionic blocker and does not gain very early entry into the CNS although we know it can cause, via the neurogenic influences in the CNS, pupillary dilation so some of it does have an effect.

To summarize the vasoactive agents, trimethaphan might be the drug to use with a closed tight head as the initial choice. Nitroprusside, nitroglycerin and hydralazine all increase ICP and have varying kinds of toxicity. It clearly makes no sense at all to potentiate this with a vasodilator, such as halothane, if one is in the operating room. At the University of Miami School of Medicine controlled hypotension, using a barbiturate, has been tried with some success, the only problem being, of course, that the patients sleep longer than they would after one of the other particular agents. The barbiturate makes sense because it increases vascular resistance, lowers metabolism and makes for a smaller brain in terms of operation.

So when faced with choosing a vasoactive agent, do not forget the early consideration that arterial hypertension may frequently be due to increased ICP. So one first takes steps to reduce the ICP with mannitol, hyperventilation, and one may not have to treat the blood pressure at all. If that does not help and one still feels the necessity to treat the blood pressure, then try trimethaphan. If that does not work, then nitroglycerin or sodium nitroprusside should be used. As our studies have shown, give it slowly. If given rapidly, the volume compensation cannot take place, and great increases in ICP will occur. If given slowly, there is time for additional buffering and there is not as great an increase in ICP.

What happens with muscle relaxants? We have often been told that they cause increases in ICP.

1. *Succinylcholine*. Previously we were told not to use it because it causes vesiculations and increases in intrathoracic pressure. We recently concluded a study at the University of California at San Diego in which we found that in the presence of barbiturate and with hyperventilation the utilization of succinylcholine is absolutely acceptable as the first-line drug for emergency intubation. It makes sense.

2. *Curare*. Used more in the ICU than in the operating room today, but it causes the release of histamine when given in large doses quickly and that results in an increase in ICP and a drop in blood pressure.

3. *Pancuronium*. This is better in the sense of avoiding histamine release, but it can lead to hypertension, and if there is poor autoregulation, that will lead to an increase in pressure. Again, if you can, give it slowly.

4. *Metabine*. Supposedly is going to be better than either of these agents because it causes less histamine release, but, in fact,

when given in an equipotent dose to obtain rapid relaxation for intubation, it is the same as curare.

Hyperventilation is good, but how much hyperventilation should one use and for how long? Certainly, acutely, in a patient who has come to us with normocapnia, a hyperventilation of 25 makes good sense. In that circumstance, we will get a reduction in ICP. However, in a patient who is chronically hyperventilated, either passively or mechanically, within a half-life of about six hours we begin to see a restitution of bicarbonate in the CSF by normal brain mechanisms that lead to CSF adaptation. This occurs in the presence of injured brain as well as normally. That means that we then have to think about changing the $PaCO_2$ further downward in order to get a better intracranial decompression. We have to do that. When we are given a patient who needs acute decompression, we institute hyperventilation. Then we give mannitol, perform surgery and perform other procedures, so that we no longer have the problem. The respirator order that is written for 25 really becomes progressively less of an order because the patient will normalize. However, there are some circumstances where ICP control can again be regained by additional hyperventilation. I think one should consider that as one goes along.

In the head injury patient CBF studies show a pretreatment phase of ischemia associated with high ICP, a posttreatment phase of hyperemia associated with high ICP and a posttreatment phase of hyperemia which occurs and suggests loss of autoregulation. Then a late phase occurs where we can have a restitution of ischemia. Certain degrees of prognosis can be made by looking at CBF characteristics. If CO_2 sensitivity is lost early, the prognosis is very grave. Early, the loss of autoregulation does not seem to relate to prognosis. Remember that if CO_2 sensitivity is lost here, one of the effective modalities for treatment is also removed. In the late stage, if autoregulation is indeed recovered, the prognosis is good and by late I mean at about one week. The therapy in this circumstance includes maintenance of oxygenation, hyperventilation, which restores autoregulation to some degree, a steady blood pressure and ICP measurement.

Concerning barbiturate protection I might mention that all kinds of other drugs are being considered in this milieu. I think sometimes the intensivists would rather turn to these drugs than their patients. The results with barbiturate protection in these three circumstances — intracranial hypertension, stroke and after cardiac arrest — are as follows: There is good laboratory and clinical confirmation that they work in terms of reducing ICP; good laboratory confirmation that they reduce the area of stroke but no clinical studies; and really a very confusing morass of information about the utilization of barbiturates after cardiac arrest. The mechanisms of head injury and stroke we think we understand in terms of how protection occurs: that is with a reduction in ICP and decreased edema formation in head injury; with improved collateral flow and decreased formation of edema in stroke; and that only when we look at the situation in postcardiac arrest encephalopathy do we need to get into all kinds of elaborate mechanisms.

In conclusion, the difficulty with this situation currently is that it has taken a long time for us to establish the concept that the use of CNS depressant drugs might be useful in the ICU. The use of that relates to our ability to determine what is going on inside the head, utilization of CBF studies, ICP studies, and now more importantly the CT scanner. If we have a patient who is sedated, and we have these various kinds of diagnostic milieus, not to leave out the EEG and evoked potentials, we can, in fact, rule out that there is an intracranial mass lesion. Therefore, when one uses a sedative drug, one can reduce the anxiety in response to noxious stimulation, as well as reduce the pressure. With stroke, more clinical trials must be done. In the case of postcardiac arrest, I think we have a situation where we might very well poison these other utilizations. Following a cardiac arrest, from my review of the literature, we have no evidence yet to indicate that one should be administering high doses of barbiturates. If we kill enough patients by doing that, then we will never be able to use it in these other situations, or in continued utilization in those situations where we have very slowly built up a rational basis for the utilization of those drugs.

References

1. Langfitt, T.W.: Pathophysiology of increased ICP. *In* Broche, M. and Dietz, H. (eds.): Intracranial Pressure. Berlin:Springer, 1973.
2. Kuramoto, T., Oshita, S., Takeshita, H. and Ishikawa, T.: Modification of the relationship between cerebral metabolism, blood flow and

electroencephalogram by stimulation during anesthesia in the dog. Anesthesiology 51:211, 1979.
3. Turner, J.M., Coroneos, N.J., Gibson, R.M. et al: The effect of althesin on intracranial pressure in man. Br. J. Anaesth. 45:168, 1973.

Self-Evaluation Quiz

1. Autoregulation is the ability of the brain's vasculature to adjust itself to a change in perfusion pressure so that cerebral blood flow remains constant.
   a) True
   b) False
2. When brain function increases, metabolism and flow will decrease.
   a) True
   b) False
3. The central tonic factor in maintaining cerebrovascular tone is the hydrogen ion concentration.
   a) True
   b) False
4. Nitrous oxide decreases intracranial pressure.
   a) True
   b) False
5. Ketamine is an excellent drug to use for a minor orthopedic procedure in patients with associated head injury.
   a) True
   b) False

Answers on page 391.

Increased Intracranial Pressure: Diagnosis, Monitoring and Treatment

Lawrence F. Marshall, M.D.

Objectives

1. To objectively identify reasons to monitor intracranial pressure.
2. To describe methods available for the treatment of intracranial hypertension.
3. To discuss the utilization of high-dose barbiturate therapy in the treatment of patients with severe brain injury and uncontrollable intracranial pressure.

Introduction

The initial phase of head injury is often accompanied by significant increases in brain bulk. This pathophysiologic process is almost always caused by brain blood volume increases rather than cerebral edema. This is seen most frequently in children and young adults, but can be seen in patients of all age groups from whatever the cause of head injury. This phenomenon in the past has been termed "brain swelling," but perhaps the term "cerebral engorgement" is more appropriate. In any case, it should not be considered cerebral edema. The fact that water increases are not important early in the course of head injury is clinically apparent when computerized axial tomographic (CAT) scanning is performed in such patients. Edema is very rarely seen during the first phase of brain injury. While it is true that increases in tissue water content do occur in head injury, this is usually a late phenomenon and is of limited significance early in the patient's course.

Lawrence F. Marshall, M.D., Associate Professor of Surgery/Neurological Surgery, University of California, San Diego.

In order to justify any invasive monitoring techniques, several requirements should be met. The first is that the parameter to be measured should be shown to be a significant factor in determining the patient's course and ultimate outcome. In patients suffering severe head injuries, Miller and Becker have demonstrated that intracranial pressures (ICP) greater than 20 mm Hg, which could not be controlled using standard methods, always proved to be fatal. Standard measures in the Richmond series included appropriate surgery, hyperventilation, thorazine sedation and high-quality intensive care. Patients dying of uncontrolled intracranial hypertension represented more than one half of all the fatalities in the Richmond series of 162 patients [1]. In 100 consecutive head injuries, Marshall et al also found that approximately one half of the fatalities were due to uncontrolled ICP [2].

It appears safe to assume, then, that of approximately 65,000 patients who survive to reach the hospital alive and subsequently die of their head injury, at least one half of these patients are dying from elevated ICP. Therefore, the first requirement for justifying invasive monitoring has been met, i.e., that intracranial hypertension is a significant factor in determining the outcome of patients with severe head injury.

The second requirement is the unavailability of a noninvasive method that can be relied upon to predict the presence or absence of intracranial hypertension. Neurosurgeons have often assumed that premonitory changes in the vital signs, the so-called Cushing or arterial pressure response, accompanies most pressure waves and could be used as a means of detecting changes in intracranial dynamics. We have shown that the classic triad of Cushing occurs less than 25% of the time in the face of pressure elevations of greater than 30 mm Hg [3]. Since the basic assumption of those who pursue an aggressive approach to the treatment of intracranial hypertension is that ICPs of greater than 15 mm Hg are always abnormal, a detection rate of less than 25% of pressures greater than 30 mm Hg is clearly unsatisfactory and indicates that some other method must be available to detect episodic changes in intracranial dynamics.

A final argument supporting ICP monitoring comes from recent data accumulated from San Diego County. Survivorship appeared to be significantly improved in patients in whom ICP was monitored when compared to patients with a matched severity of injury in whom ICP was not measured (Table 1) [4]. In patients with Glasgow Coma Scale (GCS) scores of 3-5, the mortality was significantly higher in those patients in whom ICP was not determined on a continuous basis.

Methods of Monitoring

If the foregoing arguments are found compelling for monitoring ICP, the next decision is to select a method or methods. The intraventricular cannula remains the most popular technique in university centers. It offers the most reliable means of monitoring ICP and has the added advantage of permitting cerebrospinal fluid drainage — a technique which can occasionally be life-saving in acutely brain-injured patients and frequently can be of significant benefit in controlling ICP. Case fatality rates in institutions where monitoring is done frequently demonstrate a risk of approximately one in 500. In hospitals where ICP monitoring is not routinely performed, the risks of ventricular cannulation, i.e., infection or difficulty in placing the catheter in the ventricles, will be somewhat higher. These are real disadvantages of the intraventricular cannula, particularly in hospitals where monitoring is not frequently employed.

Alternative methods, therefore, such as the subarachnoid or Richmond screw, have enjoyed increasing popularity. If the subarachnoid screw is to be used, it is critically important that

Table 1. Outcome as Related to Monitoring of ICP

	Good Recovery		Moderate Disability		Severe Disability		Vegetative		Dead		Total
	No.	%	No.	%	No.	%	No.	%	No.	%	
Glasgow Coma Score 6-7											
ICP monitored	16	49	3	9	2	6	3	9	9*	27	33
ICP not monitored	27	61	7	16	4	9	0	—	6*	14	44
Glasgow Coma Score 3-5											
ICP monitored	18	37	6	12	2	4	4	8	19†	39	49
ICP not monitored	9	24	2	6	2	6	1	3	23†	62	37

*P > .1 N.S.
†P < .05

the dura be lacerated or curetted open so that the bolt or screw rests in the subarachnoid space and not on the dura. With this proviso, the screw has been found to be reliable. It has the added advantage of avoiding penetration into the brain, and in a large series the risk from infection appears to be extremely small. We have seen no significant morbidity in over 400 patients in whom the subarachnoid screw has been used to monitor ICP.

Recently, the epidural transducer designed by Ladd has attracted increasing interest. This fiberoptic device is relatively free from drift and does not require the fluid-filled media of the subarachnoid screw. This avoids the potential danger of injecting fluid into the intracranial space. The major disadvantage of the Ladd epidural transducer is its cost, a not insignificant consideration if a large number of patients are to be monitored.

For those who are making their initial choice of a device or devices for ICP monitoring, it is necessary that they consider the possible need for more than one method. In children where the ventricular system is often collapsed following acute head injury, and in patients with severe shifts, placement of the ventricular cannula may be very difficult and alternative methods should be available. Whatever choice is made, ICP monitoring is an absolute necessity if therapy is to be rationally guided for patients with severe head injury. Unless one knows on a continuous basis what the intracranial dynamics are, the care of the brain injury, the cardiopulmonary complications and even fluid management cannot be properly integrated, particularly in the patient with multiple injuries.

Treatment

The basic goal in the treatment of intracranial hypertension is the normalization of cerebral perfusion pressure (CPP). CPP is defined as the mean systemic arterial pressure minus the mean ICP and is an approximate guide for judging the adequacy of brain nutrition. By directing care toward normalization of CPP, one can create a milieu which allows for recovery of tissues not irreversibly damaged and avoids secondary injuries to the already damaged brain. It is important to recall that the prevention of intracranial hypertension is by far easier than its treatment. Table 2 illustrates the standard method of management of patients with marked brain swelling who have a significant impairment of consciousness (GCS score of 7 or less).

Hyperventilation remains the cornerstone of all attempts to acutely reduce ICP in the severely brain injured. It is the most rapid method for reducing ICP in situations of impending disaster and in the initial resuscitation of the patient. Paramedics, therefore, should be instructed to hyperventilate all patients with significant head injuries in the field. While hyperventilation's effectiveness decreases with time, small further reductions in CO_2 tension will often achieve better control of the ICP as the patient tends to escape from the vasoconstrictive effects of a PCO_2 of from 25 to 30 mm Hg, which is the level we recommend initially. Hyperventilation below a PCO_2 of 20 to 22 mm Hg, however, should be avoided since secondary brain ischemia may occur because of the marked reduction in cerebral blood flow (CBF) that may accompany severe hyperventilation.

Osmotic Diuretics

Osmotic diuretics, particularly mannitol, continue to be extremely useful in the treatment of severe brain injury. There is some concern, however, that mannitol's role needs to be redefined in children with head injury. Bruce et al have suggested that mannitol probably should not be used on a long-term basis in children because CBF is often already increased in children, and the major effect of mannitol acutely

Table 2. Care of Patients With Significant Clinical Compromise (No Verbal Response) Because of Brain Swelling

1. Controlled ventilation (pCO_2 25 to 30 mm Hg)
2. Mannitol 0.25 gm to 1.0 gm/kg by bolus or IV infusion
3. Dexamethasone 10 to 20 mg IV q 4-6 hr
4. Ventricular drainage if possible
5. Avoid hypoxia
6. Avoid hypotonic fluids
7. Avoid halogenated anesthetics
8. Avoid systemic hypertension

is to increase CBF [5]. While the osmotic gradient created by mannitol will reduce intracranial volume by removing water from the brain, this change in water content may not be adequate in young patients to compensate for the increase in brain-blood volume that may occur with mannitol administration. In children we recommend that a smaller dose of 0.25 to 0.5 gm/kg be utilized in the emergent situation and that ICP monitoring guide further dosage. In adults, 1 gm/kg has been and will continue to be the initial form of therapy in the emergency room. This delineation is illustrative of the fact that in the future we are going to need to define specific therapies or doses for specific patients either on the basis of age or the type of injury. Chronically, smaller doses of mannitol than the previously recommended 1 gm/kg can be utilized successfully in both children and adults. We have shown that an osmotic gradient of 10 mOsm is usually sufficient to control intracranial hypertension and can be achieved with a 0.25 gm/kg dose [6]. The dangers of mannitol include severe dehydration and electrolyte imbalance. When barbiturates are subsequently introduced into the patient's therapy, and if dehydration has been severe, catastrophic hypotension can occur. It is also of interest to note that mannitol-induced dehydration and electrolyte imbalance were the most frequent causes of avoidable death in our region during a one-year, multi-institutional intensive care unit study.

The nonosmotic diuretics, particularly furosemide and ethacrynic acid, have demonstrated promise in both laboratory models and in the clinic. Although we have found the ICP response somewhat variable following the administration of these drugs vs. the relatively high level of response to mannitol, they need to be studied further. It appears that they have a direct effect on sodium transport into the brain and that they inhibit CSF production. These agents deserve trial in a controlled clinical setting and may be particularly useful under circumstances where large increases in intravascular volume must be avoided.

Glucocorticoids

Dexamethasone has been a part of every regimen introduced for the treatment of head injuries in the last ten years.

Cooper [7] and Pitts [8], however, have recently questioned the value of high-dose dexamethasone. They have suggested that dexamethasone may have only a very small role to play in the treatment of patients with head injury. The initial enthusiasm generated by the reports of Faupel [9] and Gobiet [10] must be tempered with the knowledge that the Gobiet study was not a randomized trial, but rather a report of survival in patients in succeeding years. This suggests that other influences may have played a role in the improved outcome. In the study of Faupel and Reulen, if one combines the severely damaged with those who did not survive, there is not a significant difference in outcome. We have continued to administer high doses of dexamethasone (80 mg/day) for four days and then have tapered the drug over the next week because edema does occur in head injury, albeit usually late. Nevertheless, we recognize that the value of dexamethasone in acute head injury may be extremely limited. It is important to emphasize that in circumstances other than head injury, glucocorticoids have been extremely effective. This is not surprising since in patients with primary and metastatic tumors the major causes of increased brain bulk are tumor and increased water or edema in the brain tissue. In head injury, in contrast, arteriolar engorgement is by far the most important initial factor.

Control of Systemic Arterial Pressure

High systemic arterial pressure (SAP), which we have defined as a systolic blood pressure of greater than 160 mm Hg, appears to have a deleterious effect in patients with severe brain injury and requires treatment. In the laboratory, when the systolic pressure is allowed to rise abruptly above 160 mm Hg, blood-brain barrier (BBB) damage and extravasation of proteins and other osmoles can be observed, followed by the movement of water into the brain [11]. Moreover, acute head injury is characterized by the loss of autoregulation. Thus, changes in SAP are directly reflected in the vascular bed of the brain, and hypertension will then be associated with vascular engorgement with subsequent severe intracranial hypertension triggering further systemic arterial hypertension in an attempt to return to a more favorable CPP, beginning a vicious cycle which leads to the demise of the patient.

The treatment of systemic arterial hypertension is not simple. The first step in most severely injured patients is proper sedation. We prefer morphine both because of familiarity with the drug and because of its potential reversibility. When a narcotic is combined with Pavulon in intubated patients, the obliteration of laryngeal reflexes often eliminates what appears to be systemic arterial hypertension resulting from the brain injury. If the use of sedation and induced paralysis is not successful, some direct antihypertensive agent should be utilized. The choices available include drugs that are known cerebral vasodilators such as nitroprusside and nitroglycerin. While these agents are extremely useful in other areas of neurosurgery, we have been hesitant to use them in most instances in patients with severe head injuries. Our preferences in descending order include propranolol or similar β-blockers, Arfonad, and hydralazine. The use of an antihypertensive agent can be more rationally guided with ICP monitoring. Under circumstances where other agents fail and nitroprusside must be tried, its deleterious effect on intracranial dynamics can be immediately observed and the drug discontinued if circumstances dictate. In patients with severe head injuries in whom ICP is not monitored, the use of nitroprusside and nitroglycerin is contraindicated in our view.

Additional Guidelines for the Treatment of Intracranial Hypertension

In addition to the therapies discussed briefly here, there are some general rules regarding the avoidance of complications in brain-injured patients that merit a brief mention. Siesjo has recently demonstrated that severe brain tissue acidosis has a deleterious effect on brain metabolism. Systemic acidosis which will only contribute to the acidotic state of the damaged brain must be avoided at all costs. A frequent cause of acidosis in brain-injured patients is spontaneous ventilation at a high rate. While some neurosurgeons are reluctant to utilize controlled ventilation because of the loss of the neurologic examination, it is our view that controlled ventilation is mandatory in such patients and should be instituted not only because a patient's arterial blood gases are poor or borderline, but also to avoid the potential for tissue acidosis.

Hypoxia is also a very potent cerebral vasodilator and must be avoided. PaO_2's of 60 to 70 mm Hg which are well tolerated by most normal people are unsatisfactory in brain-injured patients, and every effort should be made to obtain higher levels.

Finally, halogenated anesthetics should be avoided in patients with head injury, since they produce an increase in CBF at the same time as SAP falls. This is a bad combination when one is worried about protecting the CPP.

High-Dose Barbiturate Therapy

Barbiturates have recently been introduced for the treatment of intracranial hypertension [12]. Their major effect is a reduction in ICP. They produce a reduction in cerebral blood volume because of their cerebral vasoconstrictive effect. They also decrease the metabolic rate of the brain which in turn leads to a decreased need for CBF. In addition, it has been suggested by Bruce and Reulen that the generalized reduction in ICP produced by barbiturates may improve the resolution of edematous states. Whatever their mechanism, the drugs remain investigative and should be utilized under strictly controlled circumstances. Criteria for their use should include strict pressure criteria, and they should never be utilized if other methods can easily control ICP. An experienced intensive care unit team is also an absolute necessity. Patient monitoring must be systematic and comprehensive and should include ICP, SAP, right heart pressures and pulmonary arterial pressures. A laboratory capable of rapid serum barbiturate level determinations is also necessary.

The objectives in the administration of high-dose barbiturate therapy are to normalize the ICP and produce useful survivors. By monitoring ICP, the dose of barbiturate required can be reduced to the minimum necessary to control ICP, thus limiting problems caused from the potential side effects of these very potent drugs.

Initially, we began high-dose barbiturate therapy when the ICP exceeded 40 mm Hg for 15 minutes or more and could not be controlled with the standard methods previously outlined. Because of a trend in our data toward an improved mortality in patients with ICPs of greater than 40 mm Hg and a higher loss rate than one would have predicted in patients with pressures between 15 and 40 mm Hg, we have recently reduced the pressure criteria for the initiation of barbiturate therapy to 25 mm Hg. In addition, we have altered the method by which barbiturates are begun and terminated. An initial dose of 5 mg/kg is given as a bolus. If the mean arterial pressure (MAP) remains above 70 mm Hg and there is no effect on ICP, an additional 5 mg/kg is given 15 minutes later. This sequence is repeated until a total dose of 20 mg/kg has been administered. If no ICP response is obtained with this total dose, barbiturates will not be effective in controlling ICP, and they should be discontinued. Under most circumstances, however, satisfactory reduction of ICP will be accomplished and can then be maintained by the administration of between 100 and 200 mg of pentobarbital per hour. The dose will vary both with the age and weight of the patient. We have used as a general guideline a serum level of between 3 and 4 mg%. Although others have reported further reductions in ICP when the serum level has been greater than 4 mg%, this has not been our experience in over 70 patients. Occasionally high-dose barbiturate therapy will not be an adequate single-therapy modality. Under those circumstances, mannitol and ventricular drainage must be considered as adjuvants. The CPP should always be maintained at a level greater than 50 mm Hg. Barbiturate doses should always be withheld if the MAP falls below 65 to 70 mm Hg in an adult and below 55 mm Hg in a child.

The initiation of high-dose barbiturate therapy calls for an increase and not a decrease in patient surveillance. CAT scanning should be carried out both prior to the administration of barbiturates and when a change in the patient's pupils or ICP occurs during maintenance therapy. It must always be recalled that monitoring devices, while reliable, are not infallible and clinical judgment must be brought to bear under circumstances where there is a question as to whether a change in intracranial dynamics has taken place despite a stable tracing on the monitor. In patients where craniotomy with removal of a bone flap has been performed, particular caution should be taken in regard to relying on the ICP. We have seen patients with ICPs of between 15 and 20 mm Hg develop anisocoria and transtentorial herniation.

The routine use of the Swan-Ganz catheter in our patients reflects the fact that management of these patients, particularly when they are multiply injured, is complex and problems can result unless adequate information is available regarding intravascular volume and cardiac output. Under circumstances where mannitol in large doses has been used prior to the administration of barbiturates, pulmonary artery pressure determinations are an absolute necessity. Changes in cardiopulmonary status that occur so frequently in brain-injured patients can be better monitored and treated if the cardiac output, pulmonary arterial pressure and systemic vascular resistance can be calculated and be made available to the treating clinician.

While we have found high-dose barbiturate therapy safe and effective, other neurosurgeons have noted some problems. These include an increased incidence of hypoxia. We have reviewed our records and have found this not to be the case. High-dose barbiturates did not lead to an increased incidence of pulmonary failure. Rather, it appears that the neurosurgical community has underestimated the incidence of adult respiratory distress syndrome in patients with severe head injuries. Respiratory failure in severely brain-injured patients is a product not only of the brain-lung interaction, but also because severe dehydration produced by mannitol is superimposed on this already adverse condition.

Hypothermia in combination with high doses of barbiturates has also been noted by others to be associated with hypoxia. We deliberately avoid cooling our patients below 32 C. When the core temperature drops below this level, increases in lung stiffness and difficulty with ventilation do occur. Moreover, ventricular arrhythmias are often seen at temperatures below 30 C and can be exacerbated by high serum levels of barbiturates.

The decision to withdraw high-dose barbiturate therapy usually occurs under two circumstances. First, the ICP has risen inexorably and the patient is thought to be brain dead. Under such circumstances, four-vessel angiography can be used to determine brain death, since extremely high levels of serum barbiturates cannot depress CBF below a level of approximately 40% of normal — a level at which flow is still seen on routine angiography. It is important to remember that it is clearly unsatisfactory for the patient's family and for the personnel caring for such a patient to have that patient be maintained in an intensive care unit waiting for an EEG when four-vessel angiography can determine viability of the brain.

The second reason to withdraw barbiturates is that the patient has had successful control of intracranial hypertension and it is time for this expensive and time-consuming therapy to be discontinued. Our criteria for discontinuation of high doses of barbiturates include (1) a normal ICP of 15 mm Hg or less for at least 24 hours, (2) the absence of systemic arterial hypertension for at least 24 hours and (3) a CT scan which demonstrates resolution of major brain shifts or at least partial resolution on a scan performed not more than 24 hours prior to the beginning of the termination of barbiturate therapy.

Barbiturates should be tapered and not stopped abruptly. We have halved the dose on the first day and on the second day have increased the time interval between the doses. This same sequence is repeated until the fourth day when the drug is stopped. Intracranial hypertension of a mild to moderate degree may begin to be seen on the second and third day as the drug is being tapered. This usually reflects the return of the laryngeal reflex arcs which may require suppression if the ICP increases above 25 mm Hg. If significant intracranial hypertension with pressures continually above 30 mm Hg is seen, it is usually an indication that the process for which barbiturates were instituted has not resolved and that the patient requires immediate rescanning and reinstitution of therapy. It is important to note also that PCO_2 usually rises as barbiturates are tapered, and respiratory rate or setting adjustments need to be made to allow the PCO_2 to come up slowly.

Conclusion

There is increasing evidence that satisfactory control of increased ICP has resulted in an increased salvage rate in patients suffering severe head injury. The treatment of intra-cranial hypertension, however, must go hand-in-hand with the avoidance of secondary insults to the brain from hypoxia, hypercapnia or hypotension. The necessity of an integrated and comprehensive approach to the treatment of these very severely ill patients cannot be overemphasized. While therapies such as the use of high-dose barbiturates have a certain clinical fascination, they should be viewed as both investigational and difficult. Moreover, the need for such elaborate methods to control ICP can probably be reduced by a systematic approach to the care of brain-injured patients from the time of injury and throughout their stay in the intensive care unit setting. It must always be recalled that the prevention of intracranial hypertension is much easier than its treatment, and those concerned with the care of these patients must be ever vigilant to protect the patient from both the disease process and those iatrogenic maneuvers which can have a deleterious effect on intracranial dynamics.

References

1. Miller, J.D., Becker, D.P., Ward, J.D. et al: Significance of intracranial hypertension in severe head injury. J. Neurosurg. 47:503-512, Oct 1977.
2. Marshall, L.F., Smith, R.W. and Shapiro, H.M.: The outcome with aggressive treatment in severe head injuries. I and II. J. Neurosurg. 50:20-30, 1979.
3. Marshall, L.F., Smith, R.W. and Shapiro, H.M.: The influence of diurnal rhythms in patients with intracranial hypertension: Implications for management. Neurosurgery 2:100-102, 1978.
4. Bowers, S.A. and Marshall, L.F.: Outcome in 200 consecutive cases of severe head injury treated in San Diego County: A prospective analysis. Neurosurgery 6:337-342, 1980.
5. Bruce, D.A., Gennarelli, T.A. and Langfitt, T.W.: Resuscitation from coma due to head injury. Crit. Care Med. 6:254-269, 1978.
6. Marshall, L.F., Shapiro, H.M. and Rauscher, A.L.: Mannitol dose requirements in brain-injured patients. J. Neurosurg. 48:169-172, 1978.
7. Cooper, P.R., Moody, S., Clark, W.K. et al: Dexamethasone and severe head injury. J. Neurosurg. 51:307-316, 1979.
8. Pitts, L.H. and Kaktis, J.V.: Effects of megadose steroids on outcome following severe head injury. In Proceedings of the American Association of Neurological Surgeons Annual Meeting. Los Angeles, California, 1979.
9. Faupel, G., Reulen, H.J., Muller, D. et al: Double-blind study on the effects of steroids on severe closed head injury. In Pappius, H.M. and Feindel, W. (eds.): Dynamics of Brain Edema. Berlin/Heidelberg/New York:Springer-Verlag, 1976, pp. 337-343.
10. Gobiet, W., Bock, W.J., Leisegang, J. et al: Treatment of acute cerebral edema with high dose dexamethasone. In Beks, J.W.F., Bosch, D.A. and Brock, M. (eds.): Intracranial Pressure III. Berlin/Heidelberg/New York:Springer-Verlag, 1976.

11. Forster, A., Shapiro, H.M. et al: Influence of anesthetic agents on brain-blood barrier function during acute arterial hypertension. Anesthesiology 49:26-30, 1978.
12. Rockoff, M.A., Marshall, L.F. and Shapiro, H.M.: High-dose barbiturate therapy in humans: A clinical review of 60 patients. Ann. Neurol. 6:194-199, 1979.

Self-Evaluation Quiz

1. Increases in intracranial volume occurring early in head injury are due to:
   a) Increases in brain volume
   b) Increases in CSF production
   c) Brain edema
   d) Vascular engorgement

2. Intracranial hypertension is responsible for:
   a) At least one half of all deaths from head injury in patients who reach the hospital alive
   b) Increases in cerebral perfusion pressure
   c) An improvement in intracranial dynamics
   d) An increased survivorship in patients with head injury

3. Cerebral perfusion pressure has all the following characteristics *except*:
   a) An index of cerebral perfusion
   b) Altered by changes in blood pressure
   c) Should be considered as not an absolute reflection of the status of cerebral perfusion
   d) Is equal to the mean arterial pressure plus the intracranial pressure

4. Methods available to monitor ICP include all of the following *except*:
   a) Intraventricular cannula
   b) Subarachnoid bolt
   c) Epidural transducer
   d) Lumbar puncture

5. Standard management of brain swelling includes:
   a) Avoid hypoxia
   b) Normocapnia
   c) Hypoventilation
   d) Supine position

Matching

6. Diabetes insipidus a) Electrolyte disturbance
7. Mannitol b) Hyperosmolality
8. Hyperventilation c) Effectiveness may decrease over time
9. Dexamethasone d) May cause hypotension
10. Barbiturates e) Value in head injury questionable

Answers on page 391.

Panel Discussion

Panelist: Dr. Shapiro

Moderator: Dr. Shapiro, how important is measuring intracranial compliance when planning the management of intracranial pressure problems?

Dr. Shapiro: I think that in a situation where you are continuously measuring intracranial pressure occasional compliance measurements may be indicated, especially if you are attempting to determine which way to move therapeutically. Intracranial compliance measurements are not without risk. Other ways of obtaining the information based upon studies that have been done using compliance, for instance, would indicate that if there is any shift, as shown by CT scan or on angiography, of greater than one half of 1 cm that you can then make the assumption that compliance is low without actually making the measurement.

Moderator: What is the timing of the initation of ICP monitoring? In my view, ICP monitoring should start immediately following the CAT scan in a patient who does not have a surgical lesion. That means that the patient goes from the emergency room or wherever he has been resuscitated to the CAT scan to the operating room. We do one cut EMI scans now in trauma through the ventricular system. The first cut is a zero plane cut through the face, which allows you to look at the facial bones in addition to looking at the intracranial space. If there is a mass because of a clot, the patient's scan is discontinued and we do the scan without contrast, and the patient goes right to the operating room. We believe that in a patient with a head injury from the time he is admitted to the hospital to the time that he is in the operating room should be no more than 45 minutes. If you are going to do a full scan on one of the

171

second generation machines, then you are looking at 25 minutes just to do the scan and 15 minutes to warm it up. That is far too long. If we do not see a mass, then we complete the study. We do not do a contrast scan, unless we think there is something suspicious about the patient's clinical course. That is, could the patient have fallen down because he ruptured an aneurysm — that kind of thing. We do a contrast scan following the patient's initial stabilization and management of ICP, at four days, and we always use contrast. The reason for that is the experience of some of our colleagues showing that one may pick up bilateral subdural hematomas that were missed initially in patients who seem to have relatively difficult ICPs to control. The issue is: Should one start ICP monitoring only after two days? The ballgame is usually all over after two days, so it is very illogical to start intracranial pressure monitoring two days after a patient has suffered the head injury. Most patients, if they are going to have intracranial hypertension, have it within the first 36 to 48 hours.

Dr. Shapiro, in the treatment of systemic arterial hypertension, do you believe that one should try to reduce ICP first and therefore reduce blood pressure prior to initiating treatment for systemic arterial hypertension?

Dr. Shapiro: Yes, I do, and I stated that in my presentation.

Moderator: Do barbiturates actually increase cerebral vascular resistance? What is the mechanism of action?

Dr. Shapiro: Yes, they do increase cerebral vascular resistance. Numerous studies have shown where that derived figure can be obtained.

What is the mechanism of action? That is an entirely different situation. In my opinion and from experimental data gathered in my laboratory as well as by others, they do not act directly upon the vascular smooth muscle. They require instead a linkage between brain metabolism and the vessel itself. The linkage implies that there is either direct chemical metabolic interaction or that there is a metabolic:neurogenic interaction which involves the vasculature. In fact, when one gives high doses of barbiturates to isolated brain vessels, one gets dilation uniformly. So they require some intact brain vascular controlling mechanism in order to have their action.

Moderator: Dr. Shapiro, what methods do you use to control hypertension, that is, systemic arterial hypertension? I guess I have already answered that partially, but you might make some comments, and you may disagree with me, in the presence of intracranial hypertension following 48 hours of therapy.

Question: Do you use Aldomet?

Moderator: No, I never use Aldomet. Aldomet is a central nervous system depressant and often confuses the issue. I have already made comments about propranolol. We have used propranolol particularly in pediatrics and have been happy with it, but Dr. Shapiro, you might want to comment further about my comments about nitroprusside and nitroglycerin.

Dr. Shapiro: Is this after 48 hours?

Moderator: Yes, that is correct.

Dr. Shapiro: It depends upon whether the circumstances, one with barbiturate therapy, are ongoing or not. In the absence of barbiturate therapy, with an upward-spiralling blood pressure pattern, I would be very concerned that there was a problem intracranially and I would look to see what the ICP was and then do what was suggested by the former question, that is, do everything I possibly could to reduce the intracranial pressure. After that, I would turn to the drugs I indicated, trimethaphan and the intravenously administered drugs slowly, that is, nitroglycerin and nitroprusside, and perhaps go to hydralazine, which has the same potential for increasing ICP as I was moving into a more chronic controlled situation.

Moderator: I have three questions which I shall answer. First, regarding the Glasgow coma scale. I am going to discuss that further later when I discuss head injury. Then I shall discuss how we utilize it and discuss its importance as a triage tool. I think Dr. Daroff's comments, some of them were probably a little bit off base in my view, in terms of the evaluation of acutely brain-injured patients, but we will discuss that later.

I think mannitol is not contraindicated in children, if one uses a small dose. If one is monitoring ICP, that is, the patient is in a stable situation in the ICU, then one can use this drug, but one simply must be very careful with it — 1 gm/kg in the emergency room looks like a bad idea. That should be avoided. Use smaller doses, hyperventilate children very acutely in the ICU. In terms of maintenance fluids, what do I use? I use half-normal saline almost exclusively. The patients are often initially resuscitated with Ringer's lactate or other volume expanders. I think that is fine. We tend to use half-normal saline almost exclusively. There are considerable data from animal laboratory experiments and brain injury models, where if one uses dextrose and water, particularly in large doses, one can get astronomical brain swelling and terrible decreases in cerebral blood flow.

What do I suggest to use and what method to clear an ICP line that has become clogged? Can one have a dampened waveform from that? Yes, obviously, that is one of the major problems, particularly with the subdural screw. We disconnect it. To get bubbles out of the line is absolutely a prerequisite. We re-irrigate through the screw. I use bacteriostatic, nonpreserved saline solution, irrigate it through a needle in the screw. For the ventricular cannula, I use very small volumes of fluid to flush it. If I cannot get fluid in, I am never going to be able to get fluid out. So I use small volumes. If you cannot push it in, you cannot get it out. Sometimes you can push it in, but you cannot get it out. That is the worst possible situation. So you must be very careful. It is very important to keep air out of the system. In a patient who is being drained and redrained and is turned to monitoring and then back to redrainage, it is critical not to have a stopcock that leaks air. Many plastic stopcocks within 24 to 48 hours tend to leak a little air, the system becomes occluded and you do not have transmission of a good pulse wave. One of the real losers in intracranial pressure monitoring and where people got into trouble, particularly if they are not experienced with the subdural screw, is that they do not make a hole in the dura. There must be a hole in the dura in order to have an adequate recording. We use a large needle. Some people use a curette to make the hole. By a large needle, I mean a 12- to 14-gauge needle, through the twist drill hole, to make the hole in the dura. If you do not have that, if the system does not stay fluid-filled, you can have a very false sense of security that you are monitoring ICP and you really are not. One should never ignore the clinical examination. If the patient is getting worse, if the blood pressure is going up, even though the Cushing response is not reliable, when it happens, it means something, and the ICP trace does not look so good, trust a clinical examination. The patient should be treated, CAT scanned again. We and I think everyone has had monitoring disasters where we think the patient is fine and suddenly the pupil dilates, the ICP does not look like it is changed and what has happened is that you have a damp tracing. With experience, that happens less frequently. I think we have had one death in the last 200 patients who have been monitored, where we have had monitor failure, where I clearly felt the patient was salvageable, but the monitor failed us.

But the big trick with the subdural screw is to make a hole in the dura. If you do not have a hole in the dura, then this will not work for longer than a few hours. You must use a subdural screw as a subdural device. It must sit in the subarachnoid space and it must be fluid-filled.

Electrophysiological Recording in the ICU

R. Eugene Ramsay, M.D.

Objectives

To outline the diagnostic and prognostic usefulness of electrophysiological recordings on patients in the neurological intensive care unit. The findings in coma and the criteria for determination of electrocerebral silence are outlined. The clinical and electrographic findings in the treatment of status epilepticus are discussed as well as the use of the six major anticonvulsant drugs.

Monitoring in the intensive care units has changed dramatically in the last few years. The electrocardiogram was for many years the only physiological phenomenon which was continuously monitored. The expansion of our capabilities has taken place most dramatically in the neurological intensive care units, now with continued monitoring of arterial and venous pressures, intracranial pressures and EEG. As the patient's level of consciousness becomes depressed, we begin to lose sensitivity in the neurological examination for indexing changes in the patient condition. As this happens, the EEG and evoked responses become increasingly important to define an alteration or progression of a disease process.

Electroencephalographic Finding

The EEG findings in the normal waking and sleeping state are well defined (Fig. 1). In the waking state, a rhythmic activity occurs in the posterior portions of the brain which in

R. Eugene Ramsay, M.D., Assistant Professor of Neurology, University of Miami School of Medicine; Director, Clinical Electrophysiology Laboratory, Miami VA Medical Center.

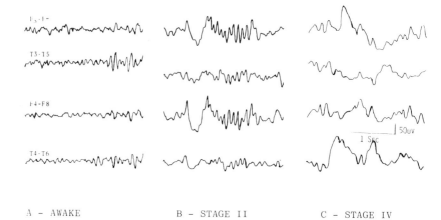

A - AWAKE   B - STAGE II   C - STAGE IV

FIG. 1. A. Normal waking and sleeping patterns: In the waking resting
state, a sinusoidal waveform of 9 to 11 Hz is seen over the occipital areas
which will block when the eyes are open. In the middle and frontal regions
of the head the activity is lower voltage and less regular. B. In early sleep
the background becomes a generalized mixture of slower activity
(predominantly 4 to 7 Hz) with superimposed low voltage and fast.
Characteristic of stage 2 sleep is the appearance of K-complexes and sleep
spindles as shown here. C. As deeper stages of sleep occur, the
K-complexes are no longer seen and the background becomes higher
voltage and very slow.

the adult ranges from 9 to 11 cps. In the frontal regions a low
voltage usually irregular, but at times rhythmic, activity is seen
which is much faster than that seen in the occipital regions.
There are two major stages of sleep which are described by the
presence or absence of rapid eye movement (REM). In
non-REM sleep a systematic change occurs and has been staged
1 through 4 with examples of stage 2 and 4 shown in Figure 1.
In response to either focal injury or generalized insult, there is
only a limited number of changes that can occur in the EEG.
These include (1) asymmetry of voltage (amplitudes), (2) increased quality of faster frequency, (3) increase in the quantity
of slow frequencies, (4) abnormal topographic distribution of
any frequency, (5) the occurrence of spike or epileptogenic
activity and (6) absence of activity. The EEG frequently can
indicate whether the process producing coma is a localized or
diffuse problem. One limitation with a few exceptions is that
the findings on an EEG are nonspecific; several processes can

result in the same EEG findings. The most common change with depressed level of consciousness is the appearance of frequencies which are slower than expected (Fig. 2). As the patient's level of consciousness becomes impaired as the result of a generalized insult (metabolic disturbance, toxin, anoxia), a progressive and usually predictable series of changes occur. With a mild insult, the normal-appearing background may persist with some interspersed slow waves (4 to 7 Hz range) (Fig. 2B). As the level of consciousness becomes progressively impaired, the normal background is lost and the slow wave component becomes more prominent and the frequency of the activity becomes progressively slower (1 to 3 Hz range) (Fig. 2C). At this stage, discharges of higher voltage delta are seen projecting bilaterally but maximally in the frontal regions (FIRDA) may be seen. Typically this pattern has been associated with metabolic/toxic disorders but can also be seen (1) with hydrocephalus and dilatation of the third ventricle, (2) with a structural lesion of the deeper midline structures (thalamus) and (3) as an interictal seizure discharge. One characteristic pattern is a frontal predominant intermittent discharge with the waveforms having a reproducible triphasic morphology (Fig. 2D). This was described first in midstage hepatic coma and less frequently can also be a result of uremia. As coma deepens, the triphasic pattern disappears as the background frequencies become progressively slower (1 Hz or less) and finally all activity becomes lower voltage and quite suppressed (Fig. 2E). Unfortunately, there is not a good correlation between the degree of slowing present on the encephalogram and the level of consciousness of any single patient. And, indeed, these changes may occur transiently in some individuals without impairment of consciousness or neurological function in response to changes such as mild hypoglycemia or hypocalcemia (Fig. 3). The reactivity or change in the EEG in response to auditory or somatosensory stimulation should be assessed. A lighter stage of coma and usually a better prognosis is associated with changes in the EEG in response to stimulation. Two further electrographic stages are seen as the patient's level of consciousness and neurological function are further depressed. The next, called suppression burst (Fig. 4), is characterized by the intermittent appearance of high voltage slow waves and/or

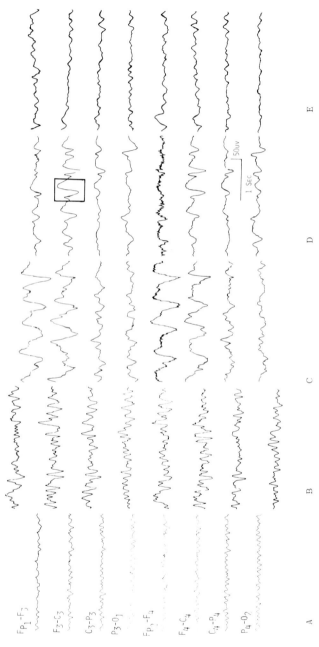

FIG. 2. The progressive change in the EEG occurs with encephalopathies. A. Normal waking EEG. B. The background alpha becomes somewhat slower and there is an interspersed activity in the theta range noted. C. Alpha frequencies are lost and progressively higher voltage slow activity in the delta range develops. D. Triphasic waves may appear which consist of a repetitive waveform having three phases which appear over both hemispheres and most prominent in the frontal regions. (Example in box.) E. In deeper stages of coma the EEG becomes lower voltage and the frequencies become progressively slower.

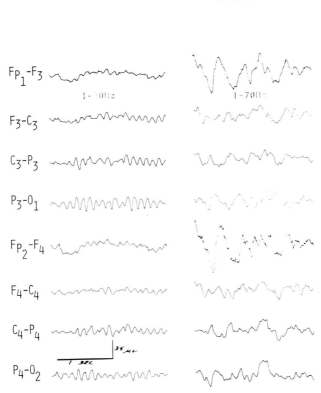

FIG. 3. Transient changes may occur in the electroencephalogram with acute changes in metabolic states such as hypoglycemia or with hyperventilation as shown here.

spikes. Between these periodic bursts, the background activity is extremely low voltage and essentially flat. Severe anoxia is the most frequent etiology of this pattern. The next stage would be complete absence of all electrocerebral activity (ECS). The suppression burst and ECS records carry extremely grave prognosis with two prominent exceptions — severe hypothermia and drug overdose. Serial recordings can provide important information as to prognosis and about the direction of the encephalopathy.

Diffuse and fairly pronounced slowing of the EEG is also seen in the postictal state but is a functional rather than an

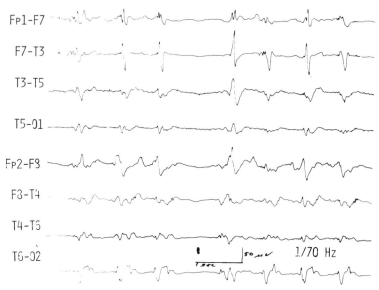

FIG. 4. Suppression-burst pattern: On a background of low voltage essentially flat activity, bursts of moderate to high voltage complexes occur which consist of spike, sharp wave and/or slow wave components. The interval between the complexes typically varies from 1 to 5 seconds. The activity may be asymmetrical over the two hemispheres as in this example. The complexes have a fairly constant morphological appearance. This is from a 49-year-old white man following a cardiac arrest and prolonged cerebral anoxia.

anatomic or toxic depression of the central nervous system. Following a grand mal seizure, the EEG findings may be similar to that of a patient who is in coma at which time the patient may not be moving spontaneously or even in response to painful stimuli. As the patient's level of consciousness gradually improves, the frequency of the EEG pattern increases back toward a normal pattern. Clinical seizures may not be apparent if the patient has received a curarizing agent or high doses of anticonvulsants. The only clue of continued seizure activity could be barely noticeable intermittent twitching of a limb, eye deviation or nystagmus and should be carefully looked for. Continued impairment of consciousness may be a result of frequent or continuous seizure activity (status epilepticus).

Status is defined as "a condition characterized by an epileptic seizure which is so prolonged or so *frequently repeated*

as to create a fixed and lasting epileptic condition." This means
that the EEG may show continued seizure activity (Fig. 5) or
the intermittent buildup and development of an epileptic
discharge following which there may be brief periods during
which the background activity is quite low voltage and slow
(Fig. 6). The recordings remain this way until the next epileptic
discharge develops. If the patient is having fairly frequent
seizures but not status, there should be change and improvement of the EEG after the seizure discharge has ceased. The
background changes from the low voltage essentially flat into a
progressively higher voltage delta activity. Progressive faster
frequency is recorded with the changes occurring over one to
several hours. This change may be the only clue that the patient
may have had a seizure if the ictal (epileptic) discharge was not
recorded.

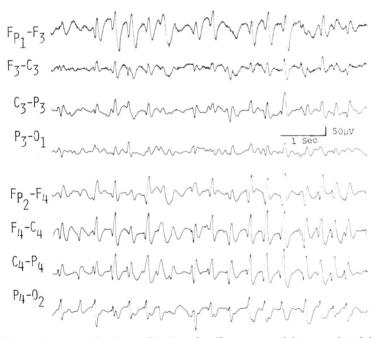

FIG. 5. Status epilepticus: Continued spike wave activity seen involving
predominantly the right hemispheric leads. This was recorded from a
patient who was comatose with continued clonic activity involving the left
hand and face.

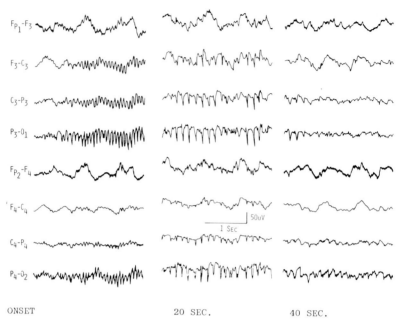

ONSET   20 SEC.   40 SEC.

FIG. 6. Status epilepticus: The frequent occurrence of seizures without recovery between the seizures is also considered status epilepticus. The buildup of bilateral predominantly posterior multiple spikes which gradually slowed and finally terminated after 40 seconds is depicted. This was recorded from a patient with a history of idiopathic epilepsy who presented having frequent generalized tonic seizures. Between the seizures she remained in coma.

There are a number of specific electrographic patterns which have been described in comatose patients. Chatrian [1] described a pattern resembling wakefulness in a patient with a brainstem infarction and clinically having a "locked-in syndrome." This has been described a number of times since then and the EEG in all respects appears to be normal. One of the characteristics of a waking EEG is that the rhythmic sinusoidal alpha activity would block when stimuli is presented to the patient and particularly when the eyes are opened. This characteristic is maintained in the patient with locked-in syndrome; however, somatosensory stimuli may not be relayed to the cortex and would not therefore produce this alerting response. In this case, only opening the eyes would produce the change. The finding of a normal EEG in these patients indicates that the patient has not sustained significant hemispheric injury and probably retains relatively normal, if not normal, higher cortical function. A second type of alpha coma pattern has been described in which the EEG has a rhythmic alpha which is similar to what is seen in a normal patient. The difference is that it occurs diffusely or in some patients more prominent in the frontal areas of the head (Fig. 7). In this case it is totally unresponsive to peripheral stimuli or opening and closing the eyes. This has been described following significant hypoxic or anoxic episodes and with drug overdose [2-6]. When resulting from hypoxia, this pattern has been associated pathologically with diffuse necrosis involving the deeper lamina of cortex. One clue that the pattern may be the result of drug intoxication (e.g., barbiturates, benzodiazepines) would be the appearance of activity in the beta frequency range (greater than 13 Hz) [6]. The frequency of the β-activity would be slower (10-16 Hz) than seen in the waking patient (20 to 25 Hz) taking these same drugs. Chatrian [7] also described a pattern resembling stage 2 sleep following head trauma. This group of patients had a better

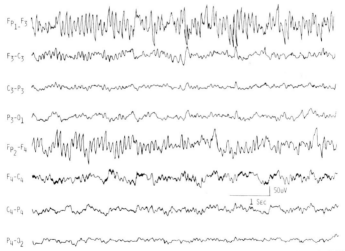

FIG. 7. Alpha coma: This pattern is most commonly a result of diffuse cerebral hypoxia but also may be seen with drug overdose. The pattern consists of a rhythmic, relatively normal-appearing alpha activity. In alpha coma, however, it is seen over all head regions or, as shown here, most prominent in the frontal portions of the head and is unresponsive to external stimuli such as opening the eyes or painful cutaneous stimuli.

prognosis which has been substantiated more recently by Naquet [8]. This pattern differs from normal sleep (Fig. 1) in that the sleep spindles occurred somewhat more frequently, are seen over all head regions, and the other stages of sleep are not clearly seen. In the initial series by Chatrian, all the patients reported "had a favorable outcome."

The determination of brain death has become increasingly important. Although there is still considerable variation between state laws governing this, the medical community has adopted a fairly uniform criteria [9-12]. The criteria for brain death are:

1. Cerebral unresponsivity: This is the state in which the patient does not respond purposefully to an externally applied stimuli, obeys no command and produces no verbal response, either spontaneously or reflexly. This is to be differentiated from spinal reflexes which may persist after all function of the cerebral hemispheres and brainstem has ceased.

2. Absence of spontaneous respirations: Assisted respiration must be stopped for a minute or more to insure adequate CO_2 buildup. Hypercapnea is a strong respiratory stimulant.

3. Absence of brainstem reflexes: This includes pupillary, corneal, oculocephalic, cileospinal, snout, swallow, pharyngeal and vestibuloocular reflexes (calorics).

4. Electrocerebral silence.

5. The absence of any potentially reversible causes of CNS depression:

     a. Hypothermia — T < 90 C

     b. Drug intoxication

     c. Severe metabolic disturbance

6. Confirmatory tests: The absence of cerebral blood flow as defined by arteriography or brain scan.

Drug intoxication and marked hypothermia have been reported to produce an isoelectric EEG and a reversible coma. A temperature of 28 C is necessary to produce a suppression burst or flat EEG which is much lower than the lower limit accepted for ECS determination (32 C). Overdose with drugs of the sedative hypnotic type (phenobarbital, doradin) has also been described as producing an isoelectric EEG with ultimate normal recovery. The quantity of drug which would be considered "significant" has not been properly addressed. The reported cases had blood levels that were well above the accepted therapeutic range. The various articles and the accepted criteria do not specifically indicate what quantity of drugs in the system would be significant. If the blood level of a drug was below the lower limits of the therapeutic range, it is unlikely that the drug could cause a significant depression and alteration in EEG. Metabolic intoxications have been reported to produce electrocerebral silence; however, there has not yet been a report of a recovery in any of these patients who otherwise meet the criteria. Again, it is difficult to assess the influence that a mild metabolic disturbance may have on the EEG of a patient with another cause for the coma. The British criteria include a statement that "metabolic and endocrine disturbances which can be responsible for or which can contribute to coma should have been excluded" [9]. This is further explained that "there should be no *profound* abnormalities of serum electrolytes, acid base balance, or blood glucose." There are obviously other metabolic disturbances which could produce alterations in central nervous system function but they are not specifically included or excluded. There is one case of hepatic coma which produced electrocerebral silence; however, this patient died 48 hours after the tracing was obtained. The question is still open as to how much of a metabolic disturbance should be considered as significant.

The American EEG Society has accepted a list of criteria for the definition and determination of electrocerebral silence. This is defined as "no electrocerebral activity over 2 μV when recorded from scalp or referential electrode pairs, 10 or more centimeters apart with inter-electrode resistances under 10,000 ohms but over 100 ohms." There are a number of other technological recommendations outlined and a copy of the guidelines can be obtained from the American EEG Society.*

Continuous EEG monitoring has now become quite feasible. Many of the intensive care unit's monitoring systems are computer-based, which will lend itself to a new method of continuously recording either the spontaneous electrocerebral activity (the EEG) [13] or activity which is produced in response to a sensory stimuli (evoked response). The spon-

---

*Executive Offices, 38238 Glenn Avenue, Willoughby, Ohio 44094.

taneous activity recorded from scalp electrodes consists of fluctuating rhythms of various frequencies. The relative quantity or "power" present in each of the frequency bands can be mathematically determined continuously by a computer and can be displayed as a series of overload graphs (Fig. 8). Figure 8 depicts the changes in the power spectrum of a patient before, six, and 24 hours after receiving a drug. In the segment before and at 24 hours after, there is a very prominent peak of activity at about 10 Hz which represents the normal resting alpha frequencies. This was markedly attenuated in the recording obtained at six hours and was replaced by much slower frequencies. This technique allows a very quick survey of a long period of time and allows individuals who have not had extensive training in electroencephalographic interpretation to detect changes which are occurring. The EEG can be continuously displayed by this technique with 24 hours of recording displayed on one or two sheets of paper. The major limitation of this technique is technical. Artifacts may not be detected as

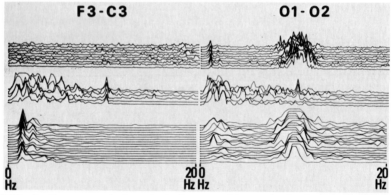

FIG. 8. Power spectral analysis is a graphic method of displaying the relative amount of various frequencies in an EEG. The higher the peak on the graph, the greater the quantity or power which is present in the frequency band which is plotted on the Y-axis. The graph displays the power spectral densities from the frontal ($F_3 - C_3$) and the occipital ($O_1 - O_2$) electrodes on a patient before (bottom portion of graph), then 6 hours (middle portion of graph) and 24 hours (top portion of graph) after ingestion of a drug. A prominent peak can be seen from the occipital leads prior to and 24 hours after the drug is given which represents the "alpha activity." The absence of this activity in the middle portion of the graph is easy to discern.

such by the computer and included in the spectral analysis producing apparent changes in the patient's condition.

Status Epilepticus

Following insults to the central nervous system, seizures and status epilepticus may result. Status epilepticus is clinically defined as either the continued occurrence of major motor seizures or frequent major motor seizures without improvement of the patient's level of consciousness in the interval between the seizures. The administration of drugs may alter the clinical manifestation and in some cases may completely inhibit the clinical expression. It must always be borne in mind that one potential reason for lack of improvement may be the occurrence of status epilepticus. Experimental studies have shown that cerebral metabolism increases three to five times during convulsion and the brain's need for oxygen and other metabolic substrates rises dramatically. Lactic acidosis from the excessive muscle activity and apnea is likely to occur and induce cerebral hypoxia. Permanent central nervous system injury can occur as a result of prolonged status. Mortality has been reported to range from 15% to 20%. The incidence of permanent neurologic deficit increases proportional to the duration of the status epilepticus. This, indeed, is a neurological emergency and should be treated as such.

Adequate respiration must be maintained (with early intubation, if necessary). Frequent arterial blood gases are imperative and O_2 must be administered at sufficient rate to prevent hypoxia. There should be sufficient padding to protect the patient from bodily harm. Careful monitoring of vital signs is important; hyperthermia and hypotension should be watched for and treated. While treatment to stop the seizure is underway, metabolic causes for status epilepticus (water intoxication, nonketotic hyperosmolar syndromes, hypoglycemia, hypocalcemia, hypomagnesemia, uremia, hepatic failure, hypoxia) should be ruled out.

The benzodiazepines have been shown to be one of the most potent classes of drugs in the treatment of status epilepticus. Like most anticonvulsant agents, these are less effective in acute cerebral disorders than in chronic ones.

Valium should be considered a first-order drug to be used immediately. The recommended dose is 10 mg IV over one to two minutes. If seizures do not stop, another 10 mg IV can be given in five minutes. Valium is not a good long-term anticonvulsant and a second drug (phenytoin) should be given even if Valium stops the seizure. Higher doses are not recommended, since CNS depression may result from the drug.

Complications of intravenous Valium. Respiratory depression and arrest have been described, particularly when administering frequent high doses or when it is used in conjunction with barbiturates. In addition, pharyngeal obstruction may occur as a result of muscular relaxation induced by the drug. Hypotension occurs very infrequently.

Intravenous phenytoin (Dilantin) is the drug of choice. If administered appropriately, phenytoin will stop a significant number of seizures and maintain control without deepening the coma of an already lethargic or unconscious patient. A dose of 1000 mg of intravenous Dilantin given at the rate of 50 mg/min will give an effective Dilantin brain level in 15 to 20 minutes in most cases. The drug should be given directly into the vein or into the intravenous tubing or can be diluted in saline, but not in glucose solutions, since it has been shown to precipitate in this mixture. A second dose of 500 to 1000 mg may be necessary if seizures continue 20 minutes after the first infusion has been completed.

Complications of intravenous Dilantin. The intravenous toxicity depends primarily upon the rate of administration. Vital signs should be monitored during the intravenous injection since cardiac arrhythmias, cardiac arrest, hypotension and apnea can occur. Hypotension and arrhythmias occur most frequently after the mid-40s. These are rate-related effects and may be treated by slowing the infusion. Patients with renal or hepatic failure may need a lower maintenance dosage of Dilantin, but the above regimen can be used to achieve adequate blood levels acutely. When toxic levels are attained, vestibulo-ocular and oculocephalic reflexes may be blocked (pupillary reflex remains normal) and may limit our assessment of a comatose patient.

Paraldehyde may be used in status epilepticus. The usual dose is 5 to 10 ml IV followed by a slow intravenous drip of 10 ml paraldehyde in 100 ml 5% Ringer's or isotonic saline. Rapid absorption occurs from the GI tract and the drug can be given per NG or per rectum. Pulmonary edema and vascular collapse may follow rapid or excessive administration.

If status persists despite adequate therapy with both intravenous Dilantin and Valium, general anesthesia via an intravenous drip of a barbiturate should be employed (short acting — sodium pentothal; long lasting — phenobarbital). These drugs should be administered only when the patient is in either the surgical or medical intensive care unit where respiratory care and vital signs can be adequately managed. The EEG should be monitored continuously (or intermittently but frequently). With higher doses of drugs, clinical manifestations of seizures may be absent while electrical seizure activity continues. Sufficient drugs should be given to stop continuous generalized electrical seizure activity.

Pentothal — 25 to 100 mg slow IV push — then 1000 mg in 500 mg Ringer's and infuse at a rate of 1 ml/min — may need up to 2 gm per day.

Phenobarbital — 1000 mg IV (50 mg/min) — then 100 mg every one to two hours. May need up to 3 gm per day.

Treatment may need to be continued for one to three days (occasionally longer) depending upon the clinical and/or EEG response.

Adjunctive Therapy

Muscle paralysis. The intravenous injection of 5 to 10 mg of d-tubocurarine chloride produces rapid muscular relaxation. This drug does not cross the blood-brain barrier very rapidly and a significant central nervous system effect probably does not occur, although the drug has been known to decrease electrocortical activity in some experimental animals. One cause of cerebral anoxia during status epilepticus is systemic anoxia induced by apnea. Paralysis is indicated if clinical seizure activity impairs adequate respiration and/or produces lactic acidosis. In this event, continuous EEG monitoring is imperative, since the clinical expression of seizure will be prevented.

Steroids. One hundred milligrams of methylprednisolone followed by 4 mg Decadron every six hours. This reduces the edema that may be associated with status. The origin of the edema is not well established and in some cases may precede the onset of the seizures.

Depressed consciousness, but not necessarily coma, may also be a result of focal, complex partial or absence status. Focal seizure activity beginning in the temporal-parietal area of the dominant hemisphere (involving Wernicke's area) may result in a functional disruption of that area of the cortex. The patient would present as a Wernicke's aphasia with total inability to comprehend any language [14]. If this is the result of an acute seizure, the symptoms would resolve over a matter of minutes to hours. I have seen this in three patients, two of whom had an electrographic finding of periodic lateralizing epileptiform discharges (PLEDS) (Fig. 9). Most patients will have a clinical seizure in association with this pattern, but the PLEDS may persist for one to two weeks without additional manifestations of seizures. However, while the EEG pattern persists, the patient may continue to manifest the aphasia. Mental dullness has been described with focal frontal lobe discharges [15]. When complex partial (temporal lobe) status or petit mal status

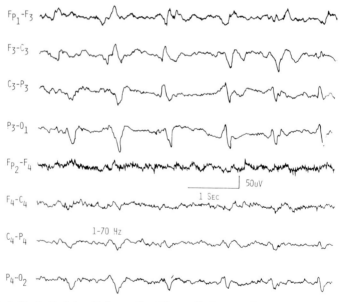

FIG. 9. Periodic lateralizing epileptiform discharges (PLEDS): This pattern consists of a lateralized periodic complex with a relatively constant morphology. The complex consists of a spike and/or sharp wave component which occurs at approximately 1 sec intervals.

occurs, prolonged behavioral disturbances and impairment of consciousness frequently result [16-21]. The behavioral disturbance may be such as to suggest a psychiatric illness. Coma is unusual in absence and complex partial status but marked depression of consciousness may result. An EEG is the only method of diagnosing these states. Generalized spike and multiple spike wave is seen in absence status. The finding in complex partial status is variable and not well agreed upon. The EEG may show diffuse slowing with additional focal abnormalities in the frontal and/or temporal areas. The focal appearance or buildup of multiple spikes or sharp slow wave activity would be indicative of an epileptic phenomenon. The changes, however, may be only the buildup of rhythmic activity without expected spike or sharp wave activity. In absence of typical epileptiform waveforms, a changing activity in one area may be the only clue that complex partial status exists. The treatment of these three types of status have some urgency but do not have the emergent nature of grand mal status.

There are six major or primary anticonvulsant drugs with which to be thoroughly familiar. The proper use of these drugs, either singly or in combination, will result in good to complete seizure control in 50% to 70% of all patients with recurrent seizures. If one is thoroughly familiar with all the drugs available, seizure control can perhaps be increased by 20% to 30%. Experience over the years indicates that in difficult cases combinations of both major and minor drugs have proven no better and in many situations not as efficacious as combinations of the major drugs.

Combinations of phenytoin (PHT), primidone (PRM), phenobarbital (PB) and carbamazepine (CBZ) are most effective in grand mal, simple partial and complex partial (psychomotor) seizures. In petit mal attacks, ethosuximide and valproic acid are the drugs of choice because of high efficiency and few side effects. Trimethadione may be equally as effective, but often carries with it troublesome side effects.

1. Phenytoin (PHT) is readily, although slowly, absorbed from the intestinal tract reaching peak plasma levels after 8 to 12 hours following a single daily dose. The plasma half-life of the drug is 20 to 24 hours, being somewhat shorter in the newborn and in early childhood. PHT distributes to all body

tissues and in the blood is approximately 90% to 95% bound to serum albumin. Rapid entry into the brain occurs with cortex concentrations reaching one and one-half to two times those in the plasma 30 minutes following an intravenous loading dose. Drug interactions are not uncommon. Valproate reduces the binding of PHT and lowers the blood level while isoniazid, disulfiram (Antabuse) and coumarin are known to interfere with metabolism resulting in toxicity in some cases. Clinical efficacy appears to correlate with plasma levels ranging from 10 to 20 μg/ml, and increasing dosage above the upper level usually does not result in enhanced seizure control. Symptoms of toxicity frequently are seen when levels exceed 25 to 30 μg/ml and are sometimes seen with levels below 20 μg/ml. Drug toxicity mainfests itself by lethargy, somnolence, cerebellar dysfunction, mental confusion, coma and rarely convulsions.

The drug is well tolerated by most patients in single daily doses of 4 to 8 mg/kg. Initiation of therapy can be done by loading the patient with a dose of 10 to 13 mg/kg (IV at 50 mg/min or PO over 12 hours in three doses). Intramuscular phenytoin tends to crystallize in the muscle and is therefore poorly absorbed. The drug is slowly absorbed over about a week so the usual oral or intravenous dosage will not produce an adequate or stable blood level when given IM. Intravenous administration is preferred if parenteral dosing is required. However, if intramuscular dosing is the only available route, then more rapid absorption can be obtained by dividing each of the injections and putting each into a different intramuscular site.

2. Phenobarbital (PB) is most commonly used in combination with anticonvulsants in the treatment of partial seizures and generalized convulsive seizures. PB is still considered the drug of choice in treating or preventing febrile convulsions and some physicians use it as the drug of choice in status. It is completely absorbed from the gastrointestinal tract, reaching peak plasma levels after four to seven hours. The half-life ranges from four to seven days. Brain accumulation of PB occurs somewhat slower than in the case of PHT. However, intravenous doses of 300 to 600 mg given slowly (50 mg/min) can rapidly modify clinical and EEG seizure activity without depressing respiration. Urinary excretion can be enhanced to tenfold by

alkalinization with intravenous sodium bicarbonate. This serves as the basis for treatment of barbiturate intoxication. The therapeutic effectiveness of PB when administered chronically to the ambulatory epileptic patient is limited by its principal toxic symptom of somnolence and slowed mentation. Chronic dosage of 1.0 to 3 mg/kg daily generally produces therapeutic plasma levels. Therapeutic levels range from 20 to 50 μg/ml with significant somnolence occurring when plasma levels exceed 50 μg/ml. Toxic signs are progressively those of inebriation, somnolence, cerebellar dysfunction and coma. Because of the long half-life, the drug is ideally suited for single daily dosing.

Intravenous PB is quite safe; however, respiratory depression or arrest may occur particularly in patients receiving diazepam. With high doses, hypotension may result, so vital signs must be monitored during and after infusion. There are few untoward reactions to chronic PB administration. The half-life of PB is such that withdrawal convulsions do not usually occur as is the case after withdrawal of rapid-acting barbiturates administered chronically.

3. Primidone (PRM) is an effective anticonvulsant agent for the treatment of complex partial seizures (psychomotor seizures). PRM should not usually be combined with PB. PRM absorption from the gastrointestinal tract is rapid with peak levels occurring one to four hours following a single dose. The half-life ranges from 6 to 12 hours. Initially, PRM is metabolized in the liver to phenyl ethyl malonamide (PEMA) and both PRM and PEMA are excreted in the urine. After several days, PB appears as a metabolite of PRM and ultimately accounts for approximately 15% to 20% of the ingested PRM. PRM and both metabolites, PEMA and PB, possess anticonvulsant activity and clinical and experimental testing indicates that greater efficacy is seen with PRM than with PB when used as a single anticonvulsant agent. Therapeutic plasma levels are thought to range between 7 and 15 μg/ml; however, the rapid absorption and half-life of PRM may make blood levels difficult to interpret. Perhaps a better indication would be assessing PB levels in patients on PRM.

When initiating PRM therapy, low dose levels should be started and gradually brought to the maintenance dose over a

10- to 20-day period. Patients often report strange initial subjective reactions to the drug as well as nausea, vomiting and gastrointestinal upset. Frequently these reactions can be avoided by premedicating the patient with PB for a week prior to starting PRM.

4. Carbamazepine (Tegretol) has recently been approved in the United States for the treatment of seizure disorders. Prior to this, it has been used successfully for the treatment of trigeminal and glossopharyngeal neuralgia. Structurally, it is a tricyclic compound similar to the tricyclic antidepressants. However, when one views the drug in a three-dimensional planar configuration and compares it to PHT, similarities exist. Carbamazepine's anticonvulsant activity is similar to that of DPH, PB and primidone in that best therapeutic results are obtained in generalized convulsive seizures, complex and simple focal seizures (more effective in complex partial seizures than in other types). This compound is a major anticonvulsant drug and not merely a supplemental medication.

Carbamazepine, when dosed chronically, is fairly rapidly absorbed from the GI tract reaching peak levels after two to four hours. The half-life of the drug after chronic administration is shorter (eight to ten hours) than after initiation of therapy, suggesting autoinduction of liver microsomal enzymes. Patients receiving carbamazepine in combination with other anticonvulsants have lower plasma levels than patients receiving comparable doses of only carbamazepine. This suggests drug interaction and enzyme induction but the effect is usually not of clinical significance.

Adverse reactions to carbamazepine therapy include aplastic anemia, leukopenia, agranulocytosis and thrombocytopenia. However, these responses are fortunately rare. One should obtain a routine blood check after initiation of therapy. Drug toxicity generally correlates with plasma levels over 10 $\mu g/ml$. Clinical signs are similar to those of other anticonvulsant drugs. Initiation of therapy should be begun slowly since many patients experience adverse reactions if started at a full calculated daily dose. The half-life of the drug is such that bi-daily dosing should be adequate to maintain stable levels. Daily dosing in the range of 10 to 20 mg/kg generally results in therapeutic plasma levels of 4 to 10 $\mu g/ml$.

5. Ethosuximide is one drug of choice in the treatment of absence (petit mal) seizures. It is ineffective in the treatment of other seizure types.

Ethosuximide is readily absorbed from the gastrointestinal tract with peak plasma levels occurring after three to four hours. With constant daily dosing, steady state plasma levels are achieved in 5 to 25 days since the plasma half-life is 50 to 60 hours in the adult and 30 to 40 hours in the child. The drug is suitable for single daily dosing; however, some patients experience nausea and gastrointestinal upset with such a regimen. The usual daily dose is 15 to 35 mg/kg. Effective seizure control is usually attained with plasma levels of 40 to 100 μg/ml. However, some patients have only obtained excellent control after plasma levels of 120 and 150 μg/ml have been reached. Ethosuximide apparently does not interact significantly with other drugs and metabolism remains constant.

Toxic reactions are unusual, even with plasma levels being maintained in the 130 to 170 μg/ml range. Minor depressions of the WBC have been observed but not enough to warrant stopping the drug. The most common side effect is nausea and vomiting. Most patients with petit mal seizures respond to ethosuximide; however, a 100% seizure control is probably not affected in over 60% of patients.

6. Valproic acid (Depakene). This drug may represent the most significant advancement in therapy since the introduction of phenytoin. It is a simple organic acid in contrast to the complex ring chemical structure of other anticonvulsant drugs. Initial studies indicate that valproic acid blocks seizure activity in the brain by altering synaptic effect of an inhibitory transmitter (GABA). The drug is very effective in absence seizures (petit mal) and myoclonus. It is effective particularly as an adjunct in the treatment of generalized tonic clonic seizures and is effective in 30% of patients with simple and complex partial seizures. The drug is rapidly absorbed from the gastrointestinal tract with peak levels occurring in 30 to 60 minutes. The half-life of the drug with chronic administration averages eight hours and necessitates three times daily dosing.

The most common side effects are nausea and vomiting. Somnolence may occur early but clears spontaneously. The drug is highly (90% to 95%) protein bound and requires high daily doses, thus interactions with other drugs can be expected. Concomitant use with phenobarbital results in elevation of phenobarbital levels and potentiation of side effects and this interaction should be anticipated. Interaction also occurs with phenytoin because of displacement from protein-binding sites, making phenytoin more readily available for metabolism. Phenytoin plasma levels initially fall, but may later return to pre-valproic acid levels because of competition for oxidative metabolism. The toxic effects are mild and appear to be dose-related. Elevation of liver enzymes and a chemical hepatitis are the most significant side effects. This has occurred only with very high doses and usually when the patient is concurrently taking other anticonvulsant drugs. Other side effects such as fine tremor, transient alopecia and weight gain are fairly specific for valproic acid. In higher doses, somnolence and unsteady gait may also be seen.

References

1. Chatrian, G.E., White, L.E. and Shaw, C-M: EEG pattern resembling wakefulness in unresponsive decerebrate state following traumatic brain-stem infarct. Electroencephalogr. Clin. Neurophysiol. 16:285-289, 1964.
2. Westmoreland, B.F., Klass, D.W., Sharbrough, F.W. et al: Alpha-coma: Electroencephalographic, clinical, pathologic, and etiologic correlations. Arch. Neurol. 32:713-718, 1975.
3. Alving, J., Moller, M., Sindrup, E. et al: "Alpha pattern coma" following cerebral anoxia. Electroencephalogr. Clin. Neurophysiol. 47:95-101, 1979.
4. Vignaendra, V., Wilkus, R.J., Copass, K. et al: Electroencephalographic rhythms of alpha frequency in comatose patients after cardiopulmonary arrest. Neurology 24:582-588, 1974.
5. Grindal, A.B., Suter, C. and Martinez, A.J.: Alpha-pattern coma: 24 cases with 9 survivors. Ann. Neurol. 1:371-377, 1977.
6. Carroll, W.M. and Mastaglia, F.L.: Alpha and beta coma in drug intoxication uncomplicated by cerebral hypoxia. Electroencephalogr. Clin. Neurophysiol. 46:95-105, 1979.
7. Chatrian, G.E., White, L.E. and Daly, D.: Electroencephalographic patterns resembling those of sleep in certain comatose states after injuries to the head. Electroencephalogr. Clin. Neurophysiol. 15:272-280, 1963.
8. Naquet, R., Vigouroux, R.P., Choux, M. et al: Etude électroencéphalographique des traumatismes crâniens récents dans un service de réanimation. Rev. Neurol. 117:512-513, 1967.
9. No author given: Diagnosis of brain death. Lancet 2:1069-1070, 1976.

10. Black, P.M.: Brain death. N. Engl. J. Med. 299:338-344 and 393-410, 1978.
11. Curran, W.J.: The brain-death concept: Judicial acceptance in Massachusetts. N. Engl. J. Med. 298:1008-1009, 1978.
12. No author given: Diagnosis of death. Br. Med. J. 1:332, 1979.
13. Bricolo, A., Turazzi, S., Faccioli, F. et al: Clinical application of compressed spectral array in long-term EEG monitoring of comatose patients. Electroencephalogr. Clin. Neurophysiol. 45:211-225, 1978.
14. Hamilton, N.G. and Matthews, T.: Aphasia: The sole manifestation of focal status epilepticus. Neurology 29:745-748, 1979.
15. Kugoh, T. and Hosokawa, K.: Mental dullness associated with left frontal continuous focal discharge. Folia Psychiatr. Neurol. Jpn. 31:473-480, 1977.
16. Markand, O.N., Wheeler, G.L. and Pollack, S.L.: Complex partial status epilepticus (psychomotor status). Neurology 28:189-196, 1978.
17. Obrecht, R., Okhomina, F.O.A. and Scott, D.F.: Value of EEG in acute confusional states. J. Neurol. Neurosurg. Psychiatry 42:75-77, 1979.
18. Mayeux, R. and Leuders, H.: Complex partial status epilepticus: Case report and proposal for diagnostic criteria. Neurology 28:957-961, 1978.
19. Engel, J., Ludwig, B.I. and Fetell, M.: Prolonged partial complex status epilepticus: EEG and behavioral observations. Neurology 28:863-869, 1978.
20. Geier, S.: Prolonged psychic epileptic seizures: A study of the absence status. Epilepsia 19:431-445, 1978.
21. Murasaki, M.: Psychomotor status: Case reports and proposal for classification. Folia Psychiatr. Neurol. Jpn. 33:353-357, 1979.

Self-Evaluation Quiz

1. An isoelectric (e.g., flat) EEG:
   a) Must be recorded twice to meet the requirement for determination of brain death
   b) May result from a body temperature of 37 C
   c) May be reversible if resulting from Doriden overdose
   d) Is not needed for the determination of brain death
2. Status epilepticus:
   a) Should be treated with high dose IM phenytoin
   b) May result from metabolic disturbances (e.g., electrolyte imbalance) and should be searched for
   c) Always is evident clinically so an EEG is not necessary for diagnosis
   d) Is self-limited; most patients survive without therapeutic intervention

3. Alpha coma:
   a) Has an excellent prognosis
   b) Infrequently results from anoxia
   c) Is frequently associated with diffuse laminar necrosis of the cortex
   d) Cannot be a result of drug intoxication
4. Complication of Depakene (valproic acid) is (are):
   a) Peripheral neuropathy
   b) Vascular collapse
   c) Hypotension and arrhythmias
   d) Hepatitis
5. Valium (diazepam):
   a) May result in respiratory arrest when given IV
   b) Is *not* a drug of choice in status epilepticus
   c) Is a good long-term anticonvulsant
   d) The standard dose in 20 mg IV given in a rapid bolus
6. Criteria for brain death include all but which of the following:
   a) Cerebral unresponsivity
   b) Absent spinal reflexes
   c) Absent brainstem reflexes
   d) Flat EEG
   e) Absence of hypothermia or drug overdose

Matching

 7. Phenytoin ___
 8. Diazepam ___
 9. Valproic Acid ___
10. Phenobarbital ___
11. Primidone ___

a) Metabolized to phenobarbital
b) Alkalinization increases urinary excretion
c) First drug of choice in status
d) Drug of choice in petit mal seizures
e) Hypotension may occur with IV administration

Answers on page 391.

Evoked Responses: Use in a Neurological Intensive Care Unit

Takashi Tsubokawa, M.D., M.D.Sc.,
and R. Eugene Ramsay, M.D.

Objectives

To discuss the clinical significance of both the auditory brainstem evoked response and the spinal cord evoked response in the monitoring of neurologically compromised ICU patients. Recording methods are described.

Since the reports by Jewett [1] and others, the use of evoked responses in the evaluation of the patient with a neurological disorder has expanded tremendously. The recording of a stimulus-related response is dependent upon two facts. One, the sensory pathways are well defined and once a neuronal response is initiated, conduction of the impulse along the pathway produces a well-defined series of potential changes. Two, the background electrical activity recorded from the brain is random. The recorded electrical activity evoked by the stimulus may be 1/20 or less than that of the resting or background activity. The technique involves adding or summing together the scalp-recorded electrical activity after each stimulus is presented to the patient. The stimulus may be in the form of a flash of light, a small shock over one of the peripheral nerves, or a series of clicks presented to the ear. Since the

Takashi Tsubokawa, M.D., M.D.Sc., Associate Professor of Neurological Surgery, Nihon University School of Medicine, Tokyo, Japan and R. Eugene Ramsay, M.D., Assistant Professor of Neurology, University of Miami School of Medicine, Fla.; Director, Clinical Electrophysiology Laboratory, Miami VA Medical Center.

background activity is random, this will tend to cancel out, and only that activity which occurs as a result of and at the same time following the stimuli will add together and become accentuated.

Recently, both the auditory brainstem (BAER) and somato-sensory (SER) evoked responses have been used in addition to the classical electrophysiological monitoring techniques in the neurological ICU. They have been shown to be of value in defining the location and severity of brainstem (BAER and SER) and spinal cord injury (SER). The results in our laboratories would agree with the reports of other authors [2-5].

Auditory and somatosensory evoked responses can be recorded at the bedside using a computer-based instrument. Its components include a stimulator, input amplifier, signal processor and an X-Y recorder. The stimulator output is a square wave pulse which is put into a set of headphones producing a click or is presented to the patient through electrodes placed over one of the peripheral nerves. The stimulator may be synchronized with, but delayed from, the R-wave component of the EKG to reduce artifacts.

Brainstem Auditory Evoked Responses

Jewett et al [1, 6] describes seven vertex positive waves of the auditory evoked response occurring within 10 msec after the stimulus. The short latency auditory evoked responses are thought to be the *farfield* reflection of sequential electrical events along successive higher levels of the brainstem auditory pathway. Direct recording at each level of the acoustic pathway has shown the correlation between the specific anatomical structures and the various waveforms described. Waves I through V are generated at the acoustic nerve (I), cochlear nuclei (II), superior olive (III), lateral lamniscus (IV), and inferior colliculus (V). Waves VI and VII are thought to be generated in the subthalamic and thalamic regions, respectively, as demonstrated by observations made during stereotaxic surgery [7]. Since reports have shown a correlation between abnormalities of the BAER and posterior fossa pathology [8, 9], we have used the technique in the neurological ICU not only to localize primary brainstem lesions but also to watch for brainstem dysfunction associated with pending and completed herniation [10].

Recording Technique

Standard EEG disc electrodes are used and positioned at the vertex and either on or behind the ear. The vertex electrode is connected to G_1 of the amplifier and the ear electrode to G_2. Auditory stimulation is presented to the patient through headphones. Standard stimulus intensity is 60 to 70 db above hearing level. Decreased hearing may alter the evoked response, so in cases where the results are questionable, maximum stimulation intensities should be used. The activity from the first 10 msec poststimulus is filtered (bandpass—100 Hz to 3,000 Hz), amplified (5×10^5) and summated. Due to the variability that may occur as a result of background activity, each response must be duplicated to insure validity of the results. The number of sweeps necessary to define an evoked response depends upon the ratio of the voltages of the response to background activity and varies from 1,000 to 4,000 sweeps for the BAER. The resulting waveforms can be printed on an X-Y plotter. Monaural stimulation should be used. Classical anatomy suggests that neurons from each cochlear nucleus contribute to the ascending pathways on both sides. However, a lateralized brainstem lesion may only affect the BAER elicited from one ear.

Five positive waveforms can consistently be identified in the normal BAER (Fig. 1). Mean latency for each wave is 1.52, 2.69, 3.75, 5.00 and 5.67 msec (standard deviation for each latency is less than .2 msec). The amplitude of each wave is not always consistent between recording sessions while the ratio of amplitudes (e.g., amplitude of V divided by amplitude of wave I) is more reproducible [11]. Whereas waves II, IV, VI and VII cannot always be distinguished in each evoked response, waves I, III and V are consistently identified in almost every recording. As the sweeps are added together, wave V is the first component to become evident. When the BAER is abnormal, this may be helpful in identifying this wave.

The technique is useful in the early diagnosis of infratentorial lesions and for determining the functional state of the brainstem. This is extremely important in evaluating the patient with possible herniation or brain death. An important charac-

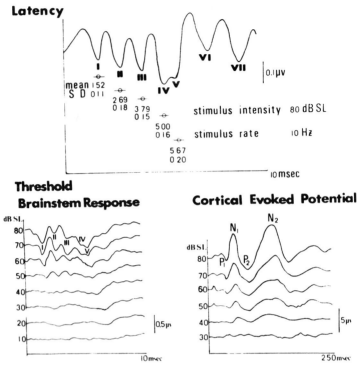

FIG. 1. Physiological characters of auditory brainstem response.

teristic of evoked responses is the relative preservation in conditions which reversibly depress the central nervous system such as marked hypothermia and deep anesthesia. Although the interpeak latencies are prolonged in these situations, the evoked response is easily obtainable demonstrating the anatomical integrity of the nervous system [12, 13]. In cases of posterior fossa pathology, the technique gives us important diagnostic clues as to damage to the brainstem. Intra- or extraparenchymal position cannot be predicted, but alteration in the BAER can be correlated with the anatomical location of invasion or compression of the brainstem defining at least the caudal extent of the dysfunction. For example, in a patient with a pontine glioma located at the caudal midbrain by CT scan, the BAER revealed waves I-II on the left and waves I-III on the right (Fig. 2). The area of involvement thus is more caudal than indicated by the CT scan. The diagnosis of extramedullary mass lesions such as

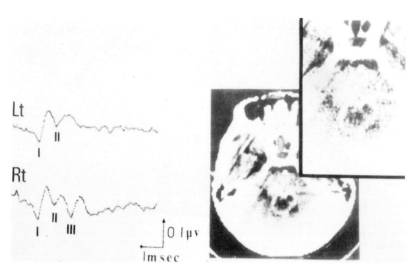

FIG. 2. Alteration of auditory brainstem responses and CT findings of pontine glioma.

acoustic neuromas may be difficult if the auditory nerve is destroyed and no evoked response is elicited. An absence response could be the result of inadequate level of stimulation (e.g., plugged external auditory canal), middle ear or cochlear disease as well as eighth nerve dysfunction. Proper recording technique and integrity of the auditory system through the eighth nerve can be assumed if at least wave I is recorded. An intraparenchymal lesion was demonstrated in the patient presenting with a left hemiparesis and left ear deafness. Normal latencies were noted for waves I and II and slightly prolonged for waves III. Wave IV-V was markedly prolonged and the amplitude was lower from stimulation of the left ear indicating involvement of the pathways in the rostral pons and midbrain region. This clearly shows that there is predominantly contralateral transmission of the evoked response to monaural stimulation at least above the level of the decasations which occur at the level of the olive.

One of the most useful applications for the recording of the BAER is in the critically ill neurosurgical patient. Sequential recordings may identify early secondary brainstem damage resulting from herniation and compression as the result of an expanding supertentorial mass. Classically, pupillary changes,

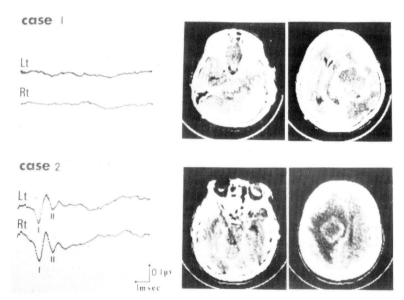

FIG. 3. Alteration of auditory brainstem responses caused by tentorial herniation. Case 1: complete herniation. Case 2: impending herniation. Note no change of such arachnoid space around the caudal midbrain in CT scan.

ocular cephalic reflexes, caloric responses and decerebrate posturing are looked for to determine if central or uncal herniation is occurring. However, all of these methods may be inadequate to demonstrate brainstem dysfunction at an early stage of herniation. Analysis of 12 cases of herniation revealed that waves VI and VII had changed early in all of the cases and was followed closely by loss of wave V. These occurred prior to the appearance of classical neurological signs or CT changes showing its utility in evaluating patients with severe head injuries [14].

Clinically, primary brainstem injury may not be detected by conventional neurological and neuroradiological examinations [15, 16]. Neuropathological studies by Crompton [17] lends support to the hypothesis that a primary brainstem injury following head trauma may not occur in exclusion to other injuries. By using both the CT scan and the BAER, primary brainstem injuries can reliably be diagnosed. The diagnostic criteria for defining a primary injury is the absence of any abnormality on CT scan with loss of components of the brainstem evoked response. We have found three cases of primary injury in 74 patients with severe head injuries. Secondary brainstem injury resulting from tentorial herniation which may be seen with acute subdural hematomas or severe contusions may be diagnosed in the early stages. Examples are shown in Figures 2 and 4 where only the first and second waves and, in one instance, wave III were preserved. In light of the anatomical origin of the waveforms, herniation in these patients resulted in loss of function of the entire midbrain and rostral and midpons. This occurred in patient 3 in the absence of any classical signs on neurological exam of herniation. This latter patient died suddenly with Cushing's phenomenon on the second day after this recording.

Results of BAERs recorded in 74 patients with severe head injury (Glasgow coma scale: less than 7) are shown in Figure 4. Thirty-three of the 74 patients had no changes in their BAER and all recovered with minimal or no neurological sequelling. Loss of all the brainstem components of the evoked response was found in 24% of the patients. Three suffered from primary and 22 from secondary brainstem injury. Seventeen of these patients died within several days after injury and eight remained in a vegetative state. Prolongation of wave V latency or

	case number	Brainstem Response		out come
		Findings	Records	
Primary Brainstem Injury	3/74	disappearance of 1st – 5th waves	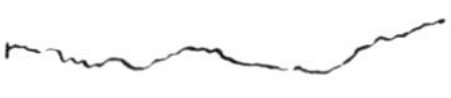	died
Secondary Brainstem Injury	14/74	prolongation of latency or disappearance of 5th wave	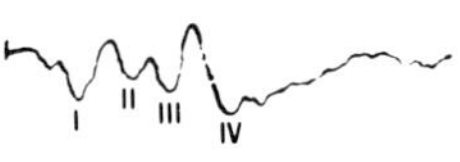	survived
	2/74	disappearance of 3rd – 5th waves	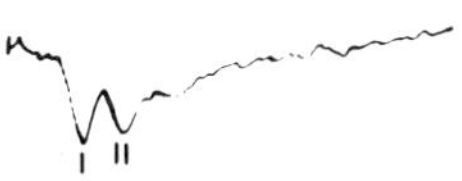	died
	22/74	disappearance of 1st – 5th waves	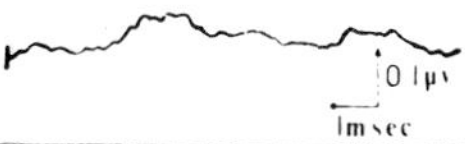	died or vegetative state

FIG. 4. Alteration of auditory brainstem response in severe head injury.

disappearance of wave V was observed in 14 cases (19%) and all recovered following treatment. Two additional patients also lost waves III and IV indicating more caudal extension of the compression and injury and these patients died several days after injury.

According to these results, alteration in BAERs not only identifies primary brainstem injury, but also is predictive of the severity of the injury and helps prognosticate the outcome.

Spinal Cord (Somatosensory) Evoked Responses

It is important to objectively determine the severity and level of injury in patients who have suffered a spinal cord injury. The H-reflex looks at the integrity of a single spinal segment. The somatosensory evoked response is recorded at the scalp and evaluates the integrity of the somatosensory system along the entire neural axis. These have been used in the past in patients with spinal cord lesions. However, the data from these techniques did not correlate well with the severity of the spinal cord injury and also could not evaluate the functioning of the descending pathways [18-21]. In contrast, recording of spinal cord evoked responses using both peripheral nerve and spinal cord stimulation allows the function of both the descending and ascending pathways to be assessed. These techniques have not been clinically utilized because of the difficulty in recording consistent responses. Recently, this difficulty has been diminished with the development and use of epidural electrodes and the refinement of a computer averaging instrumentation [22, 23]. The recording and stimulation electrodes on the spinal cord are inserted by the same technique used for epidural anesthesia. First, an 18-gauge Touhy needle is inserted into the epidural space. The active electrode which has a bare tip of 1 mm and a diameter of 0.5 mm is inserted through the Touhy needle to about 1 cm beyond the top of the needle. After the electrode has been inserted, the Touhy needle is removed. The posterior tibial nerve at the popliteal fossa or the median nerve at the wrist is stimulated through bipolar surface electrodes.

Spinal cord evoked responses are classified into two groups depending upon the relationship between the level of the spinal cord that is stimulated and the level of the spinal cord from which the recording is obtained (Fig. 5). The segmental

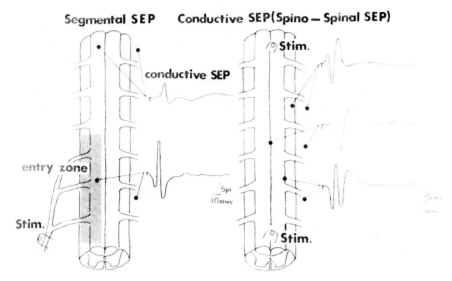

FIG. 5. The spinal cord evoked responses are divided into segmental responses and conductive responses by location of the stimulating and recording electrodes. The activity of descending pathways is tested by conductive responses (spino-spinal SEP).

response is recorded from the level at which the response enters the spinal cord while the conductive response is recorded at a distance either proximal or distal to the segment of the cord stimulated. This latter response is dependent upon the function of the descending tracts when stimulation is applied directly to the rostral portion of the spinal cord and the response is obtained in the caudal part of the cord or from the caudal aquina.

The peripheral nerve is stimulated with an 80 to a 100 volt 1 msec square wave pulse, while spinal cord stimulation necessitates only 6 to 12 volt 1 msec square wave pulse. The normal segmental response shows a positive (P1), negative (N1), positive (P2) configuration as shown in Figure 6. Normal latencies of these three components are 9.3, 11.4 and 15.6 msec, respectively. The P1 wave is a mono- or polyphasic spike potential and is thought to represent afferent volleys conducted through the dorsal root fiber. The N1 component has the highest peak potential and is followed by the slow positive P2 component which sometimes has two peaks. The descending

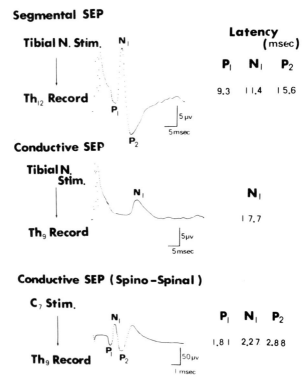

FIG. 6. The waveform and latency of each spinal cord evoked response.

conducting response has a similar configuration with the P1, N1 and P2 components. These have latencies of 1.8, 2.3 and 2.9 msec, respectively, for the stimulation and recording sites as shown but may vary as these sites are moved.

The generating mechanisms of the spinal cord evoked response is not well understood and thus the relationship between these responses and spinal cord blood flow is poorly defined. Therefore, it is difficult to correlate any change in the shape of the conducted response with pathological findings. While the disappearance of waveform clearly denotes loss of excitability of the spinal cord, the change in the amplitude of the response cannot be given any definite clinical significance at this time. In a series of 20 paraplegic or tetraplegic patients resulting from spinal cord injury, segmental and conductive responses were recorded in the acute posttraumatic state (Table

1). Fourteen patients showed a flat segmental response while a trace of low amplitude response was found in the other six. There was no difference in the neurological or neuroradiological findings in these two groups of patients. Of these 14 patients, five did not show a conductive response while the other nine showed a low amplitude conductive response. In the cases with flat, segmental and conductive responses, no improvement followed various treatments which included decompression and spinal cord cooling. Three of the cases which did not have a segmental response with preservation of low amplitude conductive response were able to walk following a similar treatment. Of the six patients with depressed amplitude of segmental response, five were able to walk following treatment and were mirrored by improvement in amplitude of their somatosensory evoked potential. These results would suggest that analysis of the SEP would aid in the identification of the patients with potentially reversible spinal cord injuries so that aggressive treatment can be given. The alteration of the spinal cord evoked response in the acute injury is useful in estimating not only the level of the injury but also for potentially predicting the

Table 1. The Alteration of Spinal Cord Evoked Responses
Following Acute Spinal Cord Injury

Pre-cooling		After Cooling	Clinical Effect		
Segmental SEP	Conductive SEP	Segmental SEP	Able To Walk	Need Help in Daily Life	No Change
	Flat 5 cases	Flat 5 cases seg. (−)	0	0	5 cases (died 1)
Flat 14 cases	Lateral (+) Dorsal (−) 6 cases	Flat 6 cases seg. (+)	0	4 cases	2 cases
	Low amplitude 3 cases	Reappear 3 cases seg. (+)	3 cases (died 1)	0	0
Trace or low amplitude 6 cases	Low amplitude 6 cases	Recover its amplitude 6 cases	5 cases	1 case	0

effectiveness of the treatment. For example, one patient presented with tetraplegia with sensory loss at the C-6,7 level (Fig. 7). Surgical x-rays showed a narrowed disc base at C-6,7 with spondylosis but without a fracture or dislocation. Head traction with Crutchfield tongs was instituted and epidural electrodes were inserted in the epidural spaces at C-2, C-4, C-5 and C-12 as illustrated. The segmental response to medial nerve stimulation was completely flat and the ascending and descending conductive response between C-7 and C-4 was also flat. A normal conductive response, however, was found between C-4 and C-2. According to these findings, it was felt that the spinal cord lesion of this patient was quite severe and that it was unlikely that the patient would recover using conventional treatment methods.

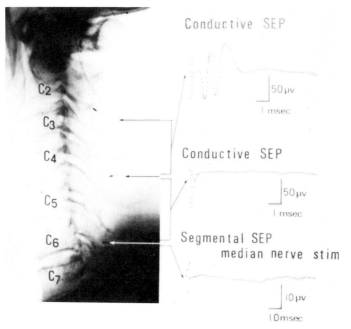

FIG. 7. Various types of spinal cord evoked response recorded in acute cervical cord injury. X-rays show no dislocation or fracture. Electrode tips are at C2-C3, C4-C5, C6-C7 epidural levels. See text.

Conclusion

The spinal cord somatosensory and the brainstem auditory evoked responses are extremely useful tools in the evaluation of the neurologically impaired patient. That technique as outlined can give objective evidence of structural lesions, even in the patient who has impaired level of consciousness. Functional loss can be demonstrated in the absence of changes on conventional neuroradiological procedures. Sequential evoked responses can be of value in prognosis since improvement or return of components of the evoked response would indicate integrity and potential recovery prior to changes on the neurological exam.

References

1. Jewett, D.L., Romano, M.N. and Williston, J.S.: Human auditory evoked potentials: Possible brainstem components detected on the scalp. Science 167:1517-1518, 1970.
2. de la Torre, J.C., Trimble, J.L., Beard, R.T. et al: Somatosensory evoked potentials for the prognosis of coma in humans. Exp. Neurol. 60:304-317, 1978.
3. Liberson, W.T.: Study of evoked potentials in aphasics. Am. J. Phys. Med. 45(3):135-142, 1966.
4. Greenberg, R.P., Mayer, D.J., Becker, D.P. and Miller, J.D.: Evaluation of brain function in severe human head trauma with multimodality evoked potentials. Part I. Evoked brain-injury potentials, methods, and analysis. J. Neurosurg. 47:150-162, 1977.
5. Greenberg, R.P., Becker, D.P., Miller, J.D. and Mayer, D.J.: Evaluation of brain function in severe human head trauma with multimodality evoked potentials. Part 2. Localization of brain dysfunction and correlation with posttraumatic neurological conditions. J. Neurosurg. 47:163-177, 1977.
6. Jewett, D.L.: Volume-conducted potentials in response to auditory stimuli as detected by averaging in the cat. Electroencephalogr. Clin. Neurophysiol. 28:609-618, 1970.
7. Tsubokawa, T., Nishimoto, H. and Moriyasu, N.: Far-field responses of acoustic brainstem potentials in thalamus and the subthalamic area. Neurol. Med. Chir. (Tokyo) 18:1-3, 1978.
8. Stockard, J.J., Stockard, J.E. and Sharbrough, F.W.: Detection and localization of occult lesions with brainstem auditory responses. Mayo Clin. Proc. 52:761-769, 1977.
9. Stockard, J.J. and Rosister, V.S.: Clinical and pathologic correlates of brainstem auditory response abnormalities. Neurology 27:316-325, 1977.

10. Tsubokawa, T.: Evaluation of brainstem damage caused by severe head injury by using far field acoustic response. Surgery 40:1163-1169, 1978 (Japanese).
11. Stockard, J.J., Stockard, J.E. and Sharbrough, F.W.: Nonpathologic factors influencing brainstem auditory evoked potentials. Am. J. EEG Technology 18:177-209, 1978.
12. Stockard, J.J., Sharbrough, F.W. and Tinker, J.A.: Effects of hypothermia on the human brainstem auditory response. Ann. Neurol. 3:368-370, 1978.
13. Stockard, J.J. and Sharbrough, F.W.: Unique contributions of short-latency auditory and somatosensory evoked potentials to neurologic diagnosis. In Desmedt, J.E. (ed.): Clinical Uses of Cerebral, Brainstem and Spinal Somatosensory Evoked Potentials. Basel:Karger, 1978.
14. Tsubokawa, T., Katayama, Y., Nishimoto, H. et al: Fatal brainstem damage caused by linear acceleration impact: Relationship between pathophysiological findings and far field acoustic response. Neurol. Med. Chir. (Tokyo) 19:287-301, 1979 (Japanese).
15. Turazzi, S., Alexandre, A. and Bricolo, A.: Incidence and significance of clinical signs of brainstem traumatic lesions. J. Neurosurg. Sci. 19:215-222, 1975.
16. Ommaya, A.K. and Gennarelli, T.A.: Cerebral concussion and traumatic unconsciousness. Brain 97:633-654, 1974.
17. Crompton, M.R.: Brainstem lesion due to closed head injury. Lancet 1:669-673, 1971.
18. Martin, S.H. and Bloedel, J.R.: Evaluation of experimental spinal cord injury using cortical evoked potentials. J. Neurosurg. 39:75-81, 1973.
19. Perot, P.L.: The clinical use of somatosensory evoked potentials in spinal cord injury. Clin. Neurosurg. 20:367-381, 1972.
20. Deecke, L. and Tator, C.H.: Neurophysiological assessment of afferent and efferent conduction in the injured spinal cord of monkeys. J. Neurosurg. 39:65-74, 1973.
21. Angelo, D., Van Gilder, J.C. and Taub, A.: Evoked cortical potentials in experimental spinal cord trauma. J. Neurosurg. 38:332-336, 1973.
22. Shimoji, K., Higashi, H. and Kano, T.: Epidural recording of spinal electrogram in man. Electroencephalogr. Clin. Neurophysiol. 30:236-239, 1971.
23. Tsubokawa, T.: The clinical significance to record spinal cord evoked responses in spinal cord injury. Clin. EEG 20:236-243, 1978 (Japanese).

Self-Evaluation Quiz

1. The normal auditory brainstem response consists of seven vertex positive waves.
   a) True
   b) False

2. The conductive response is recorded at the entry zone.
    a) True
    b) False
3. The alterations of auditory brainstem responses can identify a primary brainstem injury.
    a) True
    b) False

Answers on page 391.

Cerebral Blood Flow and Metabolism

Myron D. Ginsberg, M.D.

Objectives

1. To review certain major aspects of the normal cerebral circulation, its control and its relationship to cerebral metabolism.
2. To provide a brief description of how cerebral circulation may be affected during ischemia.
3. To indicate certain experimental approaches to the study of cerebral circulation and metabolism.

The purpose of this paper is to provide a brief, general overview of the normal cerebral circulation, along with a discussion of alterations that may occur in states of cerebral ischemia. This review is intentionally brief, since numerous exhaustive and well-referenced reviews on the subject exist in the recent literature. The reader is referred to the bibliography for detailed discussions of the points to be mentioned below.

Vascular Anatomy

The brain receives its entire blood flow from four vessels, namely, the two internal carotid arteries and the two vertebral arteries, the latter of which join to form the basilar artery. The circle of Willis provides an anastomotic connection between the carotid and basilar systems, but its degree of anatomic completeness varies considerably among individuals. Three major arteries provide blood flow to the cerebrum: the anterior, middle and posterior cerebral arteries. Anastomotic connections among the terminal portions of these vascular beds exist, but are normally small until vascular occlusion within one portion

Myron D. Ginsberg, M.D., Associate Professor of Neurology, University of Miami School of Medicine, Fla.

of the system provides the stimulus to hypertrophy of collateral circulation via these channels.

The extracranial portion of the cerebral vasculature is of particular interest to the neurologist since atherosclerosis occurs preferentially within portions of this system and serves as a major cause of stroke. Favored sites for the development of atherosclerosis include the bifurcation of the common carotid artery and the origins of the internal and external carotid arteries; the origins of the common carotid, innominate and subclavian arteries; the origins of the vertebral arteries; the initial portion of the basilar artery, etc. Atheromatous lesions may also affect the middle cerebral and other intracranial arteries at points of branching, though thrombotic occlusions at the latter sites are less common than within the extracranial vasculature.

The anatomy of the cerebral vasculature may determine the sites of preferential pathological involvement during states of diminished cerebral perfusion. Under conditions of cardiac failure or systemic hypotension, the earliest brain areas to suffer hypoperfusion are those lying between the terminal portions of the major cerebral arteries, in the "border zones" between the middle and posterior cerebral, middle and anterior cerebral, and anterior and posterior cerebral arteries. In addition, it is probable that similar border zones exist in areas lying between the terminal portions of the deep penetrating vessels to the basal ganglia and other structures. When experimental animals are subjected to profound systemic hypotension, neuropathological evidence of ischemic neuronal change is found in the cerebral border zones noted above and, on occasion, in deep cerebral structures such as the globus pallidus. Thus, the existence of deep border zone territories may in part explain the selective vulnerability of certain deep brain regions to ischemia or hypoxia.

Overall Cerebral Blood Flow and Oxygen Consumption

Although the brain constitutes only 2% of the total body weight, it receives a disproportionate amount of blood flow. Fully 15% of the body's total cardiac output perfuses the brain, providing a total blood flow of approximately 750 ml/min, or about six times the brain's blood volume. The amount of blood perfusing the brain per minute is, in fact, equivalent to fully one half of the brain's entire volume. This statistic emphasizes the extraordinary quantity of blood perfusing the brain.

The purpose of brain blood flow is to provide oxygen and glucose substrate and to remove metabolic waste products. The oxygen consumption of the brain amounts to 20% of the body's total oxygen consumption, a percentage larger than the ratio of cerebral blood flow to total cardiac output. Thus, the brain extracts a greater percentage of oxygen from each milliliter of arterial blood than does the body in general. Since the brain has no means of storing oxygen, it is dependent upon a continual supply for its metabolic needs. Glucose is the sole metabolic substrate of the brain in all but exceptional circumstances. The amount of glucose stored in the normal brain is very small. Thus, a continual supply of this substrate is needed to sustain metabolism. The aerobic metabolism of glucose results in the production of free energy in the form of adenosine triphosphate for neuronal membrane processes including neurotransmitter synthesis and ion transport, as well as for biosynthesis of other molecules and maintenance of cell structure.

Measurement of Cerebral Blood Flow

The ability to measure cerebral blood flow first became possible in man when Seymour Kety and Carl Schmidt in the 1940s developed a technique employing the inert tracer nitrous oxide, a small unmetabolized molecule capable of rapid diffusion into the brain. In this method, the concentration of the tracer is monitored in the arterial and cerebral venous (internal jugular) blood during a 10 to 15 minute period of inhalation, during which time the tracer saturates the brain and equilibrium is achieved between the arterial and cerebral venous blood. Cerebral blood flow is computed from the quotient of the equilibrium concentration and the area lying between the arterial and cerebral venous tracer concentration curves. The Kety-Schmidt method permitted overall cerebral blood flow in man to be known under normal conditions and under a variety of altered states, including depressed consciousness and administration of various pharmacological agents. However, it offered no insight into regional blood flow.

The measurement of regional cerebral blood flow in man is achieved by the use of radioactive inert tracer substances such as xenon-133. This substance is administered either by intra-carotid injection or by inhalation or intravenous administration. Brain concentration of the tracer is monitored by external radioisotope detectors placed at the numerous locations over the head. The route and manner of tracer administration determines the mathematical strategy required for analysis of brain washout curves. In general, it is attempted to resolve a desaturation curve into two components, representing "fast flow," presumably through the gray matter, and "slow flow," representing white matter blood flow. Although such bi-exponential analysis is successful in the normal brain, compart-mental analysis of this type becomes more difficult and less certain under pathological conditions. An additional factor complicating analysis of clearance curves in methods employing inhalation or intravenous administration of the tracer is the presence of tracer within extracerebral tissues overlying the brain.

Methods employing external monitoring of regional brain clearance curves have been most successful in delineating patterns of perfusion in the normal brain. Normal resting man has a mean brain flow of approximately 50 ml/100 gm of brain tissue per minute. However, blood flow is not uniform throughout the brain. Gray matter receives approximately four times the perfusion of white matter per unit weight. In addition, frontal areas of brain tend to be slightly more perfused and temporal areas slightly less perfused than average. The Scandinavian workers Niels Lassen and David Ingvar have made use of large multidetector arrays to map patterns of regional blood flow during alterations of brain function. They have clearly demonstrated that blood flow to discrete regions of the brain increases during conceptualization of movement, performance of movement, sensory stimulation and various types of mental activity. The relationship of local blood flow to local metabolism of the brain during functional activation will be discussed below.

In experimental animals, other more invasive methods of studying regional blood flow are possible. One useful method employs autoradiography. In this method, a diffusible radioactive tracer is administered to an animal in a specified manner, following which the animal is sacrificed and the brain removed. Brain sections are applied to photographic film to produce images of the radioisotope distribution within the brain. The autoradiographic images provide information as to brain blood flow in every area of a cross-section. These images may be quantitated using densitometric analysis. This method confirms that cerebral blood flow is heterogeneous in the normal animal, with gray matter structures, both superficial and deep, being much more highly perfused than white matter. Other blood flow methods applicable to the experimental animal include the use of radioactive microspheres — small carbonized particles tagged with radioactive labels, which become lodged in capillaries following intravascular administration. The relative number of particles per unit weight of brain is proportional to the amount of blood flow to that region. Microsphere methods permit multiple blood flow measurements to be performed in a single animal, but analysis requires eventual animal sacrifice and brain dissection.

Regulation of the Cerebral Circulation

Cerebral perfusion pressure, that is, the net pressure causing arterial blood to perfuse the brain, is equivalent to the mean arterial blood pressure minus the cerebral venous pressure, which is equal to the cerebrospinal fluid pressure. In distinction to many other organs, the brain is able to maintain a constant blood flow over a wide range of perfusion pressures. This phenomenon is known as autoregulation. The autoregulatory range extends from a mean arterial blood pressure of approximately 50 mm Hg to 150 to 160 mm Hg. Below this range, cerebral blood flow tends to fall passively as blood pressure declines. Above the autoregulatory range, there is a "breakthrough" of blood flow with increasing perfusion pressure. The latter phenomenon may be of pathophysiologic significance in hypertensive encephalopathy. In the chronically hypertensive patient, the entire autoregulatory range may be shifted somewhat to the right, so that the lower limit of autoregulation is attained at a blood pressure higher than in the normotensive patient. Thus, levels of moderate hypotension which are tolerated by the normotensive patient may lead to cerebral hypoperfusion in the patient who has been chronically hypertensive.

Carbon dioxide is the most potent cerebral vasodilator. In the range of 20 to 80 mm Hg, the response of cerebral blood flow to pCO_2 is described by a sigmoid curve. A reduction of arterial pCO_2 by hyperventilation to 20 mm Hg reduces cerebral blood flow to about 40% of control. Conversely, if CO_2 is retained so that arterial pCO_2 rises from 40 to 80 mm Hg, cerebral blood flow nearly doubles. Thus, whenever cerebral blood flow is being critically measured, it is of great importance that the arterial carbon dioxide tension be accurately measured and well controlled. The mechanism by which CO_2 produces arterial vasodilatation in the brain is not clearly understood, though this molecule is known to be readily diffusible and may act by producing alterations of local tissue concentration of hydrogen ion, which in turn acts directly on vascular smooth muscle.

The role of neural innervation in the regulation of cerebral blood flow is highly controversial. It is well documented that a dense sympathetic plexus arising from the stellate ganglion is found along the carotid artery and innervates the pial and even intracerebral arteries down to the level of small vessels. Using specialized histochemical techniques, one can demonstrate nerve fibers along even small arterioles. Parasympathetic, cholinergic fibers have also been demonstrated along brain blood vessels. These observations notwithstanding, the precise contribution of these nerves in regulating cerebral blood flow is not well understood. Depending upon the experimental animal preparation employed, it has been possible to demonstrate a decrease in cerebral blood flow, an increase or no effect with sympathetic nerve stimulation. More recent evidence suggests that sympathetic nerves may serve to modulate cerebral blood flow autoregulation. In animals made hypotensive by hemorrhage, cerebral blood flow autoregulation persists at lower levels of mean arterial blood pressure in animals with prior sympathetic interruption than in controls. Conversely, in animals with induced hypertension, the level of mean arterial blood pressure at which a breakthrough of autoregulation occurs is higher in animals with sympathetic trunk stimulation than in nonstimulated controls. Thus, the extrinsic sympathetic innervation of the cerebral vasculature may be of chief importance during conditions of altered cerebral perfusion pressure.

In addition to the extrinsic sympathetic system described above, recent evidence suggests that brain blood vessels may be innervated as well by an intrinsic adrenergic system originating from the locus ceruleus. Alterations of capillary permeability have been demonstrated following stimulation of this structure.

Variations in arterial oxygen tension within the physiologic range do not produce changes in cerebral blood flow. When arterial pO_2 falls into the hypoxic range (approximately 50 mm Hg or below), a significant increase in cerebral blood flow occurs. The mechanism by which this is mediated is not well understood. Under conditions of hyperbaric oxygenation (atmospheric pressure 2 to 3 atmospheres), a mild decrease in cerebral blood flow has been demonstrated.

Numerous pharmacologic agents, including anesthetic substances, have been shown to influence cerebral blood flow. Other contributors to this volume have reviewed this area in part, and several excellent reviews are available in the published literature.

Perhaps the single, most important determinant of brain blood flow at the local level is the metabolic rate of a particular brain region, which in turn is influenced by the region's level of functional activity. The recent development of an experimental method using the glucose analog 2-deoxyglucose permits the rate of glucose utilization to be quantitated at the local level. In animal studies using this method, it has been shown that the rate of glucose utilization in a brain structure is closely matched to its rate of blood flow. Local brain activation (by motor activity, visual stimulation, auditory or tactile stimuli) results in an increase in metabolism of the responsible brain region, and this is in turn coupled to an increase in local blood flow. The response of local blood flow to local functional activity of the brain has been well demonstrated by Ingvar and Lassen and their colleagues using the intracarotid injection of xenon-133 and an external radionuclide detector system.

Cerebral Circulation and Metabolism in Ischemia

As discussed above, under normal circumstances glucose is the sole metabolic substrate for the brain. When fully metabolized in the presence of oxygen, 1 mole of glucose yields 38 moles of adenosine triphosphate, the brain's chief high-energy compound. Under conditions of diminished oxygen supply, glucose tends to be metabolized anaerobically, however, proceeding only as far as the pyruvate-lactate step and yielding only 2 moles of ATP per mole of glucose, an amount insufficient to meet the brain's normal metabolic needs. In addition, anaerobic glucose metabolism produces large amounts of tissue lactate, leading to brain acidosis. Elevation of brain lactate, reduction of brain pH and depletion of high-energy compounds within brain tissue are regular accompaniments of brain ischemia, a condition resulting from diminished cerebral blood flow. Ischemia is characterized by insufficient provision of oxygen and glucose substrate to brain and impaired removal of metabolic products. Ischemia of sufficient intensity and duration results in the production of distinct cellular alterations within cerebral neurons. The earliest stage of ischemic cell change is microvacuolization of the neuron. Ultrastructurally, this corresponds to mitochondrial swelling. This stage of ischemic cell change is reversible if circulation is promptly restored. If it is not, the neuron becomes shrunken and its cytoplasm homogeneous. A still later ischemic cell alteration consists of incrustations of the neuronal membrane. The critical level of cerebral blood flow required to produce ischemic cell alterations has been examined in experimental studies. Cerebral blood flow must be reduced to approximately 15% to 20% of its normal level, or below, in order for consistent ischemic cell alterations to result. This corresponds to a flow of approximately 12 ml/100 gm of brain per minute. Blood flow reductions down to approximately 20% of control are tolerated without the consistent production of ischemic neuropathological alterations.

As cerebral blood flow falls, a variety of physiological alterations occur within the brain. In incipient ischemia, the dominant frequency of the electroencephalogram slows; with severe ischemia, the EEG rapidly becomes isoelectric. Soon thereafter, the ability to obtain evoked cerebral responses is abolished. The massive release of potassium from cells into the extracellular space occurs during severe ischemia and undoubtedly contributes to the slow and incomplete physiological recovery seen following ischemic episodes.

Alterations of regional cerebral blood flow have been noted in patients with focal cerebral ischemia and infarction (stroke). The usual finding is a focal reduction in blood flow. Paradoxical elevations of blood flow are occasionally observed peripheral to zones of diminished flow in patients with acute stroke. The latter phenomenon has been termed "luxury perfusion," signifying levels of blood flow in excess of the tissue's metabolic needs. Luxury perfusion may be due to the release of lactate from the central zone of ischemia, which produces abnormal vasodilatation in surrounding regions.

The etiology of the ischemic process in part determines its distribution and severity. Under conditions of profound generalized ischemia (e.g., cardiac arrest) the entire brain may undergo marked metabolic alterations, with lactate elevation and depletion of brain energy metabolites. However, during a threshold ischemic insult, there is a heterogeneous affection of tissue, with patchy areas of metabolic failure separated by normal zones. In experimental focal cerebral ischemia, the 2-deoxyglucose method has demonstrated the existence of a central zone of profoundly suppressed glucose utilization surrounded by a zone of higher than normal glucose utilization, possibly due to anaerobic glycolysis.

Cerebral edema may complicate brain ischemia. It arises as a consequence of impaired cellular ion-pump function and alterations in brain osmolality, as well as from damage to cerebral vasculature. Thus, ischemic cerebral edema partakes of both "cytotoxic" and "vasogenic" aspects. The consequence of cerebral edema may be an increase in tissue hydrostatic pressure, which further impairs cerebral circulation and may perpetuate and extend the ischemic process.

Among the factors modifying the brain's response to an ischemic insult is the plasma glucose level. It has been shown in several experimental studies that administration of large doses of dextrose intravenously prior to an ischemic insult markedly exacerbates the hemodynamic, metabolic and neuropathological consequences of the ischemic insult. More recent studies suggest that even smaller elevations of plasma glucose may intensify the degree of cellular injury. These observations have not yet been extended to the clinical level. An additional factor which exacerbates the outcome of ischemia is the amount of residual blood flow persisting during the ischemic insult. There is experimental evidence to suggest that preservation of small amounts of blood flow during ischemia leads to greater metabolic injury to tissue than if blood flow is completely arrested.

The ultimate degree of cerebral ischemia is seen in the "respirator brain syndrome" occurring in the setting of massive brain injury or antecedent circulatory arrest. Here, the cerebral circulation has completely ceased. Angiographic contrast material injected into extracranial vessels does not succeed in filling the intracranial vasculature.

Bibliography

Edvinsson, L. and MacKenzie, E.T.: Amine mechanisms in the cerebral circulation. Pharmacol. Rev. 28:275-348, 1977.

Ingvar, D.H. and Lassen, N.A. (eds.): Brain Work. The Coupling of Function, Metabolism and Blood Flow in the Brain. Copenhagen: Munksgaard, 1975.

Lassen, N.A. and Christensen, M.D.: Physiology of cerebral blood flow. Br. J. Anaesth. 48:719-734, 1976.

Olesen, J.: Cerebral blood flow. Methods for measurement, regulation, effects of drugs and changes in disease. Acta Neurol. Scand. 50 (Suppl. 57):134, 1974.

Paulson, O.B.: Cerebral apoplexy (stroke): Pathogenesis, pathophysiology and therapy as illustrated by regional blood flow measurements in the brain. Stroke 2:327-360, 1970.

Purves, M.J.: The Physiology of the Cerebral Circulation. Cambridge: Cambridge University Press, 1972.

Purves, M.J.: Control of cerebral blood vessels: Present state of the art. (Editorial). Ann. Neurol. 3:377-383, 1978.

Scheinberg, P., Meyer, J.S., Reivich, M. et al: Report of Joint Committee for Stroke Facilities. XIII. Cerebral circulation and metabolism in stroke. Stroke 7:212-234, 1976.

Siesjö, B.J.: Brain Energy Metabolism. Chichester:John Wiley & Sons, 1978.

Sokoloff, L.: Circulation and energy metabolism of the brain. In Siegel, G.J., Albers, R.W., Katzman, R. and Agranoff, B.W. (eds.): Basic Neurochemistry, ed. 2. Boston:Little Brown, 1976, chap. 19.

Walker, A.E.: Cerebral Death. Dallas:Professional Information Library, 1977.

Self-Evaluation Quiz

1. Cerebral blood flow is exquisitely responsive to changes of arterial blood pressure in the physiological range.

    a) True
    b) False

2. Factors of *major* importance in controlling the level of cerebral blood flow include:
    a) Arterial carbon dioxide tension
    b) Arterial oxygen tension
    c) Sympathetic nervous innervation
    d) Level of functional activity of the brain

3. Normal metabolic function of the brain requires the presence of glucose and oxygen.
    a) True
    b) False

Answers on page 391.

Panel Discussion

Moderator: Dr. Marshall

Panelists: Drs. Ginsberg, Ramsay, Tsubokawa

Moderator: Dr. Ramsay, do you believe that evoked responses are clinically useful today?

Dr. Ramsay: Yes, I think they are tremendously useful. In a comatose or traumatized patient, I think they help us at least in determining whether there is an anatomical defect. For example, in evaluating patients with acoustic neuromas, there have been some reports of 80% to 90% positive findings. I have not seen that many with acoustic neuromas come through our laboratory. I have seen only two and they both had abnormal responses.

Moderator: Dr. Ramsay, in doing the EEG, is it important to know if the patient is left- or right-handed? If so, why?

Dr. Ramsay: No, it is not important.

Moderator: Is 1 gm of dilantin given intravenously push slowly effective in controlling status epilepticus? Is 1 gm of dilantin slow intravenously push ever therapeutic?

Dr. Ramsay: Yes, it is sometimes therapeutic. One must be careful to give dilantin at 50 mg/min particularly in patients over 45 years of age since there is an increased incidence of significant hypotension that is rate-related. If you slow it down, the hypotension will not usually be a problem. If 1 gm is not enough, I would go as high as 2 gm before I proceed to another medication.

Moderator: Dr. Tsubokawa, you showed one slide of spinal cord cooling, a technique that is controversial in the United States. Please describe your technique of spinal cord cooling. Do you do a laminectomy and then infuse iced saline?

Dr. Tsubokawa: I do a laminectomy first and open the dura. I use the dura to create a reservoir and prepare 10 liters of cold saline (7 C) which is infused over the spinal cord. It takes about

229

45 minutes. After that, I record the spinal cord evoked potential and compare that with the previous preoperative study. Then if no improvement has resulted, I repeat one more 45-minute perfusion. So the maximum is 90 minutes of hypothermic perfusion.

Moderator: Are evoked responses changed during herniation gradually or suddenly? Do they precede clinical signs? There is a very good paper in the *Journal of Neurosurgery* of November 1979 that discusses that issue in great detail and looks at the various waveforms. I am afraid we do not have time to discuss that today.

Dr. Ginsberg, is hyperbaric oxygen of any use in the treatment of any kind of brain injury?

Dr. Ginsberg: Hyperbaric oxygenation is a treatment of choice in carbon monoxide poisoning. By increasing the amount of oxygen physically dissolved in the plasma, this treatment improves tissue oxygenation and hastens the elimination of CO from the blood. In cerebral vascular disorders, however, the results are far less conclusive. Hyperbaric oxygenation may produce a transient improvement in the neurologic deficit of stroke patients while in the hyperbaric chamber, but, to my knowledge, there appears to be no evidence of a sustained improvement associated with its use.

Moderator: Dr. Ginsberg, at what level of arterial hypoxia in the face of a stable CBF, that is, normal flow, but just pure hypoxic hypoxia, does ischemic cell change occur?

Dr. Ginsberg: It is very difficult both in the patient and in experimental animal models to study hypoxia without the contaminating influence of ischemia. As arterial oxygen tension is lowered to critical levels, systemic hypotension quickly results, so that cerebral hypoperfusion tends to be produced. In the physiologically best regulated animal models studied to date, the degree of arterial hypoxia required to produce ischemic cell change is quite profound. The arterial pO_2 level must be approximately 20 to 25 torr for 30 minutes. Less severe degrees of arterial hypoxia may be well tolerated in the absence of superimposed ischemia and appear not to produce ischemic cell injury.

Moderator: Dr. Ginsberg, why do CBF measurements have a confirmatory role rather than a primary role in determining brain death?

Dr. Ginsberg: CBF facilities are not always present in medical centers dealing with brain death, nor are the CBF criteria for brain death clearly established. Indeed, the key issue in the determination of brain death is the demonstration of absence of specific neurologic signs denoting brain viability. The presence of a particular level of CBF is not crucial to this phenomenon, although, of course, a prolonged period of severely reduced cerebral blood flow would be incompatible with brain survival. The radioisotopic bolus technic has been used to study the blood flow deficit associated with brain death; a recent article is by Korein and co-workers in the *Annals of Neurology*, September 1977.

Moderator: Concerning the effect of dopamine, 2 to 10 mcg/kg/minute drip, and what happens to CBF, there is really very little information available as far as I know about dopamine's effect on the cerebral vasculature. Overguard has recently written a paper, which has not yet been published, but which was presented at the European Surgical Society meeting, regarding dopamine. In the doses that are characteristically used in man for blood pressure and volume support, if you separate out the correction of hypotension and autoregulatory disturbances (which is very difficult to do), it does not appear that dopamine has much of a direct effect on the cerebral vasculature. That is a difficult question to answer.

Dr. Ramsay, some say you can have brain death with spinal reflexes, because a chicken without a head walks around. Would you care to comment on that?

Dr. Ramsay: Yes, you are correct. The persistence of spinal reflexes is not an exclusion for the determination of brain death. It is the brainstem reflexes that must be absent.

Moderator: What about the use of lorazepam, Ativan, which is a long-acting diazepam variant, made by American Hospital Corporation, Wyeth Division, in the treatment of status? We have had a contract to study the drug and so has Dr. Ramsay. Our experience with lorazepam has been very good. It has one significant advantage, not only in terms of status, but it also does not affect cerebral blood flow. Valium appears to occasionally raise intracranial pressure and not lower it. Considerable investigation is being carried on right now, particularly in Europe, of the lorazepam-diazepam variant compounds. They are probably going to be the drugs that will become considerably more important in neurological intensive care over the next ten years because diazepam receptors in the central nervous system have been demonstrated now by many groups working in Scandinavia. So I would say in the future, and I am not talking about status right now, and I shall let you answer that further, that these drugs are an area of major interest in the 1980s. We are going to be looking at variants of the barbiturates and probably in greater detail looking at Valium analogs in the future.

Dr. Ramsay: Unfortunately, of the benzodiazepines, Valium is really the only parenteral one available. Lorazepam and clonazepam are much more potent than diazepam. I do not know about its effect on cerebral blood flow. We just do not have it available in this country.

Moderator: We have lorazepam.

Dr. Ramsay: Only on an experimental basis?

Moderator: Yes, exactly.

Dr. Ramsay: I am using the same protocol, and I find it is very effective. It is just that we cannot use it routinely until lorazepam has been proven safe and effective in the present studies under way.

Moderator: Dr. Ginsberg, this question is for you, and I do not understand it and maybe the questioner can explain it: In the injured brain, where we try to engage the patient in specific activity, movement of extremities, memory and speech, is the change in CBF through their efforts to respond a more general phenomenon or is it localized?

Dr. Ginsberg: Any generalized arousal stimulus probably produces an increase in cerebral metabolism and hence cerebral blood flow. In addition, the superimposition of focal brain activity may lead to additional increases in cerebral metabolism and blood flow in the involved brain area. The sleeping brain has a lower level of blood flow than the conscious brain. A related question is whether the stimulus to increased cerebral blood flow produced by arousal or brain work is in any sense deleterious to the patient with brain injury. I am not aware of any conclusive information on this point.

Moderator: Dr. Ginsberg, if the injured brain requires glucose and cerebral edema contraindicates its use, I think they are talking about hypoglycemia data that have come from both Meyers and Siesjo, but I am not sure, what do you do?

Dr. Ginsberg: The normal as well as the injured brain, of course, both require glucose. Patients must be kept from becoming hypoglycemic from whatever cause, as hypoglycemia, if profound, may lead to neuronal injury resembling that produced by hypoxia — ischemia. The maintenance of normal blood glucose in the brain-injured patient is thus to be desired. The work of Ronald Myers as well as our own studies suggest, however, that very large amounts of intravenous glucose given in close relationship to an ischemic insult may exacerbate the degree of brain injury. Thus, we would suggest that hyperglycemia be avoided. Dr. Shapiro's point, I believe, was that one should avoid giving dextrose and water solutions or other hypotonic solutions, because they may tend to exacerbate the degree of brain swelling.

Moderator: Dr. Ramsay, first, please speak about drug intoxication aside from barbiturates and the determination of brain death with the EEG. In other words, what agents other than the barbiturates, the Valium analogs, would suppress electrical activity sufficiently to mislead one, forgetting now about hypothermia, which you discussed?

Dr. Ramsay: I think the most common ones are the drugs of the sedative/hypnotic type. Doriden, for example, has been reported to sufficiently depress the CNS to produce an EEG which is flat. This has never been reported to occur for more than 24 hours, so if a question exists a second EEG should be obtained 24 hours or more after the first. You definitely can get a totally isoelectric record that meets all of the electrographic criteria of electrocerebral silence from drugs that are commonly available.

Moderator: How do results from auditory evoked response monitoring alter care in the neurosurgical or neurological intensive care unit environment?

I would make just one comment: That is, if one has a patient who has normal evoked responses after one operates and he goes bad, one should take the patient and CAT scan him and find out why. If you look at *International Anesthesiology Clinics*, Dr. Shapiro and I have published the evoked response data next to the EMI scans on a series of patients, and you will see a large hemorrhage in a patient two days following evacuation of an acute subdural hematoma. The patient was very sick, and his evoked response went out, and the EMI scan showed a pontine midbrain hemorrhage, which obviously explained the fact that this was an irreversible change. On the other hand, in patients who get better in terms of their evoked responses, or who have normal evoked responses and who are young, from our viewpoint in head injury, it is very important to support those patients aggressively because the evoked response is a relatively good indicator of brainstem integrity, as Dr. Daroff discussed earlier. I think we are in the infancy stage of this technique, in terms of exploring it, but the potential utilization of the far field evoked response, that is, the brainstem auditory evoked response, and electrical recording in general has been underplayed. The cerebral function monitor from England which is now being extensively tested in Europe, for example, is what I would call a primitive EEG. It is a way of noninvasively monitoring electrical activity and cerebral perfusion. It has been relatively reliable and has been tested in over 1,000 patients. But I think we are just getting to the point where we process the data with microprocessors rapidly enough to make it clinically useful and that in the next ten years we are likely to see a tremendous explosion in electrical monitoring of patients because, after all, even though I do not have an aversion to ventricular catheters, and I like to operate, if there is a noninvasive way to monitor the patient, I would rather do that because it is much better for the patient and it will be much more widely utilized.

Dr. Ramsay: I think you have pretty well answered the question. One important point is, and the same thing holds for the EEG, one single evoked response may not be as important as serially following the patient because you can really tell if the patient is getting worse very quickly — much sooner than you would by your examination of the patient and from his brainstem reflexes. If someone has a normal response, we really should be much more vigorous in trying to support and maintain this patient through his acute periods.

Head Injury

Lawrence F. Marshall, M.D.

Objectives

1. To describe the care of severely head-injured patients in a systematic and organized fashion.
2. To emphasize the need for a comprehensive approach to the care of acute head injury.
3. To emphasize the importance of avoiding secondary injuries in severely head-injured patients.

Introduction

This paper discusses the care of the head-injured patient. However, head injury should be considered a prototype for the management of patients who are acutely ill from other brain insults. The care of any patient with intracerebral hemorrhage, subarachnoid hemorrhage, Reye's syndrome or head injury is similar in many respects. In each instance, a systematic and organized approach to the care of the patient is an absolute necessity.

Factors that determine the outcome of head-injured patients are not all within the control of the treating physician. It is apparent that some patients who survive to reach the hospital alive have had such severe destruction of brain tissue that their injuries are irreversible. These irreversible injuries can usually be identified by the presence of discrete neurological findings. However, the major focus of this review is to identify those factors which are within the control of the medical community and which can make the difference between a vegetative outcome and one which allows the patient's return to a useful role within his family or society.

Lawrence F. Marshall, M.D., Associate Professor of Surgery/Neurological Surgery, University of California, San Diego.

Neurosurgeons have focused the majority of their attention on what occurs in the intensive care unit setting. This focus, while not misplaced, has tended to underemphasize the importance of care delivered in the so-called prehospital phase and in the emergency room. If the major objective in the severely head-injured patient is to create a milieu in which the brain's metabolic demands can be met and further insults to an already-damaged brain can be avoided, it is apparent that the prehospital emergency room phase of care is an extremely important determinant of the patient's ultimate outcome. One can presuppose that either generalized or focal disturbances of brain function occur in head-injured patients either because metabolic demands are too great (i.e., the brain's need for oxygen and glucose exceeds the ability of the cardiopulmonary system to deliver it) as in status epilepticus or hyperthermia, or in circumstances when cerebral blood flow (CBF) is inadequate. This occurs in patients with intracranial hypertension or shock when nutrients cannot reach the brain because the cerebral perfusion pressure (CPP) is compromised. Such problems occur not 6 hours, not 18 hours, and not 48 hours following injury, but almost immediately following injury. Our emphasis, therefore, must be on a global approach to the care of these patients. With the increasing use of small vehicles and motorcycles in the United States because of fuel shortages, we are seeing a dramatic rise in the number of patients who suffer severe injury to multiple organ systems. Injuries in such patients characteristically are multiple with both-bone fractures of the lower extremities, injuries to the chest and abdomen and fractures of the upper limbs.

Patients who are injured in motor vehicle accidents suffer a much higher incidence of what Miller has called a secondary insult to the brain, which is defined as a systolic blood pressure of less than 95 mm Hg, a PaO_2 of less than 65 mm Hg or a PCO_2 of greater than 44 [1]. These do not represent at their minimum severe levels of systemic compromise, but they have been shown to be associated with a much more adverse outcome than in patients in whom none of these complications are present. In order to demonstrate that secondary insults to the brain are major determinants of the patient's course, Table 1 demonstrates the outcome of patients injured in motor

Table 1. Complications vs. Outcome in Vehicular Injury*

	Good/Moderate	Severe/Vegetative/Dead	Total
None	30 (83%)	6 (17%)	36
Complications	18 (53%)	16 (47%)	34

$$X^2 = 10.7 \ (\ p < .005)$$

*From Miller, et al [1].

vehicle accidents and compares patients in whom systemic compromise occurred and in whom it did not. In the absence of other injuries, 80% of the patients made a good or moderate recovery and only 20% were severely damaged or died. Remarkably, in patients in whom one or more of these complications were present, almost one half of the patients died or had a poor outcome.

To view the issue of secondary compromise from another perspective, one can analyze the data from our region regarding the presence or absence of multiple injuries. Such a comparison is shown in Table 2 [2]. We defined a multiple injury as one that required either a laparotomy or thoracotomy. There was a 30% mortality for the patients who did not have multiple injuries while in patients in whom multiple injuries requiring surgery occurred, a mortality of 50% was found, and the incidence of good or moderate recovery was much lower. Thus, we as neurosurgeons, nurses, intensivists and emergency room physicians must pay more attention to the prehospital and emergency room phases of the patient's management in order to reverse these systemic insults to the brain should they be present at any time in the patient's initial course.

Injuries to abdominal viscera or the chest, per se, are often not direct causes of mortality. It is the systemic consequences

Table 2. Outcome as Related to Presence or Absence of Multiple Injuries

	Good Recovery		Moderate Disability		Severe Disability		Vegetative		Dead		Total
	No.	%	No.	%	No.	%	No.	%	No.	%	
Head injury	68	48	17	12	11	8	3	2	43	30*	142
Multiple injuries	16	28	3	5	5	9	5	9	29	50*	58

*P < .01

of these injuries which result in a poor outcome. Unless we increase our concern for the organization of care at the basic level, i.e., from the field to the hospital, the quality of care in the ICU setting will become less and less relevant because the outcome will already have been determined for many of our patients.

Inherent in the concern about the prehospital and emergency room phases of care is that the neurosurgeon make his desires clear to all personnel who care for these patients in that environment. It is too often assumed that the paramedics and the emergency room physicians know exactly what the neurosurgical community expects, but this is not a correct assumption. Direct instructions regarding intubation, fluid management, the use of CAT scanning and the position in which the patient should be transported all need to be communicated to these other providers of care.

Regional Plan

An optimal triage plan for head-injured patients is a regional-dependent phenomenon. The geography and demography of a particular area should be a determinant of the plan for that area, and the plan should not be superimposed from one region to another simply because it has worked in an area that may be completely different. San Diego County has a relatively low population density and covers a large geographic area. A plan for the care of patients in our region, which would centralize the care for head- and spinal cord-injured patients to one hospital, not only would be economically unfeasible, but would also lead to unnecessarily long triage times. Thus, it appears more logical in our region to designate those hospitals that can deliver a high level of care and have the Regional Trauma Center at University Hospital act as a teaching and coordinating arm for such a plan.

In this way, a high level of care should be available within a few minutes of the accident scene. Our system is predicated upon a median paramedic response time of ten minutes. If what we presently believe is true, i.e., that care in the field is a critical determinant, then the organization of care around that philosophy naturally follows. In our region, criteria for hospitals to be eligible to receive patients with head and spinal cord injury have been developed based on the demography and geography of our area. They include:

1. A CAT scanner be available immediately at the hospital facility.

2. A dedicated neurosurgical service at that institution.

3. An experienced ICU team.

4. A minimum of 35 neurosurgical operative procedures performed a year within the hospital.

5. An emergency room physician on call 24 hours a day trained in advanced life support and capable of endotracheal intubation even under circumstances where the patient has severe multiple injuries.

These criteria must be recognized as arbitrary although they do incorporate what appears to be the plan of the American Association of Neurological Surgeons for minimum hospital standards.

Once one has developed a triage plan for hospitals, one needs triage criteria for patients. We have used the Glasgow Coma Scale score shown in Table 3 in combination with examination of the pupils and a search for the presence or

Table 3. Severe Head Injury: Glasgow Coma Scale Score of 7 or Less Persisting for Six Hours or More

Glasgow Coma Scale		
Eyes open	Never	= 1
	To pain	= 2
	To speech	= 3
	Spontaneously	= 4
Best verbal response	None	= 1
	Garbled	= 2
	Inappropriate	= 3
	Confused	= 4
	Oriented	= 5
Best motor response	None	= 1
	Extension	= 2
	Abnormal flexion	= 3
	Withdrawal	= 4
	Localizes pain	= 5
	Obeys commands	= 6
	Total score	=

absence of lateralizing signs as an index for the rapidity of evacuation and the urgency of intervention. In patients with Glasgow Coma Scale scores of 7 or less, our regional plan calls for intubation or the placement of an esophageal obturator in such patients and for acute hyperventilation. There should be no exceptions to this principle.

Jennett and his colleagues have shown that the mortality in those patients with Glasgow Coma Scale scores of 7 or less exceeds 50% [3]. If one does not have a systematic and somewhat rigid plan for the care of this high-risk group, one is likely to have patients deteriorate in the field, upon admission to the hospital or during scanning. Such outcomes are potentially avoidable with a systematic and nonarbitrary triage plan.

The neurological examination in the emergency room facility should be brief. It should include the Glasgow Coma Scale score, the presence or absence of lateralization, status of the pupils and the oculocephalic responses. In addition, a lateral cervical radiograph should be obtained which demonstrates all of the cervical vertebrae. Routine skull radiographs in patients who are this severely injured (Glasgow Coma Scale scores of 7 or less) are not necessary, since CAT scanning will give adequate detail of the bone structures of the skull, and skull radiographs are really only an index of the severity or force to which the brain has been subjected and not the major focus of interest in such patients.

This emphasis on brevity does not mean that the patient should not undergo a thorough neurological examination. However, if one accepts the premise that the more rapidly a space-occupying lesion is removed, the more likely the patient is to do well, time is of the essence. Thus, a more detailed examination can be postponed until the CAT scan is completed. In general, no more than 45 minutes from the time of arrival in the emergency room to the patient's arrival in the operating room (including the performance of a CAT scan) should elapse. In that period the brief neurological examination has been performed, appropriate management instituted and CAT scan completed. This is a guideline and not an absolute rule. Things do go wrong — CAT scanners break down, anesthesiologists and neurosurgeons may need to delay acute surgical intervention — but the point is that this is a guideline to aim for.

When the CAT scan is performed, higher cuts through the ventricular system should be done first in order to define the presence or absence of an extraparenchymal, supratentorial or superficial supratentorial hematoma. If no surgical mass is seen, the rest of the study should then be completed. Contrast should be administered only if there is some doubt as to the etiology of the patient's sudden neurological deterioration. It should never delay the evacuation of significant extraparenchymal or superficial intracerebral hematomas.

Once the patient's emergency room evaluation, CAT scan and initial therapy are completed and operative intervention has been carried out in those who need it, the patient is transported to the ICU setting. All ICU facilities should be using some type of time-oriented record, and most do. Unfortunately, much of the recordkeeping in ICU facilities is irrelevant and time-wasting. Pages of nursing notes and progress noted are often meaningless and do not convey information that should be readily transferable from one provider of care to another. Since we have begun to work on data collection through the National Traumatic Coma Data Bank, much of our efforts have been devoted toward the development of time-oriented and event-oriented data collection instruments that are more meaningful. The use of a time-oriented record, as shown in Figure 1, illustrates one possible approach toward a patient's ICU data collection. When something changes for the worse in a patient one is interested in (1) what associated changes have occurred, (2) can they be the cause or are they also the effect of what has been seen and, most importantly, (3) what can be done to reverse the situation.

Thus, data flow sheets should be continuous and must be interchangeable between the ICU setting, the operating room, and any other facility where the patient may go. It is also imperative that the system used to follow the patient can be reliably used by all personnel involved in patient care. This is one major advantage of the Glasgow Coma Scale where interobserver reliability has been shown to be approximately 95%. Paramedics, emergency room technicians, emergency room physicians and ICU teams have found the scale both satisfactory and useful. There may be limitations to it as a keystone in the ICU setting, but I believe it is the one scale that

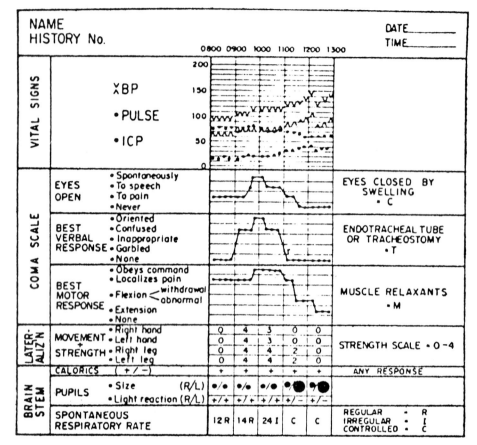

FIG. 1. Time-oriented record.

should be used in the foreseeable future until a better one is available. The Glasgow Coma Scale has the significant advantage of defining the patient's condition in terms of response to external stimuli. It does not include terms such as stuporous, comatose or lethargic which are poorly understood from one observer to another.

To demonstrate the importance of a continuous time-oriented record, an example of an interesting clinical observation from our Regional Trauma Center is demonstrated in Table 4. One observation that puzzled neurosurgeons for many years was the fact that patients with severe head injuries often

Table 4. Temporal Pattern of Intracranial Hypertension (n = 21)

	No.	Percent	Probability
Episodes of ICP > 30 mm Hg	185		
Episodes between 4:00 a.m. and 9:00 a.m.	124	67	
Episodes between 9:00 a.m. and 4:00 a.m.	61	33	<0.01
Early morning episodes responsive to barbiturates*	104/124	84	
Other episodes responsive to barbiturates*	35/61	57	<0.01

*ICP reduced to <15 mm Hg.

appeared to deteriorate in the late night and early morning hours. This observation was terribly disturbing and also poorly explained. When a retrospective analysis of the patients' records was carried out, it was obvious that almost 70% of severely head-injured patients with intracranial hypertension had the majority of their pressure waves (ICP greater than 30 mm Hg) in the early morning hours. However, since the PCO_2's were not recorded on the record at the same time that these observations were made, it was felt that these occurrences of intracranial hypertension were attributable to increases in PCO_2. However, when a time-oriented and event-oriented data collection system was instituted, it became clear that these diurnal changes were not a response to changes in CO_2, but rather reflected increases in brain-blood volume which were causing severe intracranial hypertension in a considerable number of patients [4]. Observation and therapy were altered in these patients so that they were directed more intensively toward this time frame.

Specific Patient Management

Cardiopulmonary

Hyperventilation is a foundation stone in the management of brain-injured patients. Not only is it the most useful method for reducing intracranial pressure acutely, but also the respiratory alkalosis that is induced may benefit brain tissue acidosis, an almost invariable accompaniment of severe head injury.

It is true that as hyperventilation is continued for longer periods of time, the CO_2 responsiveness of the cerebral vasculature falls. However, one can often maintain adequate control of intracranial pressure by pushing the CO_2 a bit lower over time. Continual hyperventilation for more than three to five days is routine in our unit.

Patient Position

All severely head-injured patients should be managed in the head-up position with one exception: the patients who are in shock. Furthermore, the head should be kept in the neutral plane with respect to the body. If the neck is turned to the left or right, severe increases in ICP can occur, and pressure waves can be precipitated in patients where brain compliance is already low. The head-up position is often particularly beneficial when positive end expiratory pressure (PEEP) is utilized. The increased venous volume that occurs in the superior portion of the body with PEEP can be significantly mitigated by having the head up, thus permitting hydrostatic forces to return blood to the chest. All neurosurgeons should recognize that good chest care is of critical importance in patients with head and multiple injuries. However, such care must be delivered with a high level of recognition of the effects chest physiotherapy has on intracranial dynamics.

When one carries out procedures that have a potentially deleterious effect on intracranial volume, nursing personnel should be instructed to look at the ICP monitor. If the ICP exceeds 30 mm Hg, chest physiotherapy should be immediately stopped and not reinstituted until pressures fall to below 15 mm Hg.

Many of these problems can be avoided by the use of adequate amounts of sedation and hyperventilation when one is planning to suction a patient, perform bronchoscopy or other respiratory care maneuvers. It is critical to coordinate the protection of the brain with the treatment of the respiratory tract.

General Sedation and Paralysis

We sedate and paralyze every severely head-injured patient with an endotracheal tube in place. The use of paralyzing agents alone is not adequate to protect patients from the reflex arcs that occur from laryngeal stimuli and which often result in systemic arterial hypertension. Since changes in systemic arterial pressure (SAP) are not only reflected in brain-blood volume but can also aggravate blood-brain barrier disturbances, they should be avoided if at all possible. Often simple sedation will greatly aid in preventing unacceptable rises in SAP.

The choice of a paralyzing agent and narcotic is primarily one of personal preference. Pancuronium (Pavulon) has been routine in our unit. An hourly dose of 2 mg in an adult 70 kg man is usually sufficient. We also have utilized morphine as a primary sedative agent. Small doses of between 1 and 3 mg intravenously per hour are almost always adequate. Pupillary dilatation will still occur in patients if tentorial herniation occurs in the face of such doses. Morphine is a reliable agent with a rather minimal effect on cardiac output in the great majority of head-injured patients. If severe dehydration is part of the management plan, however, the dose of morphine must be reduced.

Fluid Management

Chronic fluid management in the head-injured patient is different from the fluid management of other critically ill patients. Dextrose in water is a poor choice in patients with preexisting brain injuries because experimental models have demonstrated rather dramatic exacerbations of brain edema in animals with preexisting brain injuries. The ideal fluid is lactated Ringer's or normal saline. However, salt loading may become a problem if such fluids are used. Half-normal saline, with or without dextrose, is the solution of choice in adults.

In the pediatric age group, ¼-normal saline is usually most appropriate. Fluid balance should be judicious. Severe dehydration, while recommended as a management tool by some, often leads to grave problems and the long-term benefits have yet to be demonstrated. If one is considering the use of thiopental or pentobarbital, the presence of severe dehydration when these drugs are introduced can lead to catastrophic and irreversible falls in cardiac output. Severe dehydration should be avoided unless one is prepared to rapidly rehydrate such patients.

Fever

Hyperthermia from whatever cause dramatically increases brain metabolic rate and has a deleterious effect on patients with severe brain injury. The cause of the fever should be rapidly searched for, but the fever must also be rapidly treated. A combination of rectal Tylenol or aspirin and a cooling blanket should be instituted if the temperature exceeds 101 F. Ideally, normothermia should be striven for, but it is often impossible to achieve temperatures below 36.5 C. Patients should not be allowed to become severely hyperthermic while waiting to obtain blood or other cultures. The prophylactic prevention of hyperthermia in brain-injured patients is absolutely critical.

Seizures must also be prevented, if at all possible. We have seen patients who have made very nice recoveries from severe head injury who have subsequently deteriorated and not recovered again following one or two motor seizures. The prophylactic administration of diphenylhydantoin in an initial loading dose of 8 to 10 mg/kg over several hours followed by a daily dose regimen is appropriate unless there is an allergy to phenytoin. Under those circumstances, phenobarbital can be substituted.

Outcome

The methods of care in our region with the exception of the management of intracranial hypertension which has been described elsewhere have been outlined. One must inquire whether the approach described here has yielded a satisfactory outcome for the patients. Table 5 describes the outcome statistics for our region and is displayed according to the patient's Glasgow Coma Scale score six hours following admis-

Table 5. Outcome of 200 Consecutive Study Patients With a
Glasgow Coma Scale Score of 7 or Less Persisting for 6 Hours or More

Glasgow Coma Score	Good Recovery		Moderate Disability		Severe Disability		Vegetative		Dead		Total
	No.	%	No.	%	No.	%	No.	%	No.	%	
7	29	63	5	11	4	9	1	2	7	15	46
6	26	48	7	13	5	9	2	4	14	26	54
5	13	50	2	8	4	15	–	–	7	27	26
4	10	24	5	12	1	2	4	10	21	51	41
3	6	18	1	3	2	6	1	3	23	70	33

sion. The Glasgow Outcome Scale score has been used by Jennett and Bond to indicate the outcomes.

The overall mortality was 36%, significantly below that of the multinational study reported by Jennett et al. These data indicate that this systemic approach has a beneficial effect on outcome for head-injured patients. Although patients who are decerebrate or unresponsive to deep pain at six hours did poorly in our region, 30% still survived — a significant improvement over previous results reported and indicative of the fact that vigorous and aggressive therapy may well transform some of these patients into useful survivors.

Concerns that aggressive care might result in the production of an increased number of patients who remain in a vegetative state or are severely disabled appear to be unfounded based on our experience and that of our colleagues at the Medical College of Virginia who manage their patients similarly [5].

With no new therapeutic breakthroughs on the horizon, it appears necessary to consolidate the gains made over the last decade. The introduction of the CAT scanner and more routine monitoring and management of ICP, coupled with the general measures described here, can be utilized in almost every region of the United States and should have a beneficial effect on the outcome of treatment of patients suffering severe head injury.

References

1. Miller, J.D., Sweet, R.C., Norayan, R. et al: Early insults to the injured brain. JAMA 240:439-442, 1978.
2. Bowers, S.A. and Marshall, L.F.: The outcome in 200 consecutive cases of severe head injury in San Diego County: A prospective analysis. Neurosurgery 6:337-342, 1980.
3. Jennett, B., Teasdale, G., Galbraith, S. et al: Severe head injuries in three countries. J. Neurol. Neurosurg. Psychiat. 40:291-298, 1977.
4. Marshall, L.F., Smith, R.W. and Shapiro, H.M.: The influence of diurnal rhythms in patients with intracranial hypertension: Implications for management. Neurosurgery 2:100-101, 1978.
5. Becker, D.P., Miller, J.D., Ward, J.D. et al: The outcome from severe head injury with early diagnosis and intense management. J. Neurosurg. 47:491-502, 1977.

Self-Evaluation Quiz

1. Care of the severely head-injured patient must be comprehensively organized because of all the following reasons *except*:

a) The quality of ICU care determines the outcome for most patients
b) The prehospital phase is often critical in determining the ultimate outcome of the patient
c) Significant systemic compromise is a major determinant of survivorship from head injury
d) The avoidance of secondary complications following brain injury may influence the outcome

2. Systemic compromise is defined as the presence of all of the following *except*:
   a) PaO$_2$ of less than 65
   b) Systolic blood pressure of less than 95
   c) PCO$_2$ of greater than 44
   d) Diastolic blood pressure of less than 70

3. Regional triage plans should have all of the following characteristics *except*:
   a) Should be tailored to fit a region
   b) Need to be developed as part of the entire effort in emergency medical services
   c) Should aim for emergency medical technicians or paramedic response times of less than 15 minutes
   d) Should be of one design and utilized in all regions

4. Prophylaxis for seizures is desirable in head-injured patients and may be associated with the prevention of secondary insults to the brain.
   a) True
   b) False

Match the Following

5. Halothane	a)	Preferred
6. Head-up position	b)	To be avoided
7. Glasgow Coma Scale	c)	Needs aggressive treatment
8. Fever	d)	Uses external stimuli
9. Hyperventilation	e)	Less effective over time

Answers on page 391.

Acute Spinal Cord Injury: Emergency Room Care and Diagnosis, Medical and Surgical Management

Barth A. Green, M.D. and K. John Klose, Ph.D.

Objectives

To provide a rational approach and protocols for the multidisciplinary team triage and care of acute spinal cord injury victims from their arrival at the emergency room through the various diagnostic and therapeutic components of the acute care program. These include (1) emergency room triage, (2) neurological as well as orthopedic and general assessments, (3) neuroradiological assessment battery, (4) medical and surgical protocols and (5) intensive care management.

Emergency Room Management

When a patient suspected of having a spinal or spinal cord injury arrives at the ER, the same priorities as established for the accident scene must be initiated, i.e., (1) respiratory stabilization, (2) cardiovascular stabilization and (3) splinting the patient, i.e., immobilizing the entire spine in a neutral supine position.

The key to ER care is the multidisciplinary team triage. While the nurse takes the basic vital signs, the physician should

Barth A. Green, M.D., Chief, Acute Spinal Cord Injury; Associate Professor, Department of Neurological Surgery and K. John Klose, Ph.D., Director, Central Nervous System Trauma Programs, University of Miami School of Medicine, Fla.

Partially supported by grants from NINCDS NS 14468-03 and RSA 13-P-59258/4-02.

Parts of this chapter are taken from *Neurological Update* with permission of Peritz Scheinberg, Editor.

obtain a careful detailed history and perform a complete physical and neurological examination. The history has a special significance in these injuries, not only regarding therapeutic decisions, but also from a medical-legal standpoint. The majority of these cases become involved in litigation. Therefore, a careful history regarding mechanisms and forces involved in the injury is of importance. The victim as well as the witnesses and rescue personnel should be interviewed and their remarks included in the history on the chart. Past medical history and allergies and surgical history are significant with regard to developing a therapeutic plan.

The physical examination should be performed by the ER physician or trauma surgeon and should include a detailed assessment of the chest and abdomen as well as the extremities. If there is any suspicion of abdominal visceral injury, a peritoneal lavage should be performed by the appropriate team member. The extra 10 to 15 minutes it takes to clear the abdomen of suspected injuries is well invested, considering the dire consequences of an undiagnosed acute abdomen.

The neurosurgeon and orthopedic surgeon, usually together, examine the patient's spinal areas. The neurological examination should be comprehensive because of the significant association between head and spinal cord injuries. One of the most important aspects of the neurological assessment is the rectal examination because of the concept of sacral sparing. Any sparing of motor or sensory function in the perianal area classifies the patient as an incomplete deficit which changes the prognosis to one of probable functional improvement. The most significant assessment parameters are the motor and sensory evaluations. The presence or absence of reflexes has not been a reliable predictor of prognosis or of diagnosis of complete or incomplete lesions. A complete injury should be defined as a complete loss of motor and sensory function below the level of injury. An incomplete lesion should be defined as any sparing of motor or sensory function below the level of injury. As a general rule, patients with an incomplete lesion will show some degree of neurological recovery and patients with a complete lesion rarely show any degree of neurological recovery.

The majority of patients falling into the incomplete category show mixed motor and sensory pictures rather than falling into classical syndrome categories. The Brown-Sequard syndrome presents with an ipsilateral motor and dorsal column function loss from the level of injury down and a contralateral pain and temperature loss starting slightly below the injury level. This syndrome may be associated with a spinal cord hemisection, often from a penetrating injury such as a gunshot or stab wound or a rotational injury. The anterior spinal cord syndrome is usually associated with a flexion injury and is hypothetically related to interruption of the anterior spinal artery blood supply. In these cases, patients present with loss of pain, temperature and motor function below the level of injury but retain touch, vibration and position sense. The central cord syndrome is usually associated with a hyperextension injury in patients in the middle or older age groups often with severe spondylosis and spinal canal stenosis. This syndrome often presents in patients without spinal column disruption, although it can occur in cases of spinal fractures. These patients usually suffer damage to the central part of the spinal cord in the low cervical area and present with a neurological picture of motor and sensory deficit greater in the upper than in the lower extremities and most pronounced in the distal upper extremities. Such patients usually improve spontaneously, but often plateau neurologically with residual deficit most pronounced in the distal upper extremities. The acute cervical spinal cord syndrome is associated with a sympathectomy-like response to cervical or upper thoracic injury. These patients present with bradycardia, hypotension and hypothermia. They often have a blood pressure of 70 systolic, a pulse below 60 and a temperature below 94 F. The question of whether to treat this physiological imbalance pharmacologically is best answered with a Swan-Ganz catheter to monitor the cardiac index. Adjustments should be made on an individual basis according to the degree of cardiovascular function compromise.

The syndromes described in the preceding paragraph are most often associated with mid to low cervical injuries, coinciding with the most mobile and frequently injured spinal column levels. The thoracolumbar junction ranks second in the degree of spinal column mobility and is the second most commonly injured level. These injuries are often associated with a conus medullaris syndrome which may involve a combination of upper and lower motor neuron findings, often symmetrical, with severe compromise of bowel and bladder function. The cauda equina syndrome is associated with injuries below the first lumbar level and most cases present with an incomplete motor and sensory lesion, often asymmetrical, which carries a fairly good prognosis for recovery (i.e., involves peripheral nervous system tissue with a better potential for recovery). It should be emphasized that the majority of patients do not fit into any of these classical syndromes, but usually present as mixed motor-sensory deficits, best recorded as such with careful differentiation between the various sensory modalities and assessment of motor function using the classical 0-5 scale. It is our opinion that the presence or absence of bulbocavernosus reflex, cremasteric reflex, abdominal reflex, Babinski reflex or withdrawal reflex is not a reliable sign with regard to prognosis and should not be considered to be as significant as motor or sensory sparing.

Spinal shock is usually synonymous with a complete lesion where there is loss of motor, sensory and reflex function below the level of injury. Initially, the patient is flaccid below the level of injury and presents as a lower motor neuron type of preparation. In a matter of 6 to 12 weeks these patients often develop manifest spasticity with increased reflexes and hypertonicity, heralding the end of the state of spinal shock. It has been suggested that the true neurological status of a patient cannot be assessed until after the stage of spinal shock, but it is our opinion that spinal shock is not as significant a prognostic factor as establishing whether the lesion is associated with a complete or incomplete deficit.

Spinal cord concussion is defined as a transitory alteration of spinal cord function, i.e., motor or sensory, which resolves within 24 hours following injury. Within the first 24 hours following injury, it is impossible to differentiate between a concussion and a more permanent injury. All acutely injured patients should be treated aggressively even when presenting with complete lesions, because they might evolve as a concussion syndrome, i.e., regain some degree of function within the first 24 hours, changing their entire prognosis. It is rarely possible to differentiate between a physiological and an anatomical transection of the cord, the latter being very rare.

While the physical and neurological status is being evaluated, a large bore catheter is placed into one or the other forearm veins and blood samples drawn for baseline CBC, electrolytes, coagulation studies, liver enzymes, cardiac enzymes, serum amylase, serum creatinine and serum osmolality, as well as for typing. The blood is usually typed and held rather than cross-matched until a decision is made to operate or transfuse the patient. Through the same large bore catheter, intravenous fluids, either Ringer's lactate or 5% dextrose in half-strength saline, is administered. A Foley catheter is inserted into the bladder and urine is sent for baseline analysis. If any gross blood is noted, an emergency IVP is performed. The baseline laboratory chemistries and urinalysis are repeated every 8 hours for the first 24 hours, then every 12 hours for the first 72 hours following injury, and after that at least daily for the next seven days. An electrocardiogram is performed for baseline assessment and repeated only as required by changes found initially or if stressful interventions such as surgery are anticipated. Baseline arterial blood gases are obtained in the ER; then a 40% O_2 humidity mask is placed on each patient and blood gases are repeated, with minimal acceptable levels of at least 100 PO_2 and below 45 PCO_2. When airway problems are significant enough to require intervention, tracheostomy should not be considered. With the use of a fiberoptic scope and nasotracheal intubation, there is rarely justification for performing a tracheostomy in the ER. Patients can tolerate endotracheal tubes for days and weeks without developing the complications which uniformly accompany tracheostomies, in particular Pseudomonas colonization. A tracheostomy also eliminates the availability of the anterior cervical approach when decompression and/or stabilization is required. The fact that a patient has good skin color and seems to be breathing adequately is not evidence of adequate oxygenation. Daily arterial blood gases should be obtained during the first week and then on a PRN basis as required by each patient's status.

Each patient with an acute spinal cord injury should have a central line inserted. In young, uncomplicated, healthy patients, a central venous pressure line is placed with x-ray localization into the right atrium. In multiple trauma patients or in older age group patients with complicated medical histories, it is preferable to insert a Swan-Ganz catheter and obtain baseline cardiac index parameters, including cardiac output and pulmonary artery wedge pressure. These catheters should be placed by experienced personnel with x-ray confirmation and be changed, as all central lines, every three to five days with special attention paid to the sterile management of the entrance site.

Once baseline physical and neurological examinations and laboratory tests are performed, the patient is taken to the x-ray department where a chest x-ray, abdominal x-ray and AP and lateral views of the entire spinal column are obtained. As part of this general survey, special attention is focused on areas of concern as indicated by the neurological and physical examinations. The entire spinal column is surveyed because the incidence of multiple level injuries is significant, i.e., approximately 20%. When indicated, skull x-rays or extremity x-rays are obtained. It can be most difficult to obtain good quality plain spinal films in acutely traumatized patients, especially in obese or muscular patients. Special views in these cases are indicated, such as swimmer's views of the cervical-thoracic junction. Pillar or oblique views of the cervical spine often provide additional information regarding spinal column disruption or stability.

On radiological examination, an initial determination of spinal stability must be made. Parameters of instability include severe disruption of the anterior and/or posterior elements at any level. In the cervical spine additional parameters for instability include subluxation of more than 3.5 mm or an angulation between adjacent bodies of greater than 11 degrees. Open-mouth views of the odontoid process are an essential part of the spinal survey. If the plain survey does not reveal any abnormalities, further scrutiny is directed to areas under suspicion after the physical and neurological examinations. *Under the neurosurgeon's and/or orthopedic surgeon's close supervision*, flexion and extension films are obtained at levels in question. Motion views often add critical information regarding stability and do not endanger the patient as long as they are performed with the required skill and under close physician supervision.

Patients complaining of pain with movement during such maneuvers should be returned to a neutral position immediately. Traction should never be applied in the pre-hospital phase or in the ER until baseline spinal surveys are taken and appropriate indications established.

If a neurological examination reveals a deficit, the authors recommend that 1 gm of methylprednisolone sodium succinate (i.e., Solu-Medrol) be given intravenously over a ten-minute period immediately in the ER. Theoretically, steroids are used as anti-inflammatory and anti-edema agents to stabilize ultra-structural membranes, to increase spinal cord perfusion and to minimize the effects of ischemia. These mechanisms are questioned by many authors with regard to therapeutic effectiveness. It is these authors' opinion that the general systemic benefits of high-dose intravenous steroids in these acutely traumatized and often shocky patients are sufficient enough to justify administration. It is well documented that the spinal cord provides an important feedback pathway for the endogenous cortisol response to stress. This pathway is often interrupted, especially in severe spinal cord injuries, thus providing additional rationale for endogenous cortisol administration during the first minutes, hours and days following trauma. As a prophylaxis to gastrointestinal hemorrhage, each patient is given a dose of 0.1 mg of Robinul (an anticholinergic with specific inhibiting action on gastric acid secretion) with each dose of steroid and a nasogastric sump tube is inserted in the ER and connected to a low continuous Gomco suction apparatus whether or not an ileus is present. Each patient is kept NPO for a minimum of 48 hours following injury.

Simultaneous with steroid administration, 500 ml of 20% mannitol is administered intravenously over a 30-minute period. This hyperosmolar diuretic acts quickly to reduce edema with a response time in minutes rather than the hours necessary to obtain sufficient tissue cortisol levels from exogenous steroids. Mannitol causes massive diuresis, which requires careful monitoring of the intake-output balance, electrolyte balance and Foley catheter drainage at all times. *Mannitol should be used only with great caution in the face of shock*; however, it may actually be of benefit in shock because of its characteristic support of renal function. In shocky conditions, the Swan-Ganz catheter should be inserted and fluid replacement determined on a quantitative basis with serial cardiac index determinations.

Spinal cord injured patients are initially started on IV fluids at a rate of 125 ml/hr for an average-sized adult; appropriate volumes for children are calculated on a volume per weight basis. They should not be maintained in a dehydrated state as is the case with head injuries. Solu-Medrol, mannitol, and Robinul are administered IV every six hours. The only other medication given in the ER is 1 gm of Cefadyl as prophylaxis for the central line and Foley catheter and other invasive procedures. Wider spectrum IV antibiotic coverage is added in cases of grossly compounded or contaminated wounds. During the entire program of ER care, the patient should be maintained supine in a neutral position, sandbagged and taped (unchanged from his arrival status in the ER). Only after all baseline x-rays and tests and stabilizing procedures are performed should any change in position be considered. Patients should never be lifted, and any special manipulations or procedures should be performed under the close supervision of the neurological and/or orthopedic surgeons. Position changes should only be accomplished using a log roll maneuver.

Before leaving the ER, all cases of spinal instability from the C-1 to T-1 levels should be placed in a cervical traction apparatus. The easiest and quickest available is the Gardner-Wells tongs which requires shaving the scalp approximately two finger-breadths above the anterior aspect of the ear and preparing the area with Betadine followed by infiltration of the scalp with 1% Xylocaine. The tongs are then inserted into the outer table of the skull as determined by a meter, which should protrude 1 mm from one of the tong handles, indicating proper depth of placement. Once in position, attached bolts should be tightened with pliers to prevent displacement at a later time. An AP skull x-ray should be taken to insure proper placement into the outer layer of the skull. The area of entrance of the tongs should be dressed with Betadine ointment and this dressing changed and cleansed with antiseptic solution on a daily basis. The tongs may be placed 2 cm anterior to this location in cases where additional extension is required for optimal reduction and 2 cm posterior in cases where additional flexion would benefit fracture reduction. A new type of apparatus called the Heifetz tongs is now available; it has three-point fixation to minimize the AP rotation of the skull and maximize the capability of reduction in certain degrees of extension or flexion.

In cases where the surgeon anticipates the application of a halo either as primary treatment for the fracture or as supplementary support to surgical stabilization, the halo ring should be inserted in the ER instead of the Gardner-Wells or Heifetz tongs. This procedure takes a few additional minutes, but ultimately saves time and minimizes the chance of secondary injury if application of halo jacket cervical traction is anticipated. We suggest keeping a supply of various sizes of halo rings in the ER. Custom polypropylene jackets can be ordered and delivered on a 24-hour basis to complete the halo traction apparatus. These authors prefer the custom-made polypropylene jackets with sheepskin linings to conventional plaster jackets. The halo jacket should not be applied in the ER before the neuroradiological assessment and therapeutic program decisions have been made. These jackets should never be applied before a central line, either CVP or Swan-Ganz catheter, is in place. In critical patients, the halo jacket presents an added risk if cardiopulmonary resuscitation, i.e., external massage, is a possibility. In these cases, the jackets should not be applied until the patient is stabilized and ICU discharge is anticipated.

Cervical traction should not be applied until x-ray control is available, i.e., never in the pre-hospital phase. The basic rule of thumb is to start with 5 lb per interspace. For example, a C3-4 dislocation usually requires between 15 and 20 lb and a C6-7 between 30 and 35 lb of traction. There are many exceptions to this rule, the most important being in cases of severe spinal disruption when even a lower cervical spinal column injury could be overdistracted by as little as 5 to 10 lb of traction and result in increased neurological deficit.

During the entire ER triage, the patient should be monitored constantly for cardiopulmonary and neurological parameters. Cardiopulmonary complications represent the major cause of morbidity and mortality in the first weeks of hospitalization following injury. Wireless telemetry is optimal in these cases because of patient movement between various areas within the hospital center setting. In the ER and during the neuroradiological procedures it is imperative that a nurse or physician be present at all times, because of the physiological lability that characterizes these injuries. After being evaluated and stabilized all patients with neurological deficits are moved to the neuroradiological suite for further diagnostic evaluations. The only exception to this rule is the multitrauma patient who has a life-threatening injury such as a ruptured viscus. Such complicating injuries take priority over the neurological injury when necessitating a life-saving procedure, i.e., abdominal exploration because of a drop in blood pressure or hematocrit or positive peritoneal lavage. In those cases the neuroradiological protocol is delayed until deemed feasible by appropriate consultants of the multidisciplinary team.

There are two significant pathophysiological factors in spinal cord injuries: (1) Intrinsic factors include hemorrhage, edema, ischemia, hypoxia and biochemical alterations within the spinal cord. These changes are being treated by the steroid-mannitol-oxygen regimen as well as by providing optimal perfusion of the injured tissue by maintaining physiological parameters as close to normal as possible. At this time, there is no agent or combination of agents or procedures which have been proven to be effective in reversing such intrinsic damage. (2) Extrinsic factors include any bone or soft tissue compressing the spinal cord secondary to spinal column disruption or pre-existing spinal cord stenosis. We believe that extrinsic factors, including compressing bone or soft tissues, can and must be dealt with immediately within the first minutes and hours following injury if there is to be any hope of reversing or limiting the intrinsic pathophysiological process.

Neuroradiological Procedures

At this time, the protocol for determining whether the spinal canal is patent (i.e., if there is any impingement by extrinsic factors upon spinal cord tissue) includes metrizamide myelography followed by computerized axial tomography. All patients are given 5 mg of Valium IV and 5 mg IM as a muscle relaxant as well as an anticonvulsant because of the possibility of seizure during or following metrizamide myelography. Using this protocol, there have been no reports of seizures over the last 24-month period in spinal cord injured patients.

The myelogram is performed using the following technique. The area around the mastoid process on either the left or right side is shaved and prepped with Betadine and draped. The area approximately 1 cm behind and below the mastoid process is then infiltrated with Xylocaine (1%) and a #20 spinal needle is inserted at the C1-2 interspace perpendicular to the spinal column and directed to enter the spinal column between the anterior and middle thirds of the spinal canal (i.e., if imaginary lines divided the spinal canal into three equal sections, then the junction of the anterior and middle thirds is the optimal point for needle placement for myelography). AP and lateral x-rays should be taken to insure the proper direction and degree of penetrance of the needle into the subarachnoid space. Fluoroscopy can expedite needle placement. Once the needle is in place, spinal fluid is withdrawn (3 ml) and 10 ml of metrizamide is injected slowly into the subarachnoid space with the patient's head at approximately 30 degrees reverse Trendelenburg to prevent the dye from defusing into the head. (The entire myelography procedure should be performed with the patient immobilized either on a plywood board or other appropriate orthosis. The O'Heir splint is a radiolucent polypropylene device recently made available which is optimal for patient immobilization during various phases of this protocol.) The head of the patient should be elevated slowly until the dye runs down to the point of suspected injury regardless of spinal level. Once the dye is pooled in this region, AP and cross-table lateral views are taken. In certain cases, special views may be obtained by manipulating the x-ray tube and x-ray plate without compromising the patient's splinted position. If the contrast material moves past the area of the lesion and there is no block or evidence of extrinsic compression, the metrizamide is then run up and down the spinal column to insure that no extrinsic compression exists at any other spinal level. The procedure is then terminated and the patient transferred to the computerized body scanner for views at the level of the lesion as well as other levels under suspicion.

If there is a complete block on the myelogram, before the patient is moved there is a further attempt to realign the spinal column. In the C-1 through T-1 level cases additional weights may be added to the cervical spine traction apparatus. In the past we have advocated the use of weights up to 100 lb. Recently, however, we have found that the key to reduction and realignment in these cases is the use of higher doses of muscle relaxants rather than excessive (do not use over 60 lb) weights for distraction. Since soft tissues stabilize the spinal column in a dislocated position, it is logical to treat the primary cause of the refractory subluxation, i.e., use additional doses of Valium under close observation of respiratory function. In difficult cases one may use as much as 10 mg IV and 10 mg IM (always given in 5-mg increments). In those rare cases in which the muscle relaxants and increased weights (not over 60 lb) do not reduce the dislocation, an anesthesiologist should be consulted and the patient intubated, ventilated and completely paralyzed to expedite spinal column realignment. Less than 1% of the blocks on cervical myelography (i.e., secondary to subluxations) have not responded to this protocol (in the C-1 through T-1 levels). Such reduction should always be performed under x-ray control and the reassessment of areas of previous blockage should be repeated after these manipulations. The rare cases of refractory block are usually due to pre-injury existing cervical stenosis from spondylosis or congenital causes. Rarely does intramedullary hemorrhage and edema account for a complete block in the absence of spinal canal stenosis. In cases of refractory blocks, immediate open (surgical) spinal cord decompression is indicated. Extravasation of contrast material during myelography can indicate dural disruption or avulsion of nerve roots as they exit the spinal cord. Dural disruption usually occurs only in penetrating wounds or in cases of severe distraction injuries. Nerve root avulsions have a classical myelographic appearance, especially at the level of the brachial plexus.

In cases of thoracic or lumbar dislocations, reduction by external manipulation can be performed with the patient in a supine position by carefully placing a pillow under the chest or back under fluoroscopic control. A certain degree of manual distraction on the shoulder girdle and pelvis can be of benefit in closed manipulations. We believe that only minimal efforts at closed reduction should be made, because only rarely will cases of thoracic or lumbar disruption and instability respond to manipulation. More aggressive attempts can result in further spinal distortion and secondary neurological injury. The addition of intravenous analgesics, as a supplement to muscle relaxants, is often of additional benefit. Manipulations should be performed only under the close observation of vital signs and neurological function.

After the myelogram is completed all patients are taken to the body scanner where computerized axial tomography (CAT) is performed while the patient remains immobilized on the spine board or other appropriate radiolucent splint. This study provides significant additional information regarding the degree of spinal column disruption and the integrity of the spinal canal and any compression of its contents. The CAT scan following metrizamide myelography yields greater information than either test individually. The recent updating of such computerized equipment adds the capability of longitudinal reconstruction, which provides additional information which can aid in determining the need for surgery or the type of surgery required. In certain cases, conventional tomography can be of benefit in evaluating spinal areas of difficult access or questionable involvement. These authors are of the opinion that such conventional tomography will soon be outdated by the increased availability and further refinement (i.e., increased speed and resolution) of computerized tomography.

If the patient has a history of iodine allergy, after a loading dose of steroids, they receive a C1-2 puncture and the injection of 4 cc of pantopaque into the subarachnoid space. This agent is not significantly absorbed and, therefore, has not presented a problem with regard to anaphylactic reactions. Another advantage is the fact that it is easier to visualize in patients with obesity or excessive musculature. This contrast material also remains available for postoperative myelographic reassessment. If there is not a complete block, additional pantopaque can be injected for a more detailed study and can be removed at a later date. These authors still prefer metrizamide as the agent of choice because of the decreased chance of delayed arachnoiditis and because of its greater solubility. In addition, metrizamide complements the capability of CAT, while pantopaque creates artifactual distortion in the CAT scan studies. Myelography is usually unnecessary in cases of penetrating injuries from gunshot and stab wounds where immediate surgical intervention is most often indicated. In such cases one must question what myelography could add to the information available from the plain x-rays and CAT scan.

Under optimal circumstances, the entire myelogram and CAT scan should require no more than one hour, time well invested in establishing a logical therapeutic plan for each case. Spinal cord angiography should be restricted to suspected vascular injury. In such cases spinal angiography with magnification (using subtraction techniques) can often provide useful information; however, for the average case of spinal cord injury such studies involve risks that outweigh any potential benefits. At this time the use of spinal cord evoked responses remains experimental. It has been our experience that patients who have incomplete clinical deficits may have absent evoked responses and, conversely, occasionally patients with clinically complete lesions have shown the presence of evoked responses. In contrast to the use of the well-defined evoked responses for auditory or visual function, spinal cord evoked responses require further refinement before becoming acceptable as a basic clinical tool. These authors are continuing to evaluate the use of evoked responses and are optimistic that technological advances may soon develop this method into a valuable diagnostic and prognostic instrument (not to mention the value for intra-operative monitoring of spinal cord function).

Therapeutic Pathways

Spinal cord injury patients who have completed the baseline assessments including the neuroradiological protocol are placed into one of five categories.

1. Patients with myelogram and CAT scan revealing no extrinsic pressure on the spinal cord (i.e., patent canal) and no spinal fractures or instability. Those patients are transferred immediately to the ICU to receive the standard acute care protocol with no indications for immediate or delayed surgery.

2. Patients with no evidence of extrinsic pressure on myelography or CAT scan, but with radiological evidence of spinal instability. These patients are transferred immediately to the ICU, where they are started on the standard acute care protocol. Seven to ten days after injury, they are taken to the OR for surgical fusion or placement in the halo apparatus or both.

3. Patients with myelographic and/or CAT scan evidence of a refractory block (i.e., extrinsic spinal cord compression which traction or manipulation has failed to relieve). All of these patients who arrive at the center within the first 24 hours are taken immediately to the OR where surgery is performed to reestablish the integrity of the canal (realign the canal), i.e., to decompress the spinal cord and/or its nerve roots and simultaneously stabilize the thoracolumbar injuries and only rarely cervical injuries.

4. Patients with penetrating wounds are taken immediately to the OR after ER and radiological procedures are completed. Their wounds are surgically debrided and all foreign bodies are removed and dural tears repaired.

5. Patients with life-threatening injuries that take priority over their neurological injury are not entered into protocol categories 1 through 4 until deemed safe by the appropriate multidisciplinary team members.

In rare cases when neurological deterioration occurs after the patient's initial examination a radiological reassessment is performed before any consideration is given to surgical intervention. In most cases readjustment of splinting and traction (i.e., spinal realignment) in conjunction with administration of extra doses of the steroid-mannitol regimen has been effective in reversing such changes which formerly were thought to require surgical intervention.

After surgery all patients with spinal instability are splinted by a Philadelphia cervical collar, halo traction apparatus or polypropylene thoracolumbar jacket as required by their level of injury and type of surgical procedure.

Intensive Care Protocol

After completing the ER and neuroradiological protocols and in some cases postoperatively, patients are taken to the ICU where they are placed on the Kean Roto-Rest Mark I bed. Each patient is rotated (continuous motion) for at least 20 out of each 24-hour period, being stopped only for feeding, hygiene, physiotherapy, respiratory therapy, diagnostic tests and x-rays. It is our opinion that the Roto-Rest bed is the only equipment presently available which effectively immobilizes patients with unstable spinal columns during all phases of acute care. Its continuous motion decreases the complications associated with the state of immobility experienced by paralyzed individuals. The system of hatches and flaps allows nursing and other allied health personnel access to all areas of the body without compromising spinal stability. The majority of spinal surgery procedures can be performed on the Roto-Rest, thus providing a continuum of kinetic therapy and spinal immobilization throughout preoperative, intraoperative and postoperative phases. Patients remain on the Roto-Rest bed during their entire intensive care stay. After discharge from the ICU, each patient remains on the bed as long as necessary to treat or prevent associated cardiopulmonary or other system complications. It has been well documented that the alternative devices sometimes used, i.e., the Stryker frame and Circo-Electric bed, are not safe or effective in the treatment of such patients because of their inability to maintain spinal stability as well as the compromise of respiratory function which may occur with the patient in a prone position. It must be emphasized that the Roto-Rest does not diminish the amount of time that intensive care nurses spend caring for each patient. Instead, it allows them to concentrate their efforts on more skilled nursing activities such as assessments and treatments rather than on patient lifting and turning.

All ICU patients are placed on routine orders including vital and neurological signs every hour and careful intake and output charting. Sump nasogastric tubing is connected to a low gumco suction for a minimum period of 48 hours. At that time, if a patient has good bowel sounds, the sump tube is removed and a clear liquid diet is started and slowly advanced. Once a general diet is tolerated, each patient is started on a medication program including daily stool softeners and laxative suppositories every other day. In addition, they are given vitamin C, 500 mg qid, and a multivitamin bid. Macrodantin, 100 mg qid, for prophylaxis against urinary sepsis is started when Cefadyl is discontinued after the tenth day of acute care. Foley catheters are retained for the entire ten-day period while patients remain on the steroid-mannitol protocol. Urine samples are sent for culture and sensitivity every three days while the indwelling Foley remains in place. After the tenth day, the Foley is discontinued and an every four hour intermittent catheterization program is instituted with weekly culture and sensitivity determinations. IVP, cystogram and urodynamic baseline studies are performed after the intermittent catheterization is started.

After their initial ER dose of steroids, 1000 mg, each patient receives 250 mg of Solu-Medrol and 0.1 mg of Robinul q6h for ten days. After the initial dose of 500 ml of 20% mannitol the patient receives 100 ml q6h for ten days, at which time this regimen is stopped abruptly without dosage tapering. There has been no evidence that dosage tapering is necessary in stopping these medications after only a ten-day treatment course. The reason for the ten-day treatment program with the steroid-mannitol protocol is because of evidence that central nervous system edema, although peaking by the second and third day, often remains significant at one week and can be present even as long as ten days following injury. The use of such high-dose steroids and diuretics during this short period has not been associated with any significant morbidity in these authors' experience.

The acute care medication regimen requires daily monitoring of blood chemistries including CBC, urinalysis and electrolytes as well as serum osmolality, urine osmolality, serum creatinine, serum glucose and serum amylase. Pancreatitis, whether clinically or only chemically evident, is common in spinal cord injured patients and may be associated with many factors, including multiple trauma with direct pancreatic injury, steroid administration or the spinal cord injury itself. When evident, this condition requires continuous sump nasogastric drainage and daily monitoring of serum amylase. In our experience in these cases it has never been necessary to discontinue the steroid regimen. Glucose levels also require careful monitoring in patients on the steroid-mannitol regimen. Daily serum glucose determinations are made in addition to urine testing every six hours for sugar and acetone. Each patient is covered with a regular insulin sliding scale, with treatment for a plus three or four sugar or acetone.

In cases where the patient remains physiologically stable, the Swan-Ganz catheter is usually removed between the third and fifth day and replaced by a central venous pressure line. All central lines are replaced at least every five days, but either a Swan-Ganz catheter or central venous pressure line is in place during the entire ten-day postinjury period. During this time each patient receives Cefadyl (1 gm IV every six hours) as prophylaxis for these lines (and for the indwelling Foley catheter). Maintaining good cardiovascular function and vital organ perfusion is a basic element in any program directed at maximizing neurological recovery as well as patient survival.

Each patient is provided with padded foam boots and full-length pressure gradient hose and receives full range of motion maneuvers of all four extremities during each nursing shift. Daily hygiene for the patient as well as for the Roto-Rest bed is required and includes chest physiotherapy treatments and jet nebulizer treatments as well as pulmonary exercise programs conducted by respiratory therapists. Postural drainage can be accomplished easily on the Roto-Rest bed. Chest x-rays and serial spinal x-rays are obtained at least every other day during the intensive care stay. These x-rays are taken through the radiolucent hatches and pads without compromising spinal stability. Miniheparin or aspirin has not been required while patients are on the Roto-Rest and receiving kinetic therapy. A review of the last 150 cases has revealed no occurrences of thrombophlebitis or pulmonary emboli in these kinetically treated patients. All patients being transferred from the Roto-Rest to a conventional bed when leaving ICU or postoperatively are placed on a regimen of either miniheparin (5000 units every 12 hours subcutaneously) or aspirin (10 grains orally or by rectum every 12 hours) until they achieve a state of increased daily mobility.

When arriving at the ICU each patient should again be informed (as in the ER) of the diagnosis and prognosis. Family and/or close friends should be an integral part of such discussions. Social service should be consulted on each case early during the ICU stay along with the other rehabilitation team members. Early communication creates optimal relationships between patient, family and the treating team and serves to expedite transformation into the next phase of treatment (rehabilitation center). Daily ICU contact in the form of treatments by other rehabilitation team members, i.e., physical and occupational therapists, is also of benefit in easing this often traumatic transformation from the ICU to the rehabilitation environments.

Most spinal cord injured patients experience various psychological phenomena following paralysis. The first phase includes *denial* of their paralysis and/or its permanency. This denial is often despite daily communication with physicians and other team members. The second phase is characterized by *anger* which is usually indiscriminately directed toward staff as well as the patient's family and friends. The third phase of *depression* often includes suicidal overtures, if not actual attempts. Patients often withdraw from the treating team, their family and friends. The first two phases usually last only a matter of days, whereas, the depression can last weeks, months and, unfortunately not too rarely, even years. Passing from the depressive stage is heralded by a patient's apparent decision to try to "cope" with his disability. It must be stressed that no paraplegic or quadriplegic will "accept" his paralysis. We have never encountered a paralyzed patient who doesn't wish to walk again at any price. Recognition and understanding of the psychology of spinal cord injury with its component phases can aid the physicians, allied health team, family and friends to better relate to these individuals during the acute postinjury phase. Programs directed at patient, family and staff education help to create an acute care experience most rewarding for all concerned.

It is not within the purview of this paper to discuss the next two phases of spinal cord injury system care which include rehabilitation and lifelong follow-up. Involvement with team members from both of these phases is of great benefit to those participating in the acute care protocol. Rehabilitation phase care should be performed by a multidisciplinary team of physicians and allied health personnel. Physicians include specialists from physical medicine and rehabilitation, neurological surgery, orthopedic surgery, psychiatry and urological surgery with consultants occasionally required from other medical specialties. In this country most physicians caring for these patients still retain their identification as members of certain medical specialties. Recently, there has been a movement toward establishing a medical specialty in paraplegia. Allied health team members include staff rehabilitation nurses as well as nurse clinicians, physical therapists, occupational therapists, recreational therapists, educational therapists, respiratory therapists, psychologists, social service specialists, vocational rehabilitation specialists, work evaluation specialists, peer counselors, dietitians, driver education instructors, urological technicians and various administrative personnel. It must be emphasized that only a part of the rehabilitation process is directed toward physical restoration. The total process also includes psychological, social, sexual and vocational rehabilitation, all of which are significant program components. The overall goal of this rehabilitation phase is to return each patient to society with the maximum degree of neurological function possible as reflected by their independence and mobility. Toward this goal, half-way houses (transitional living facilities) and communal living facilities have been created to ease patient movements between the rehabilitative phase of care and a more normal life within their previous family and community setting.

Lifelong follow-up care is a necessary part of a spinal cord injury system because of the importance of regular check-ups with regard to long-term patient survival. It has been estimated the average spinal cord injured individual, after surviving the first year following injury, has a life expectancy within 10% of that expected for the able-bodied population. Patient clinic follow-up visits should include evaluation by rehabilitative team members, not only of the patient's physical status, but also his general psychosocial skills. The major causes of death in the rehabilitative and lifelong follow-up phases of care are renal failure and decubitus ulcers. To prevent these complications and achieve the potential longevity that has recently been projected, it is necessary to insure that all patients leaving a rehabilitation institute be affiliated with a well-organized follow-up clinic care program. Whereas, few spinal cord injured veterans from World War I survived to World War II, today, spinal cord injured Americans are filling leadership roles in local and national businesses, professions and politics and have emerged as an effective part of our society.

Bibliography

Benes, V.: Spinal Cord Injury. Baltimore:Williams and Wilkins, 1968.
Green, B.A. and Callahan, R.: A radiological approach to acute spinal cord injury. *In* Radiographic Evaluation Of The Spine: Current Advances

With Emphasis on Computed Tomography. Massoon Publishers Inc., 1980.

Green, B.A., Khan, T. and Klose, K.J.: Comparative study of large doses of two commonly used steroids in the treatment of acute spinal cord injury. Surg. Neurol. 13:91-97, 1980.

Guttman, L.: Spinal Cord Injuries: Comprehensive Management and Research, ed. 2. Oxford:Blackwell Scientific Publications, 1976.

Ruge, D.: Spinal Cord Injuries. Springfield, Ill.:Charles C Thomas Publisher, 1969.

Yashon, D.: Spinal Injury. New York:Appleton-Century-Crofts, 1978.

Self-Evaluation Quiz

1. Which of the following is the most important part of the neurological examination with regard to prognosis in the acute spinal cord injured patient?
   a) Cremasteric reflex
   b) Bulbocavernous reflex
   c) Anal wink
   d) Sacral sparing
   e) Withdrawal reflex

2. The Brown-Sequard syndrome is most often associated with:
   a) Flexion injuries
   b) Extension injuries
   c) Penetrating wounds of the spinal cord
   d) High speed automobile accidents
   e) Diving accidents

3. The anterior spinal cord syndrome is usually associated with:
   1. Dorsal column function sparing
   2. Spinal thalamic function sparing
   3. Flexion injuries
   4. Extension injuries
   5. Cortico-spinal function sparing
   a) Only 4
   b) 1 and 4
   c) 1 and 3
   d) 3 and 4
   e) 4 and 5

4. The acute cervical spinal cord syndrome is classically associated with:

      1. Tachycardia
      2. Bradycardia
      3. A sympathectomy-like syndrome
      4. A vagal block
      5. Hypotension
      a) Only 4
      b) 2, 3 and 4
      c) 2, 3 and 5
      d) 3 and 5
      e) 4 and 5

5. A good prognosis for recovery is usually associated with:
      1. A complete lesion
      2. An incomplete lesion
      3. A cauda equina syndrome
      4. A conus medullaris syndrome
      5. Spinal cord transections
      a) 1, 3 and 4
      b) 2 and 3
      c) 1 and 5
      d) 2, 3 and 4
      e) 4 and 5

6. Pancreatitis may be associated with:
      1. Spinal cord injury
      2. Fractured extremity
      3. Blunt trauma to the abdomen
      4. Fractured pelvis
      5. Steroid therapy
      a) 1, 3 and 5
      b) 2 and 4
      c) 3, 4 and 5
      d) All of the above
      e) None of the above

7. The following are indications for immediate surgery in the first hours following spinal cord injury:
      1. Penetrating wounds of the spinal cord
      2. Neurological deterioration
      3. Patients with refractory myelography blocks after adequate trial of traction and manipulation with muscle relaxers and analgesics
      4. Patients with patent spinal canals on myelography or with spinal instability

    5. A ruptured spleen
    a) None of the above
    b) 1 and 2
    c) 3 and 4
    d) 1, 3 and 5
    e) All of the above

8. The most mobile and commonly injured levels of the spinal column include:
    1. High cervical level
    2. Sacral level
    3. Low cervical level
    4. Midthoracic level
    5. Thoracic-lumbar junction
    a) 1 and 2
    b) 2 and 4
    c) 1 and 4
    d) 3 and 5
    e) All have equal mobility

9. The two major causes of death in the acute in-hospital phase include:
    a) Respiratory and cardiovascular complications
    b) Renal failure and decubitus ulcers
    c) Aspiration and shock
    d) Pancreatitis and liver failure
    e) Gastrointestinal hemorrhage and shock

10. Spinal cord concussion is a transient loss of neurological function following a spinal cord injury with function returning within:
    a) 1 hour
    b) 12 hours
    c) 24 hours
    d) 1 week
    e) 6-12 weeks

Answers on page 391.

Cerebrovascular Disease: A Neurosurgeon's Perspective

Arthur L. Day, M.D.

Objectives

To concentrate on the pathophysiology and management of ischemic and hemorrhagic cerebrovascular disease. Areas to be discussed include relationship to arteriosclerosis, selection of patients for surgery, carotid endarterectomy, EC-IC bypass, the acute ischemic event, aneurysms and AVMs.

Stroke is the primary neurological disease and third leading cause of death in the United States. There are currently 2 million people in America alive after suffering a cerebral vascular insult, and the majority of these patients are below the age of 65 years. Because rehabilitation of patients with completed strokes is limited, the central aim of therapy in this disease is prevention [1].

Strokes may be subdivided into ischemic and hemorrhagic varieties (Table 1), based on the site and type of blood vessel injury. Ischemic strokes follow occlusion or thrombosis of the blood vessel lumen, causing impairment of blood flow beyond this obstruction. Nearly two thirds of patients with stroke disease will have this variety. In hemorrhagic stroke disease, blood escapes from the blood vessel, causing either a focal clot within the brain substance (intraparenchymal) or a diffuse layering of blood over the surface of the brain (subarachnoid).

Arthur L. Day, M.D., Assistant Professor, Neurological Surgery, University of Florida, Gainesville.

Table 1. Types of Stroke

1. Ischemic		
	A. Thrombotic	55%-65%
	B. Embolic	10%-15%
2. Hemorrhagic		
	A. Subarachnoid	10%-15%
	B. Intraparenchymal	10%-15%

Ischemic Stroke Disease

Most ischemic strokes are affiliated with arteriosclerosis, producing cerebral symptoms by one of several mechanisms. First, ulceration of the atheromatous arterial wall may act as a source of emboli (fibrin, platelets or cholesterol), which dislodge and travel up the cerebral circulation to occlude distal vessels. Arteriosclerosis may act as a substrate for thrombosis, acutely reducing cerebral blood flow and often causing infarction in the distribution of the involved vessel. Third, gradual luminal occlusion by atherosclerosis may progressively reduce cerebral perfusion. Combinations of these mechanisms frequently occur within the same patient.

Arteriosclerosis is a disease that primarily affects large arteries, with relative sparing of the distal vessels of the brain. The degree and distribution of arteriosclerosis is proportional to the blood pressure and the radius of the involved vessel. By eliminating (or bypassing) these proximal obstructive or ulcerative lesions, a reduction in the morbidity and mortality of ischemic stroke disease may be accomplished.

The resultant symptoms of ischemic cerebrovascular disease may be divided into several clinical categories. A TIA (transient ischemic attack) implies by definition a transient neurologic deficit lasting less than 24 hours and usually only for a few minutes. Deficits which reverse over longer periods of time are called RINDs (reversible ischemic neurologic deficits). Other clinical categories include a deficit which does not totally resolve (completed stroke) or chronic cerebral ischemia, usually secondary to multiple large vessel occlusion.

The presenting patient is immediately classified into one of these clinical groups, allowing the subsequent speed and choice of management to be more appropriately selected. The asymptomatic bruit may be approached somewhat leisurely, while patients with TIAs are more urgent. A high frequency or crescendo pattern of TIAs would be evaluated rapidly. Patients with acute completed infarction are generally not immediate operative candidates, and surgery in such patients is usually postponed for four to six weeks to allow the deficit and cerebral damage to stabilize. Chronic cerebral ischemia is a less well-defined entity, and its management is somewhat controversial at this time. This clinical syndrome usually follows multiple large vessel occlusions, with resultant gradual dementia or multifocal decline in cerebral function. Under these circumstances, distinction from degenerative diseases may be quite difficult.

A more focal example of chronic cerebral ischemia, however, may occur in some patients who do not recover satisfactorily following a completed stroke. The extent of functional recovery following cerebral infarction is generally attributable to the development of compensatory brain mechanisms or the recovery of neurons in the periphery of the infarcted areas. However, the relatively high late neurologic recovery rates reported following bypass procedures in patients with completed stroke support the hypothesis that a pool of "chronically sleeping neurons" surrounds many infarctions and that procedures designed to augment cerebral blood flow may restore function to some of these cells [2].

If a patient is judged to be an operative candidate (based upon his present clinical category and other associated medical risk factors), an arteriogram is performed. This study should include fluoroscopic visualization of the aortic arch, two views of each carotid bifurcation, and total intracranial circulation assessment. At least one vertebral and possibly selective internal and external carotid injections should be performed. Thus, the blood supply of the symptomatic hemisphere from primary and collateral sources can be evaluated.

Once the pathology is accurately identified, the subsequent management (medical versus surgical) can then be more properly selected. The chosen therapy is directed at the suspected mechanisms responsible for the patient's symptoms. Prevention of emboli or thrombosis may be accomplished by either medical or surgical therapy. Medical treatment includes cardiac stabilization and the use of anticoagulation (minor or major), while surgical treatment would include carotid endarterectomy. Improvement in cerebral blood flow by medical treatment is not directly effective, although thrombosis may be prevented for an interval sufficiently long enough to allow collateral circulation to develop. Surgical treatment to improve cerebral blood flow includes carotid endarterectomy and EC-IC (extracranial-to-intracranial) bypass.

Indications for medical therapy include severe major medical risk, recent major cerebral infarction, bilateral disease while awaiting a second procedure and mild-to-moderate ulcerative disease without evidence of stenosis. Angiographic abnormalities which may be helped by endarterectomy include carotid stenosis and/or ulceration, contralateral carotid stenosis and/or ulceration with an ipsilateral occlusion (with good intracranial cross-over) and external carotid stenotic lesions. Patients with carotid occlusions or associated intracranial lesions may benefit from bypass surgery.

Carotid Endarterectomy

Our anesthetic technique of carotid endarterectomy utilizes general anesthesia (halothane) and normocarbic blood gases. A shunt is used routinely, allowing the atheroma to be dissected more leisurely and providing excellent educational benefits. The arteriotomy is always extended beyond the termination of the atheroma if possible, thus minimizing embolism possibilities during shunt insertion. EEG monitoring, with our neurologist in the operating room, provides several advantages to the surgeon [3]. During the endarterectomy, focal abnormalities on the EEG may reflect shunt occlusion. In addition, focal electrical changes reflecting hemispheric ischemia will occur in some patients with a functioning shunt in place, and this response is frequently abolished by elevating the blood pressure 10 to 20 mm Hg. Mild hypertension is also routinely used during the periods of carotid clamping.

Postoperative monitoring is primarily aimed at blood pressure control and is achieved by radial artery cannulation. The manipulation of the atheromatous carotid bifurcation frequently impairs the carotid sinus regulation of blood pressure, especially in the early postoperative period. Uncontrolled hypertension may lead to rupture of the carotid artery or to intracerebral hemorrhage, especially in those patients who have had a previous mild cerebral infarction. Therefore, systolic blood pressure is maintained in the range between 120 to 180 mm Hg for at least 24 hours after surgery. Patients are not allowed to leave the operating room without prepared IV solutions of nitroprusside and neosynephrine to control their blood pressure at all times.

The risk of endarterectomy is largely limited by the other associated medical conditions (Table 2) [4]. Many patients also have similar degrees of arteriosclerosis affecting the coronary vasculature, producing angina, previous myocardial infarction or dysfunction and congestive heart failure. Patients with certain associated heart conditions should probably not receive carotid endarterectomy until the coronary arteries have been revascularized, either simultaneously or during staged procedures [5]. Even without concomitant or prior cardiac symptoms, endarterectomy patients would receive close cardiac monitoring during the early postoperative course to minimize myocardial consequences.

Certain endarterectomy candidates, including the asymptomatic bruit and the mild-to-moderate ulcerative lesion without stenosis, require special comment. The decision to angiogram a patient with an asymptomatic bruit is based on the risks of such a procedure at individual institutions, the location and character of the bruit and the associated medical risks of the patient. Noninvasive studies, such as ultrasonic arteriography or flow-

Table 2. Medical Risk Factors —
Endarterectomy

1. Angina
2. Myocardial infarction within six months
3. Congestive heart failure
4. Hypertension > 180/110 mm Hg
5. Diabetes mellitus
6. Peripheral vascular disease
7. Hyperlipidemia
8. Chronic obstructive pulmonary disease
9. Smoking
10. Age > 70
11. Severe obesity

directional doppler, may be useful adjuncts in this patient group. Endarterectomy is usually recommended for those patients with high-grade internal carotid artery stenosis (greater than 70% luminal reduction) or severe sinus ulceration (Fig. 1) [6]. Lesser lesions, or mild-to-moderate ulcerations in symptomatic patients, are usually treated with aspirin (10 grains bid). If symptoms break through on this regimen, surgery is then performed. All endarterectomy patients receive postoperative aspirin as soon as they can begin oral medications, and continuance of this medicine is generally recommended for as long as it is safely tolerated.

Microvascular Anastomosis (EC-IC Bypass)

At least one third of patients receiving arteriograms for ischemic cerebral vascular symptoms will have lesions which are not amenable to carotid endarterectomy [7]. This group of patients may now benefit from augmentation of cerebral blood flow by extrancranial-to-intracranial anastomotic procedures. A microvascular bypass should be considered when the angiogram identifies disease distal to the cervical carotid bifurcation or occluding it. Angiographic candidates for this procedure include occlusion of the common or internal carotid artery; stenosis of the internal carotid artery at the base of skull, siphon, or distally; middle cerebral stenosis or occlusion; and selected vertebrobasilar stenosis or occlusion (Table 3) [8]. EC-IC bypass may also be useful when an intracranial vessel must be sacrificed during tumor removal or aneurysm ligation and resection [9]. Thus, bypass surgery is able to circumvent large proximal obstructive lesions to augment deficient intracranial collateral circulation.

The clinical indications and risk factors for EC-IC bypass closely parallel those of carotid endarterectomy. Clinical categories include TIAs, RINDs, mild completed strokes with or without fluctuating neurologic deficits, generalized low perfusion syndromes and progressive or slow strokes. Clinical distinction of this group of patients from the endarterectomy group is impossible, and high quality pancerebral arteriography is essential.

The presence of an inaccessible intracranial lesion is not an automatic indication for EC-IC bypass. This operation has its

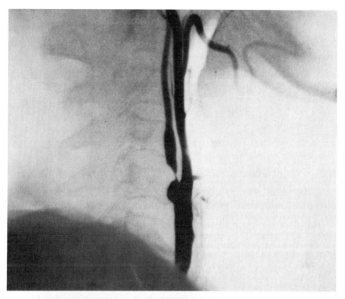

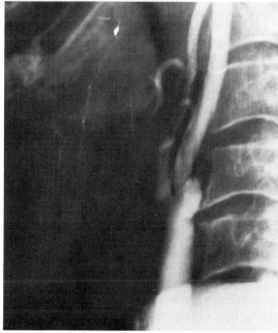

FIG. 1. Endarterectomy. *Top*, High grade, focal right carotid sinus stenosis. *Bottom*, Large posterior ulcer crater originating from internal carotid artery.

Table 3. Angiographic Indications for EC-IC Bypass

1. Occlusion of internal or common carotid artery in the neck
2. Stenosis of the internal carotid artery at the siphon or distally
3. Occlusion or stenosis of the middle cerebral artery
4. Selected vertebrobasilar artery occlusions
5. Planned occlusions with aneurysm or tumor resection

greatest effectiveness and patency rate when the offending lesion significantly reduces distal cerebral perfusion (Fig. 2). Ulcerative lesions are probably better managed with anticoagulation. In addition, many apparent intracranial or inaccessible stenotic lesions will resolve without surgery and probably occur following dissection, embolism or subintimal hemorrhage into a previously minor atheroma. Symptoms from high cervical, petrous and distal carotid siphon lesions, as well as many middle cerebral artery lesions, may be due to emboli rather than cerebral perfusion reduction [10-13]. A careful search for proximal disease (heart or carotid sinus) should always be performed prior to bypass consideration.

The postoperative management of EC-IC patients is also quite similar to endarterectomy, and careful attention to associated risk factors is mandatory. Complications with this procedure are often related to blood pressure, and this parameter is carefully controlled for the initial 48 hours after surgery with pressor or vasodilator agents as indicated. Hypotension, or compression from external sources (tight head dressing, glasses, nasal O2 cannula), have been implicated in some cases of graft thrombosis. Uncontrolled hypertension may lead to intracerebral hemorrhage at the fresh anastomotic site.

The emergency use of either of these procedures is rarely justifiable. Exceptions include fresh carotid occlusions during angiography, sudden loss of bruit with or without associated symptoms, thrombus identification within the vessel lumen, or inadvertent damage to an intracranial vessel. When one of these conditions is present, immediate barbiturate loading is recommended followed by the appropriate vascular procedure. Significant delays (greater than four to eight hours) in reconstitution of flow often lead to irreversible deficits or catastrophic hemorrhage into freshly infarcted tissue.

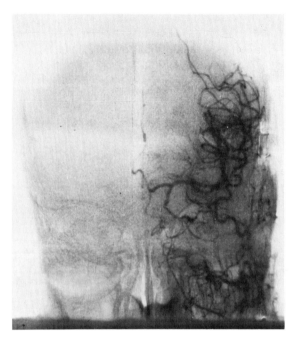

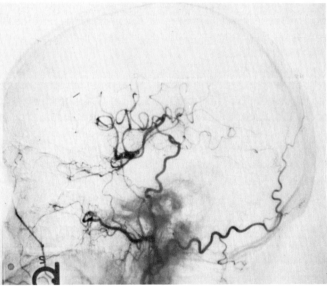

FIG. 2. EC-IC bypass. Postoperative angiogram in patient whose initial angiogram showed left ICA occlusion, trace left MCA filling from opposite anterior communicating collateral channels. *Top,* AP view. *Bottom,* Lateral view.

Hemorrhagic Stroke Disease

Intracranial hemorrhage may be divided into two broad categories, dependent upon the site and usual source of blood accumulation. The superficial location of aneurysms and arteriovenous malformation (AVMs) predisposes these lesions to bleed into the subarachnoid space, with diffuse layering of blood over the surface of the brain. Intraparenchymal hemorrhages, although sometimes associated with aneurysms and AVMs, are more often due to hypertension and are often deep in location. This discussion will center primarily around the perioperative management of subarachnoid hemorrhage, as largely practiced at the University of Florida.

Aneurysms

Most aneurysms present with subarachnoid hemorrhage and are unsuspected clinically until this event occurs. Survival from this initial catastrophe is limited by the site and extent of hemorrhage and its effects on the vital CNS life-supporting centers for cardiovascular and pulmonary function. Once the diagnosis is suspected, the care of these patients may be divided into preoperative, operative and postoperative phases, each with its own special hazards.

The preoperative management of subarachnoid hemorrhage is outlined in Table 4. A history suggesting this diagnosis should be confirmed with a lumbar puncture. A computerized tomographic (CT) scan is ideally performed prior to spinal puncture, especially in patients with significant deficits, to avoid potential complications from an associated intraparenchymal hematoma. Once xanthochromic spinal fluid is obtained, immediate measures are initiated to prevent bleeding while preserving maximal cerebral function. A detailed history and physical exam will disclose any associated risk factors which must receive special consideration. Particular attention is given to blood pressure, cardiopulmonary stability, electrolyte balance, hematocrit, state of hydration and prior medications.

After the initial evaluation, the neurologic condition of each patient is classified according to the Hunt modification of the Botterell System (Table 5) [14]. In the absence of significant intracranial hematoma, the level of consciousness is probably the most sensitive indicator of cerebral perfusion, and such a

Table 4. Preoperative Management of Subarachnoid Hemorrhage (SAH)

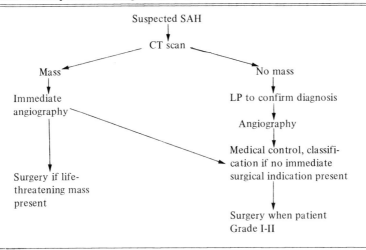

system is clinically useful in assessing the effects of the hemorrhage on the brain. A declining grade may indicate cerebral hypoperfusion, edema, or infarction or may reflect irregularities in oxygenation or electrolytes. A stable or improving level, especially in grade I and II patients, is usually an accurate indicator that the brain can tolerate the manipulation required to surgically obliterate the aneurysm.

Table 5. Hunt Modification of Botterell System of Aneurysm Grading

Category*	Criteria
Grade I	Asymptomatic, or minimal headache and slight nuchal rigidity
Grade II	Moderate to severe headache, nuchal rigidity, no neurologic deficit other than cranial nerve palsy
Grade III	Drowsiness, confusion or mild focal deficit
Grade IV	Stupor, moderate-to-severe hemiparesis, possibly early decerebrate rigidity and vegetative disturbances
Grade V	Deep coma, decerebrate rigidity, moribund appearance

*Serious systemic disease (hypertension, diabetes, severe arteriosclerosis, COPD and severe angiographic vasospasm) results in placement of patient into the next less favorable category.

Detailed cerebral angiography is usually performed on the earliest daytime slot available, except when life-threatening clot has been identified by CT scan. Transfemoral catheterization and selective injection of all four major cerebral vessels is preferable, with special views and subtraction techniques to accurately define the neck of the aneurysm and its relationships to adjacent vessels. Close correlation of the size, shape and location of the aneurysm with CT scan will usually identify the correct bleeding site when multiple lesions are present [15] (Fig. 3).

Until a suitable clinical status for surgery is achieved, awake patients are kept at bedrest in a quiet, darkened room with minimal stimulation. Neurologic function, blood pressure and pulse are checked every two to four hours, with particular attention to the level of alertness. Fluid restriction and sedation-seizure prophylaxis (with phenobarbital) often lower any associated hypertension, but antidiuretics, Aldomet or Apresoline may be necessary supplements. Antifibrinolytic agents, such as E-amino caproic acid (Amicar), are also advocated to postpone dissolution of the clot surrounding the aneurysm. Dosages of 36 to 48 gm/day are administered by continuous intravenous infusion via a Harvard pump [16].

Although the timing of surgical intervention remains contro-versial, patients with grade I or II classifications are certainly better operative risks than higher grades, and it is often our practice to operate on such patients as soon as this clinical grade is reached, especially when the aneurysm arises from the internal carotid or middle cerebral arteries. Midline basal (anterior communicating and basilar) and other posterior fossa aneurysms are more often postponed for 10 to 14 days, since earlier intervention at these sites may be accompanied by an increased incidence of postoperative neurologic deterioration.

Preoperative measures are continued until the patient enters the operating room on the morning of surgery. A slack brain is ensured by the use of steroids, lumbar drainage and osmotic agents. Deep hypotension using sodium nitroprusside is often employed during the dissection and clipping of the aneurysm. Once the offending lesion is removed from the circulation, blood pressure is returned to normal and the clip is carefully watched to ensure that its position is maintained. The patient is

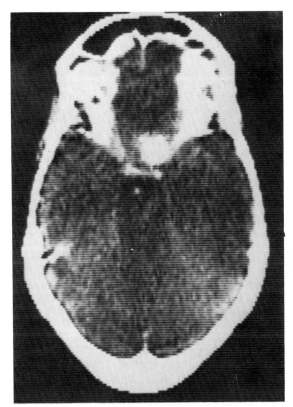

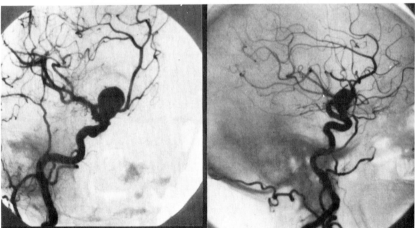

FIG. 3. Aneurysm. Right carotid-ophthalmic artery aneurysm producing visual loss, subarachnoid hemorrhage. *Top*, CT scan reveals contrast-enhancing lesion overlying right anterior clinoid process. *Bottom*, Oblique, lateral arterial phase angiography reveals 1.5 cm lesion.

then transfused with several units of packed red blood cells to improve circulating blood volume toward normal ranges.

Intensive care is maintained for the first 24 to 48 hours following aneurysm surgery to ensure adequate oxygenation, hydration and neurologic observation. The level of alertness remains as the most reliable indicator of adequate cerebral perfusion during this period.

Progressive neurologic deterioration is common in patients with aneurysms and subarachnoid hemorrhage and may occur in the pre- or postoperative period. Although vasospasm is the most likely cause for this deterioration, other common and more treatable factors may be identified, including hyponatremia, hypoxemia, seizures, hydrocephalus and recurrent intracranial hemorrhage. If an obvious systemic abnormality is identified, corrective measures are instituted immediately. If the cause of the decline is not evident, a CT scan is recommended. In the absence of clot, this study should be followed by arteriography to definitely identify the presence of vasospasm.

Once vasospasm is diagnosed, vigorous measures aimed at improving cerebral perfusion should be initiated. The patient is immediately transferred to the intensive care unit, where continuous monitoring of arterial blood gases, blood pressure, pulmonary wedge pressure and intracranial pressure are begun. Circulating blood volume is increased by the addition of whole blood, dextran, or crystalloid to elevate pulmonary capillary wedge pressure to high-normal levels (15 to 18 mm Hg). In preoperative patients, blood pressure is allowed to reach high-normal levels by the volume replacement and the reduction of hypertensive medication dosages. Induced hypertension (mean arterial pressure 110 to 120 mm Hg), using vasopressors, may be useful in patients whose aneurysms have already been removed from the circulation [17]. Oxygenation and carbon dioxide levels are maintained at normal levels, and any worsening ($\downarrow PO_2$, $\uparrow pCO_2$) is an indication for intubation and total respiratory control. High-dose steroids are administered intravenously to combat cerebral edema. Monitoring of ICP is accomplished by an intraventricular catheter, allowing removal of CSF to further improve cerebral perfusion pressure.

Further pharmacologic manipulation of the vasospastic vessels is controversial and unproven, although the failing and refractory course of some patients often justifies such desperate measures. Isuprel and aminophylline by constant intravenous infusion is currently the most promising pharmacologic treatment available [18]. This regimen is limited by frequent cardiovascular problems and its ineffectiveness on more chronically established vasoconstriction.

Prevention of vasospasm is theoretically more attractive than treating an already established case, and the combination of prophylactic kanamycin and reserpine has lowered the incidence of this entity in one large series [19]. Although circulating serotonin levels were reduced, similar clinical success has not been reported by others [20].

AVMs

Arteriovenous malformations may present with headaches, bruit, congestive heart failure, macrocephaly, hydrocephalus, seizures, progressive neurologic decline or hemorrhage. The progressive neurologic loss is often attributed to "steal," but the frequent operative identification of small, old hemorrhages suggests that subclinical bleeding may contribute to this phenomena.

The indications for surgery are based on the severity of the presenting complaints and the location of the offending lesion. AVMs producing hemorrhage-related episodes, regardless of location, should be strongly considered for surgery. Less severe symptoms require individual judgments based on the likelihood of further surgically induced neurologic loss. A superficial right frontal lobe lesion should be more aggressively approached than peri-Rolandic lesions of the dominant hemisphere (Fig. 4).

The subarachnoid hemorrhage from AVMs is usually milder than that associated with aneurysms and is rarely accompanied by any vasospastic complications. In the absence of mass-related life-threatening intraparenchymal hemorrhage, therefore, the initial course of most AVMs is benign. The long-term outlook for AVMs, however, is often discouraging, since major neurologic morbidity and mortality occur from recurrent hemmorhage, steal or seizure-related complications [21, 22]. To successfully reduce these long-term consequences, operative intervention must completely eradicate the lesion. A gliotic pseudocapsule often surrounds AVMs, and resection is often possible without neurologic worsening [23].

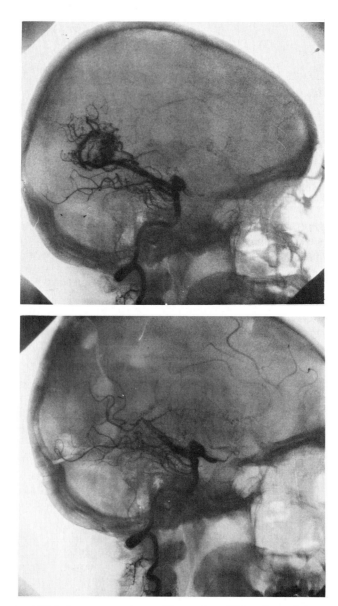

FIG. 4. AVM. Large vascular malformation filling from left posterior cerebral artery, producing visual loss, alexia, ataxia (hydrocephalus) from successive hemorrhages. *Top*, Preoperative view — AP-lateral. *Bottom*, Postoperative view — AP-lateral.

Interventional radiology using catheter injection of adhesives or emboli has not been shown to convincingly reduce morbidity from these lesions, although some authors feel that preoperative embolization reduces blood loss at surgery [24-26]. While sclerosing radiation may be useful in isolated cases, its beneficial responses may not become apparent for several years. Therefore, surgery should be considered in all accessible cases, regardless of presenting symptoms, because total surgical excision is the only proven effective treatment modality.

References

1. Chater, N., Mani, J. and Tonnemacher, K.: Superficial temporal artery bypass in occlusive cerebral vascular disease. Calif. Med. 119:9-13, 1973.
2. Lee, M.C., Ausman, J.I. and Geiger, J.D.: Superficial temporal to middle cerebral artery anastomosis, clinical outcome in patients with ischemia or infarction in internal carotid artery distribution. Arch. Neurol. 36:1, 1979.
3. Chiappa K.H., Burke, S.R. and Young, R.R.: Results of electro-encephalographic monitoring during 367 carotid endarterectomies: Use of a dedicated minicomputer. Stroke 10:381, 1979.
4. Sundt, T.M., Sandok, B.A. and Whisnant, J.P.: Carotid endarterectomy: Complications and pre-operative assessment of risk. Mayo Clin. Proc. 50:301, 1975.
5. Ennix, C.L., Lawrie, G.M., Morris, G.C. et al.: Improved results of carotid endarterectomy in patients with symptomatic coronary disease: An analysis of 1,546 consecutive carotid operations. Stroke 10:122, 1979.
6. Thompson, J.E. and Talkington, C.M.: Carotid surgery for cerebral ischemia. Surg. Clin. North Am. 59:539, 1979.
7. Hass, W.K., Fields, W.S., North, R.R. et al. Joint study of extracranial arterial occlusion. II. Arteriography, techniques, sites, and complications. JAMA 203:159, 1968.
8. Chater, N. and Popp, J.: Microsurgical vascular bypass for occlusive cerebrovascular disease: Review of 100 cases. Surg. Neurol. 6:115, 1976.
9. Gelber, B.R. and Sundt, T.M.: Treatment of intracavernous and giant carotid aneurysms by combined internal carotid ligation and extra-to-intracranial bypass. J. Neurosurg. 52:1, 1980.
10. Friedman, W.I., Rhoton, A.L., Day, A.L. et al.: Dissecting aneurysms of the internal carotid artery. Presented at the Southern Neurosurgical Society, Savannah, Georgia, March, 1980.
11. Day, A.L., Rhoton, A.L. and Quisling, R.G.: Resolving siphon stenosis following endarterectomy. Stroke. (In press.)

12. Hinton, R.C., Mohr, J.P. and Ackerman, R.H.: Symptomatic middle cerebral artery stenosis. Ann. Neurol. 5:152, 1979.

13. Day, A.L. and Rhoton, A.L.: Middle cerebral artery obstruction: The value of repeat arteriography. In preparation.

14. Hunt, W.E., Meagher, J.N. and Barnes, J.E.: The management of intracranial aneurysms. J. Neurosurg. 19:34, 1962.

15. Kendall, B.E., Lee, B.C.P. and Claveria, E.: Computerized tomography and angiography in subarachnoid hemorrhage. Br. J. Radiol. 49:483, 1976.

16. Tovi, D.: The use of antifibrinolytic drugs to prevent early recurrent aneurysmal subarachnoid hemorrhage. Acta Neurol. Scand. 49:163, 1973.

17. Gianotta, S.L., McGillicuddy, J.E. and Kindt, G.W.: Diagnosis and treatment of post-operative cerebral vasospasm. Surg. Neurol. 8:286, 1977.

18. Fleisher, A.S., Raggio, J.F. and Tindall, G.T.: Aminophylline and isoproterenol in the treatment of cerebral vasospasm. Surg. Neurol. 8:117-121, 1977.

19. Zervas, N.T., Candia, M., Candia, G. et al.: Reduced incidence of cerebral ischemia following rupture of intracranial aneurysms. Surg. Neurol. 11:339, 1979.

20. Blumenkopf, B., Wilkins, R.H. and Feldman, J.M.: Cerebral vasospasm and delayed neurological deficit after aneurysm rupture despite administration of reserpine and kanamycin, in cerebral arterial spasm. In Wilkins, R.H. (ed.): Proceedings of the Second International Workshop. Baltimore:Williams and Wilkins, Co. (In press.)

21. Forster, D.M.C., Steiner, L. and Hakanson, S.: Arteriovenous malformations of the brain: A long-term clinical study. J. Neurosurg. 37:562, 1970.

22. Troupp, H., Marttila, I. and Halonen, V.: Natural history of arteriovenous malformations. Presented at Symposium on Aneurysms, Arteriovenous Malformations and Carotid Cavernous Fistulae. 50th Anniversary, University of Chicago, November, 1977.

23. Kunc, Z.: Surgery of arteriovenous malformations in the speech and motor-sensory regions. J. Neurosurg. 40:293, 1974.

24. Kerber, C.W., Bank, W.O. and Cromwell, L.D.: Calibrated leak balloon microcatheter: A device for arterial exploration and occlusive therapy. A.J.R. 132:207, 1979.

25. Luessenhop, A.J. and Presper, J.H.: Surgical embolization of cerebral arteriovenous malformations through internal carotid and vertebral arteries: Long term results. J. Neurosurg. 42:443, 1975.

26. Stein, B.M. and Wolpert, S.M.: Surgical and embolic treatment of cerebral arteriovenous malformations. Surg. Neurol. 7:359, 1977.

Self-Evaluation Quiz

1. Hemorrhagic stroke disease, in which blood escapes from a blood vessel causing either an intraparenchymal or subarach-

noid clot, is more common than ischemic stroke disease in which a vessel is occluded from within.
a) True
b) False

2. The risks of surgery in ischemic stroke disease patients are best defined by transfemoral four-vessel cerebral arteriography.
a) True
b) False

3. The selection of the appropriate surgical procedure in patients with operative ischemic stroke disease can usually be made on the basis of the clinical signs and symptoms.
a) True
b) False

4. Re-establishment of cerebral blood flow by endarterectomy or EC-IC bypass usually results in improvement of the chronic neurologic deficit from previous infarction.
a) True
b) False

5. EC-IC bypass procedures have their greatest effectiveness and patency rate when the offending lesion:
a) Is located in the middle cerebral artery distribution
b) Produces certain characteristic clinical signs and symptoms
c) Significantly reduces distal middle cerebral perfusion
d) Serves as a source for recurrent embolic events
e) Does not compromise collateral circulation channels

6. Most hemorrhagic stroke disease in adults arises from undiagnosed arteriovenous malformations.
a) True
b) False

7. The surgical microscope has greatly improved the surgical mortality in grade IV and grade V aneurysm patients.
a) True
b) False

8. Cerebral vasospasm (following subarachnoid hemorrhage) is usually easily distinguishable from other causes of progressive neurologic deterioration on the basis of clinical findings.
a) True
b) False

9. The most critical indicator that cerebral perfusion is inadequate (following subarachnoid hemorrhage) is probably:
   a) A dilated pupil
   b) Blood pressure elevation
   c) Level of consciousness alteration
   d) Angiographic demonstration of vasospasm
10. Symptoms arising from cerebral atherosclerosis may be favorably altered by surgery because of all of the following reasons *except*:
    a) The disease primarily affects large vessels, with relative sparing of the distal brain vessels
    b) Sources of emboli may be eliminated
    c) The disease is largely confined to the cerebral vasculature
    d) Completed stroke is often preceded by transient deficits (TIAs)

Answers on page 391.

The Early Management of Cerebrovascular Disease: A Neurologist's Perspective

Steve D. Wheeler, M.D. and
Peritz Scheinberg, M.D.

Objectives

An approach to the assessment and management of the patient with acute stroke is presented. Emphasis is on the differential diagnosis, medical complications, "stroke in progression" and available therapeutic modalities. The physiologic objectives of therapy are described along with the types of edema seen in cerebral infarction.

There are about 500,000 new strokes in the United States each year [1]. Of these, approximately 40% of the patients die within the first 30 days. Of those patients who survive, 40% will require special care, 40% have a mild disability and 10% have no disability. Thus, it is clear that the provision of adequate facilities and care for these patients is a major public health problem. The aggressive acute management of these patients conceivably could alter the necessity for prolonged care if their deficits were minimal or reversed.

In recent years there has been a substantial decline in the incidence of stroke and its associated mortality in the United States [2]. This probably is in part a result of a change in cigarette smoking habits and the identification and aggressive treatment of hypertension, hypercholesterolemia and obesity. Indeed, the reduction in mortality from stroke is probably not

Steve D. Wheeler, M.D., Resident in Neurology and Peritz Scheinberg, M.D., Professor and Chairman of Neurology, University of Miami Medical Center, Fla.

only related to the changing incidence, but also reflects the considerable improvement and increased sophistication in the techniques of diagnosis and care of the acutely ill patient.

During the early 1950s there was a renaissance in cerebrovascular disease, with major contributions made by such pioneers as C. Miller Fisher, Clark Millikan and Michael DeBakey [3-8]. They provided major impetus into the study of carotid and vertebral artery disease, anticoagulation and carotid endarterectomy. Recently, there has been considerable interest in the physiology and biochemistry of the cerebral circulation. Hopefully, this approach will suggest reasonable pharmacological interventions which might alter progression of the ischemic process.

The management of acute stroke is often a difficult problem and, unfortunately, there has not been much recent progress; however, there are several basic principles which govern the initial assessment and treatment of the patient with an acute stroke. Foremost, the etiology of the underlying disorder must be established. Second, the primary medical problems or their complications must be identified and treated. Here particular emphasis must be placed on the prevention of pulmonary aspiration. Third, progression of the neurological deficit must be determined. Finally, therapeutic intervention with pharmacological agents must be initiated when indicated.

Consideration of the differential diagnosis of the stroke syndrome brings a wide array of medical and neurological disorders into focus. Those who are intimately involved in the care of these patients realize that, on occasion, the problem is altogether different from a cerebral infarction. For example, patients with intracranial metastases may present with the sudden onset of focal signs which may represent hemorrhage into tumor. On the other hand, both primary and metastatic brain tumors can present with localized signs which insidiously develop over 24 to 36 hours. In part, this is related to increasing mass effect as a result of either attendant edema or enlarging tumor. Todd's postictal paralysis can simulate stroke, particularly when there is no previous history of epilepsy. Focal neurologic signs may be present in the metabolic encephalopathies. Thus, such disorders as hypoglycemia, hypo- and hyperosmolar states, hepatic and uremic encephalopathy must be considered, although the presence of postural tremor, multifocal myoclonus and asterixis may help suggest an underlying metabolic derangement [9-11]. Unrecognized head trauma must be considered, since these individuals may be confused, amnestic or aphasic and simply unable to give an accurately complete history. The hemorrhagic disorders may be confused with cerebral infarction because they may progress; however, the management of subarachnoid hemorrhage, subdural hematoma and intracranial hemorrhage differs so drastically from that of stroke that they must be identified early.

Once it has been decided that the patient does not have one of the previously mentioned disorders the issue of thrombotic versus embolic stroke must be settled. The clinical profile of large artery thrombosis is different from that of embolic stroke. Thrombosis usually presents with the gradual, stepwise or stuttering onset of a neurologic deficit whereas a sudden or fluctuating onset is more typical of embolic stroke [12]. Emboli are responsible for approximately 35% to 40% of all strokes admitted to hospitals in the United States today. These in major part are a consequence of cardiac and carotid artery disease. Atrial fibrillation is said to increase the incidence of stroke fivefold and if it is accompanied by valvular heart disease there is a seventeenfold increase in the incidence of stroke [13]. Similarly, the sick sinus syndrome, also known as the brady-cardia-tachycardia syndrome, when associated with tachycardia, may present with stroke. In this syndrome strokes are either manifestations of profound bradycardia and inadequate cerebral perfusion or embolic phenomena associated with atrial fibrillation. Cerebral embolic phenomena in the setting of myocardial infarction occur secondary to either mural thrombus or ventricular aneurysm. A ventricular aneurysm may produce stroke by the generation of clot either within the aneurysm or adjacent to a hypokinetic ventricular wall. Additionally, atrial myxoma and mitral valve prolapse may predispose to stroke.

There is controversy concerning the issue of whether the incidental finding of mitral valve prolapse is reponsible for a significant number of cerebral emboli. There is no doubt that the true prolapsed mitral valve which is associated with myxomatous degeneration of the valve, progressive heart failure and arrhythmias may be associated with embolic phenomena.

Recently Barnett et al [14] reported the incidence of mitral valve prolapse in two groups of patients with cerebral ischemia, one above 45 years of age and the other below. Of those patients over 45 years, 8 of 141 (5.7%) had prolapse, but 24 of 60 patients (40%) below the age of 45 had prolapse, thus suggesting that in younger patients this entity may play a role in cerebral ischemia.

Needless lives are lost if there is inadequate management of the medical complications of stroke. Particular attention must be paid to the cardiac arrhythmias which occur in the setting of subarachnoid hemorrhage and cerebral infarction [15]. These often necessitate continuous electrocardiographic monitoring in an acute care unit. Otherwise, 24-hour ambulatory electrocardiographic monitoring can be used to identify less malignant arrhythmias and diagnose the sick sinus syndrome. Atrial fibrillation, endocarditis, myocardial infarction, ventricular aneurysm, mitral valve proplase, cardiomyopathy and atrial myxoma may predispose to further systemic and cerebral embolization. Low cardiac output states must be treated since they may potentiate cerebral ischemia. Urosepsis following urinary retention must be avoided.

The major emphasis in the management of pulmonary aspiration is prevention. Good nursing care is essential. The patient who is lethargic or who has had a vertebral-basilar stroke must be watched for the risk factors associated with aspiration. The head of the bed must be elevated, the patient's ability to handle oropharyngeal secretions assessed and the status of the gag reflex noted. If the patient is unable to manage oropharyngeal secretions adequately because of obtundation or an absent gag reflex, timely consideration must be given to prophylactic endotracheal intubation, otherwise intubation may become a necessity as the patient progressively becomes hypoxemic. Once aspiration occurs it adds significant morbidity by prolonging hospitalization and can be a cause of death in a significant number of patients.

During the first 12 to 24 hours following an acute stroke the progression of the neurologic deficit must be closely monitored with frequent vital signs and neurological examinations. It is these initial hours which are exceedingly important simply because it is impossible to adequately predict the degree of recovery that an individual may make; thus, if there is a role for therapeutic interventions, they must certainly be initiated prior to the onset of completed stroke, brain herniation or death. Even though there is no indication for anticoagulation in completed strokes, there is evidence which suggests that it is beneficial in progressive strokes [16]. Progression of a previous neurological deficit does not, however, imply extension of a cerebral infarction. The possibility of increasing mass effect secondary to peri-infarction edema must be considered. Unrecognized, this can eventuate in transtentorial herniation. Hemorrhage into an infarction or intracerebral hemorrhage also gives the appearance of "stroke in progression"; however, computerized tomography has decreased the morbidity that would have been associated with heparin anticoagulation of these lesions. Indeed, on clinical grounds alone it is occasionally difficult to distinguish hemorrhagic from nonhemorrhagic strokes. Although headache and moderate alterations in level of consciousness were once thought to occur with hemorrhagic strokes, recent observations suggest that this is not always true [12]. Thus, computerized tomography is the final arbiter and, when possible, every patient should have this study.

Therapeutic intervention in the management of acute stroke centers around the theme of preventing, reversing or minimizing progression of the ischemic state. In order to achieve this there are basically three physiological objectives of management: (1) to increase collateral circulation, (2) to decrease the rate of energy utilization and (3) to reduce brain edema.

Although the notion of increasing cerebral blood flow to the ischemic brain is relatively simple, it has not been easily accomplished. Earlier work suggested that since the cerebral vasculature vasodilated in response to falling pH, a concomitant rise in cerebral blood flow might be expected. Since carbon dioxide inhalation results in a prompt increase in cerebral blood flow, it was hoped that it would be of some clinical use. What actually happened, however, was that ischemic brain was further deprived of blood as the increased circulation was diverted to uninvolved normal brain. The consequence of this is a perpetuation of the ischemic process.

There are several clinical situations in which there is impairment of cerebral autoregulation, and cerebral ischemia is the most common of these. In this circumstance, instead of blood flow remaining relatively constant around 750 ml/min it tends to vary linearly with mean arterial pressure. Thus, if blood pressure falls precipitously, cerebral blood flow will fall concurrently resulting in the enhancement of any underlying ischemic process. Conversely, there is experimental evidence which confirms the impression that by increasing mean arterial pressure cerebral blood flow is increased [17]. Nonetheless, the methods used to induce elevated blood pressures have required vasopressors as potent as angiotensin, norepinephrine and metaraminol. Certainly, this technique would not be without considerable morbidity in an elderly population at risk for coronary artery disease. At any rate, there is presently no reasonably safe method of increasing cerebral blood flow; on the other hand, drastic blood pressure reductions should be avoided.

The concept of diminishing the rate of energy utilization by ischemic tissue presupposes that ongoing metabolism in injured tissue is harmful and that there is a critical period during which adequate collateral circulation develops. Hypothermia was originally employed as a method of reducing brain metabolism, but the risks of significant hypothermia are substantial. Subsequently, barbiturates were used for this purpose. It has been shown that pretreatment with barbiturates reduces the size of cerebral infarction in small animals whose middle cerebral or internal carotid arteries have been ligated [18]. The major action of barbiturates is probably on the cellular and subcellular membrane [19, 20]. It is a free radical scavenger and may inhibit the lipid peroxidation of the mitochondrial membrane, sparing mitochondrial swelling and certain cell death. Although theoretical considerations suggest that barbiturates should be useful in preventing ongoing cerebral ischemia, the clinical evidence thus far is unimpressive.

Cerebral edema associated with infarction can present a wide spectrum of clinical manifestations. These may vary from a mild progression of the original focal deficit to stupor, coma or a full-blown syndrome of tentorial herniation. Early in stroke cytotoxic edema occurs, but this is soon followed by vasogenic edema [21]. Cytotoxic edema represents swelling of all cellular elements following ischemic injury with failure of the ATP-dependent sodium pump, and rapid intracellular accumulation of sodium as water obligately follows to maintain the osmotic equilibrium. If the endothelial cells are so involved, they may swell to such an extent that they compromise the capillary lumen. Vasogenic edema, on the other hand, is characterized by increased capillary endothelial cell permeability. As edema fluid escapes there is a tendency to compress capillaries, thus the capillary lumens are more encroached upon and perfusion to the ischemic areas further limited. These considerations suggest, therefore, that the goal of anti-edema therapy should be to prevent the excessive intracellular accumulation of water and to prevent the diminished cerebral perfusion which accompanies capillary compression. These processes underlie cellular dysfunction and can eventuate in massive hemisphere swelling, brain compression and herniation.

Treatment modalities for brain edema have consisted of hyperventilation, corticosteroids and hypertonic solutions. There is no question that hyperventilation-induced hypocapnia in the range of 25 to 30 torr will diminish cerebral blood flow, resulting in a dramatic reduction in intracranial pressure [22]. Nevertheless, this response is temporary and acclimatization occurs within 24 to 48 hours. On the contrary, there is no consistently convincing evidence that corticosteroids are of any benefit in cerebral infarction [23], although there is some clinical suspicion that infarct-associated symptomatic edema, as demonstrated by computerized tomography, may respond to high-dose dexamethasone.

Osmotherapy relies on the principle that an osmotic gradient must exist between blood and brain to result in a water shift that produces a decrease in brain volume; however, there are several issues which must be considered when hypertonic solutions are utilized. The plasma osmolality must increase approximately 30 mOsm/kg H_2O above normal before there is a loss of brain water. Since equilibrium concentrations are reached in a few hours, the final result is only a temporary change in brain edema. As a consequence of vasogenic edema "shrinkage" occurs in normal brain where normal capillary permeability exists and does not occur in the edematous regions. Additionally, in view of the fact that the hyperosmolar solute is not excluded from the edematous tissue, there may be a rebound in edema formation. This rebound phenomenon particularly occurs with mannitol and urea and does not occur with glycerol. This is probably a manifestation of brain metabolism of glycerol to glucose, whereas the other hypertonic solutions are nonmetabolizable.

This presentation has addressed the principles involved in the early management of the acute stroke, emphasizing the importance of skilled and frequent observation of the patient's neurologic and cardiovascular status. Early treatment of ischemia is essential if infarction is to be minimized or prevented. The ideal pharmacologic agent has not yet been discovered, but continued studies of the biology of ischemia will certainly lead to a scientific rather than empiric form of therapy.

References

1. Stallones, R.A., Dyken, M.L., Fang, H.C.H. et al: Epidemiology for stroke facilities planning. *In* Sahs, A.L. and Hartman, E.C. (eds.): Fundamentals of Stroke Care. DHEW Publications No. (HRA) 76-14016, 1976, pp. 5-13.

2. Garraway, W.M., Whisnant, J.P., Furlan, A.J. et al: The declining incidence of stroke. N. Engl. J. Med. 300:449-452, 1979.

3. Fisher, C.M.: Occlusion of the internal carotid artery. AMA Arch Neurol Psychiatry 65:346-377, 1951.

4. Fisher, C.M.: Occlusion of the carotid arteries. AMA Arch Neurol Psychiatry 72:187-204, 1954.

5. Fisher, C.M.: The use of anticoagulants in cerebral thrombosis. Neurology 8:311-332, 1958.

6. Millikan, C.H., Siekert, R.G. and Shick, R.M.: Studies in cerebrovascular disease. III. The use of anticoagulant drugs in the treatment of insufficiency or thrombosis within the basilar arterial system. Proc Staff Meet Mayo Clin 30:116-126, 1955.

7. Millikan, C.H. and Siekert, R.G.: Studies in cerebrovascular disease. IV. The syndrome of intermittent insufficiency of the carotid arterial system. Proc. Staff Meet. Mayo Clin. 30:186-191, 1955.

8. DeBakey, M.E., Crawford, E.S. and Fields, W.S.: Surgical treatment of lesions producing arterial insufficiency of the internal carotid, common carotid, vertebral, innominate and subclavian arteries. Ann. Intern. Med. 51:436-448, 1959.

9. Montgomery, B.M. and Pinner, C.A.: Transient hypoglycemic hemiplegia. Arch. Intern. Med. 114:680-684, 1964.

10. Pearce, J.M.S.: Focal neurological syndromes in hepatic failure. Postgrad. Med. J. 39:653-657, 1963.

11. Raskin, N.H. and Fishman, R.A.: Neurologic disorders in renal failure. N. Engl. J. Med. 294:143-148 and 204-210, 1976.

12. Mohr, J.P., Caplan, L.R., Melski, J.W. et al: The Harvard Cooperative Stroke Registry: A prospective registry. Neurology 28:754-762, 1978.
13. Wolf, P.A., Dawber, T.R., Thomas, H.E. and Kannel, W.B.: Epidemiologic assessment of chronic atrial fibrillation and risk of stroke: The Framingham Study. Neurology 28:973-977, 1978.
14. Barnett, H.J.M., Boughner, D.R., Taylor, D.W. et al: Further evidence relating mitral-valve prolapse to cerebral ischemic events. N. Engl. J. Med. 302:139-144, 1980.
15. Weintraub, B.M. and McHenry, L.C.: Cardiac abnormalities in subarachnoid hemorrhage: A resumé. Stroke 5:384-392, 1974.
16. Genton, E., Barnett, H.J.M., Fields, W.S. et al: XIV. Cerebral ischemia: The role of thrombosis and of antithrombotic therapy. Study group on antithrombotic therapy. Stroke 8:150-175, 1977.
17. Hope, D.T., Branston, N.M. and Symon, L.: Restoration of neurological function with induced hypertension in acute experimental cerebral ischaemia. Acta Neurol. Scand. 56 (Suppl 64):506-507, 1977.
18. Smith, A.L., Hoff, J.T., Nielsen, S.L. and Larson, C.P.: Barbiturate protection in acute focal cerebral ischemia. Stroke 5:1-7, 1974.
19. Flamm, E.S., Demopoulos, H.B., Seligman, M.L. and Ransohoff, J.: Possible molecular mechanisms of barbiturate-mediated protection in regional cerebral ischemia. Acta Neurol. Scand. 56 (Suppl 64):150-151, 1977.
20. Demopoulos, H.B., Flamm, E.S., Seligman, M.L. et al: Antioxidant effects of barbiturates in model membranes undergoing free radical damage. Acta Neurol. Scand. 56 (Suppl 64):152-153, 1977.
21. Katzman, R., Clasen, R., Klatzo, I. et al: IV. Brain edema in stroke. Study group on brain edema in stroke. Stroke 8:512-540, 1977.
22. Harper, A.M. and Glass, H.I.: Effects of alterations in the arterial carbon dioxide tension on the blood flow through the cerebral cortex at normal and low arterial blood pressures. J. Neurol. Neurosurg. Psychiatry 28:449-452, 1965.
23. Anderson, D.C. and Cranford, R.E.: Corticosteroids in ischemic stroke. Stroke 10:68-71, 1979.

Self-Evaluation Quiz

1. Both primary and metastatic brain tumors can present with localized signs which develop over 24 to 36 hours.
   a) True
   b) False

2. Cerebral embolic phenomena in the setting of myocardial infarction occur secondary to either mural thrombus or ventricular aneurysm.
   a) True
   b) False

3. In recent years there has been a substantial increase in the incidence of stroke and its associated mortality in the United States.
    a) True
    b) False
4. Todd's postictal paralysis can simulate stroke, particularly when there is no previous history of epilepsy.
    a) True
    b) False
5. Management of intracranial hemorrhage, subdural hematoma and subarachnoid hemorrhage is the same as that for stroke.
    a) True
    b) False

Answers on page 391.

Panel Discussion

Moderator: Dr. Green

Panelists: Drs. Day, Marshall and Scheinberg

Moderator: The first questions are directed to me.

Question: Do you recommend the use of steroids in the field by the paramedics in the patient who has a Glasgow scale of less than 7 or a CNS spine injury?

Yes, I do.

Question: What do you do when you encounter your first seizure secondary to metrizamide in a cord-injured patient?

I hope we will not encounter such a patient; however, if we do, we would probably try to give intravenous Valium, establish the airway and remember our other priorities. Immobilizing the spine could be quite a problem if it did occur.

Question: Do you myelogram central cord syndromes?

Yes, we myelogram anyone with a neurological deficit who comes in within the first 24 hours except for penetrating wounds to the spinal canal. If the patient has the central cord syndrome but has a complete block with signs of extrinsic pressure on the spinal cord, then we do something about it acutely. Most of the patients with central cord syndromes are not blocked myelographically.

Question: What about prophylactic decompressive laminectomies?

We rarely do laminectomies anymore. A laminectomy is not appropriate in the majority of spinal cord injuries to decompress the spinal cord. In the thoracolumbar area, the Harrington rods realign, stabilize and decompress the cord. Usually, very little if any bone needs be removed. In the cervical area, if decompression is necessary, it is usually best attained by the anterior approach and should be combined with stabilization. But we do not do laminectomies with any frequency anymore.

303

Question: Do you operate on all gunshot wounds to the spine?

Yes, we do for those who come in within the first 24 hours who do not have general surgical complications which would contraindicate it. In other words, if this is the major injury, then we operate, but if the patient has a life-threatening abdominal wound or chest wound, that would take priority.

Dr. Marshall: Please address the issue of operative versus nonoperative management of the patient because I think there are at least 30 questions that deal with that issue. There is considerable misconception in the audience about what you in Miami do in patients who have complete spinal cord injuries.

Moderator: We operate on complete spinal cord injuries to realign the spinal canal and to stabilize them for early mobilization. We do not operate to make them be able to walk again. That is the principle behind our management, i.e., early stabilization for early mobilization. We do not always operate in order to accomplish it. Sometimes, we use the halo. But if instability requiring surgery exists, we do operate to stabilize. We usually use rods in the thoracolumbar and wires in the cervical area to stabilize. Decompression usually occurs with removing little or no bone, if one realigns the canal no matter what level is involved. We must stress that principle. Laminectomy is really useless in most cases. All it does is to potentially cause a secondary injury by making the spinal column unstable. We do not operate on patients unless they are unstable or incomplete further along following the early acute period.

Dr. Marshall: Dr. Green, do you use spinal cord cooling?

Moderator: I did a laboratory study as a resident that showed that spinal cord cooling is a sound concept except that it does not work because it preferentially cools the exposed part of the spinal cord. The body does a better job of heating the spinal cord than we can do of cooling it at this point. The problem is that there is a temperature gradient from dorsal to ventral. We did a great job of cooling the dorsal columns. In fact, clinical reports confirm this because people who went out and started pouring saline on patients' backs actually reported some dorsal column sparing. I think cooling has a very exciting potential, but we just do not have the technology to apply it at this time to make it a useful clinical tool, although it is being used by many people. I am sure Doctors Albin, White and others might disagree with me. I used spinal cord cooling eight years ago on one patient who did not change clinically. But I do think this technique has potential for the future if sophisticated.

Dr. Marshall: Dr. Green, why do you myelogram complete spinal cord injuries?

Moderator: Because, as I explained earlier, I do not know what a complete spinal cord injury is. Maybe someone can tell me.

Dr. Marshall: Completely out, motor, sensory, no reflexes, why do you myelogram him?

Moderator: You missed my point. The point is that I do not think a physiological short-circuiting of the spinal cord indicates that there is a physical transection, i.e., an irreversible lesion. It is my experience that within the first 24 hours, you cannot make that determination, and I do not think it is reasonable to deprive these patients of the potential benefits of early aggressive therapy with the idea of treating both the intrinsic and extrinsic pathological factors. I personally am unable to differentiate a patient with a spinal cord concussion from one with a total irreversible lesion.

Comment: I would like to make the comment that you are not the only institution which myelograms all complete spinal cord injured patients.

Moderator: At the University of Maryland, where Dr. Saul works, they have a very similar approach to trauma. It is one of the finest trauma centers in the country, and not because they do things similar to the way we do things at the University of Miami.

Dr. Marshall: I shall read the question and then answer it. The first question is: Do you increase your chance of making intracranial hematomas worse by administering mannitol prior to CT scanning?

That is one of the old issues in neurosurgery. If one has a patient whose neurologic status is deteriorating, one should treat the potentially treatable lesion, and that is intracranial hypertension, and I think the patient should have mannitol. As to the issue of whether one can make an intracranial hematoma worse, I think that is unsettled. One point that is important is I think all patients with significant head injuries should be treated with anticonvulsants. A very good study which will be published in the very near future on the use of prophylactic anticonvulsants in patients with severe head injury was done at the University of Kentucky. It is a triple-blind trial of diphenylhydantoin versus phenobarbital versus placebo in patients with severe head injuries. The incidence of late seizures was much higher in the patients who were treated with placebo, and a significant number of patients who were treated with either phenytoin or phenobarbital at six months could be removed from anticonvulsant therapy, having had no seizures and having done very well. I think that is a very important study. The other point concerns the patients who were treated with barbiturates. I certainly agree with Dr. Scheinberg, I think there is no evidence in stroke patients that barbiturates are of any use in man. The laboratory models are now coming into question. But using barbiturates to treat intracranial hypertension is a very different indication and they should be given prophylactic anticonvulsants concomitantly with that. We use dilantin because patients with severe head injury are at risk for seizure, and it is one of the preventable secondary injuries to the brain.

Dr. Day: *Question:* Why do you not use local anesthesia for endarterectomy, since it allows you to talk to the patient during surgery and to better monitor his function?

There are obvious advantages, of course, to monitoring neurologic function during endarterectomy, but I believe that EEG under light general anesthesia is also quite useful. Endotracheal general anesthesia assures maximum control of oxygenation and other parameters, while the EEG recording will identify most untoward intraoperative perfusion problems. EEG recording also allows a much more relaxed operating room situation, especially at a training institution, where residents perform many of the operations.

Question: If I have a patient who shows focal EEG abnormalities consistent with ipsilateral hemispheric ischemia that does not resolve with insertion of the shunt, what do I do with regard to protecting the brain? Would I give the patient barbiturates?

Under most circumstances, elevation of the patient's blood pressure will resolve the EEG changes, especially if they are due to hypoperfusion rather than emboli. If these changes did not resolve, then I would consider barbiturates. I do not know, however, of its effectiveness from personal experience.

Dr. Scheinberg: I have been asked to comment on the usefulness of or dangers of angiography for acute thrombotic stroke.

The fact is that if the patient has a significant neurologic deficit after an acute thrombotic stroke, we do not do angiography. Angiography is reserved for that period when the patient has recovered sufficiently hopefully that he might be a candidate for carotid endarterectomy, if in fact he has a carotid stenosis. So in the patient who already has the completed stroke, unless the neurologic deficit is minimal, angiography would not be considered. The dangers of angiography, of course, vary from one institution to the next. In those places where the people who are doing them are highly skilled, the morbidity is extremely low. But this is a procedure which has a very definite morbidity. Unfortunately, it also has a small mortality even in the best of hands and even under the most benign of circumstances.

Question: What is the role of anticoagulation in thrombotic stroke and embolic-ischemic stroke?

I wish I could answer that as simply as the question was phrased, but I cannot. This is a controversial issue. A number of studies have been done which pertain to the use of anticoagulants. Unfortunately, most of them have been poorly controlled. My response to that would be based upon my experience and what I believe to be the case and it would be very difficult to substantiate it from the literature. I do believe that there are patients, particularly with vertebral-basilar disease and/or intracranial vascular disease, who have had a definite transient ischemic attack or "small stroke" and who have significant viable brain tissue, whom I think are at considerable risk for the recurrence of a stroke. Therefore, I feel they should be on anticoagulants. I believe that the key to proper anticoagulation therapy is that it is done well, which means that the patients have to be followed extremely carefully, that prothrombin times have to be done regularly, just as anticonvulsant blood levels have to be done regularly because they can vary considerably. The reasons why anticoagulants have been in disfavor I think relates primarily to the fact that they have been poorly used. The patients have been allowed to go for weeks, months and sometimes longer without getting proper anti-coagulation and being properly observed. So, yes, I do believe that there are definite indications for the use of anticoagulants but I believe they have to be individualized.

Question: Why is aspirin effective in reducing stroke in the male and not in the female? Is aspirin a natural drug?

It obviously is. There is no question about the implication of Dr. Barnett's study — there was a 48% reduction in morbidity and mortality from all causes, particularly cardiovascular causes, in the men who took two aspirin tablets twice a day but not in women. The reasons are certainly not understood. But I think those reasons are potentially extremely interesting because they may offer us another view into what the differences and the problems are in the occurrence of those changes inside the vascular system which produce strokes in both sexes. But it is true that at the moment aspirin is not considered to be effective in women.

Dr. Marshall: I have a question about stimulating patients to maximum as a determining factor in gauging their level of consciousness. Is that still an acceptable method of evaluating the patient?

It depends upon what you mean. Masters' and Johnson's definition of maximum stimulation is certainly different from mine. I think if you look at Neil Lassen's pictures of what happens when you ask a patient to perform a very simple task, for instance, to squeeze your hand or to see what happens when you stimulate patients with a painful stimulus and you see what happens to cerebral blood volume, the changes can be absolutely fantastic. We like to monitor the patients who are paralyzed and ventilated with sufficient frequency so that their neurologic status can be assessed but with insufficient frequency that they are not stimulated every 15 or 20 minutes. So the patients on my service in general are examined three to four times per day, once by me and three times by the nurses, in an attempt to have a relatively good idea of their status. This does not mean we do not look at the pupils, it does not mean that we do not look at their caloric responses once daily, and it does not mean that they do not have a neurological examination. It does mean that we do it carefully and we do not stimulate the patient excessively.

Another question was about sedation, in terms of chest physiotherapy, what do I do?

As I said earlier, what is appropriate in one institution may not be appropriate in another. I believe that in many instances a little hyperventilation which not only primarily reduces cardiac output and does not change the PCO_2 prior to suctioning will blunt many problems. If one uses small doses of morphine, I think that is fine. The Europeans right now like an anesthetic agent called althesin for respiratory care and it is also used as an anesthetic in neurosurgery. I do not think the agent one uses is important. The basic principle that is important is that chest physiotherapy be guided by the ICP and one should take steps to prevent those things which will hurt the patient. What will hurt will be to hyperventilate them excessively, so you should sedate them with whatever drug you like.

Dr. Scheinberg: I would like to comment about what Dr. Marshall has just said. He mentioned that Dr. Neil Lassen and Dr. David Ingvar's beautiful study using computerized regional cerebral blood flow technique showed that there are regional blood flow changes in the brain with physiologic stimuli. Of course, that is true and I think it has been suspected for a long time. But what is also true is that there is no total increase in cerebral blood flow. There is simply a redistribution of blood flow. So in fact I am not sure that one has proven by this that it makes any difference whether or not one stimulates the patient in terms of how much blood one delivers to his head.

Dr. Marshall: I think the difficulty with that is that in a patient without a brain injury that is true. But at a meeting on cerebral vascular disease we were presented data from four places, including Lund and Copenhagen, looking at changes in brain-blood volume using the positron tomography device that Neil Lassen has, showing rather dramatic increases in patients who have an increase in intracranial volume, that is, patients with gliomas. There is a massive increase in cerebral blood volume just in patients who are moderately sick, whose ICP may not be very elevated, asking them to squeeze their hand or to raise one finger. So I think probably the difficulty has always been in CBF to go from normal brain where the compartmentalization of flow is normal, to the situation where it is abnormal in the patient with severe head injury, where you really do not know what you are looking at. I think there is relatively good evidence now that you are seeing big increases in blood volume because I cannot explain the change in ICP on any other basis.

Moderator: I think the answer would be probably not sedation and not rigorous chest physiotherapy, but to place these high-risk patients on a Roto-Bed. It does not affect the ICP and you can prevent respiratory complications and treat preexisting ones kinetically.

Dr. Day: *Question:* What is the role of aspirin, and where do we use it in the surgical management of patients? Do I routinely order aspirin in the patient who is having endarterectomy or do I use other agents?

I routinely use aspirin on all patients undergoing endarterectomy both pre- and postoperatively. The preoperative vessel wall may have less adherence of blood products that might embolize during the operation. Since the exposed postoperative vessel wall is potentially thrombogenic, I do not immediately reverse the heparin, but let it taper off. As soon as the patient is taking oral medications, aspirin is initiated in all patients who can tolerate the medication. Female patients are also given Persantine. Both these drugs are inexpensive and safe, and I currently recommend continuance for the remainder of life unless side effects intervene.

In addition, virtually all bypass patients are on a similar aspirin and Persantine regimen. The coagulation products in the small blood vessels of the anastomosis seem stickier under the microscope in some patients who have not been on aspirin, which, theoretically, may affect patency rates of the anastomosis.

Dr. Marshall: Many people have asked about vasospasm, and it might be useful to talk about the various therapies that are presently being used.

Dr. Day: Vasospasm is a very complicated constrictive reaction of cerebral blood vessels that usually follows aneurysmal subarachnoid hemorrhage. Although its cause is poorly understood, the catastrophic end result is brain ischemia and infarction. To date, there is no universally effective treatment of vasospasm. Medical measures that enhance oxygen-carrying capacity or flow are certainly logical in this hypoperfusion state, and there are accumulating anecdotal reports that oxygenation, volume expansion, blood transfusions and controlled hypertension may reverse neurologic deficits in some patients. This may be difficult, however, in the patient whose aneurysm is still in the circulation, since he may have increased rebleeding risks when such measures are instituted.

Kanamycin and reserpine can effectively deplete circulating serotonin levels, but this may not be the only agent or mechanism responsible for this disease. Certainly other institutions have not reported similar successes as those reported by Dr. Zervas with this regimen. Isuprel and aminophyllin also have received recent literature boosts, working by direct vessel relaxation and antagonism of phosphodiesterases. We have had some gratifying results with both of the above regimens, but of no statistical significance at present. Other causes of progressive neurologic deterioration are usually much more responsive to therapy and should be carefully searched prior to institution of any "vasodilator" therapy.

Pediatric Intensive Care: General Considerations

Bernard H. Holzman, M.D.

Objectives

Pediatric intensive care medicine has recently made major advances in monitoring and treating critically ill children. A broad overview of the field is presented with discussion of newer monitoring techniques, description of major differences between adult and pediatric physiology and an outline of newer therapies. The area of treatment of acute cerebral insults is emphasized.

The main objective of intensive care is to provide maximal surveillance and support of vital organ systems in patients with acute, but reversible life-threatening diseases [1]. In pediatric intensive care, this is of special significance because of the many useful years which can be added to the child's life. The key phrases here are "maximal surveillance and support," and "acute but reversible." In an intensive care unit, as much equipment and personnel as is required is utilized for each patient. Only if the second key phrase "acute, but reversible" is kept in mind, can such an enormous expenditure be justified.

In order to provide optimal intensive care, there are several requirements [2]. There must be a medical director whose primary interest and responsibility is the organization and administration of the unit and who assumes the role of overseer and coordinator of all patient care. This is especially important in pediatric intensive care, where the patients span a wide range of ages and, consequently, require different care. Additional

Bernard H. Holzman, M.D., Director, Pediatric Critical Care Medicine; Assistant Professor of Pediatrics, University of Miami School of Medicine; Director, Pediatric Intensive Care Unit, Jackson Memorial Hospital, Miami, Fla.

24-hour physician availability in Anesthesia, Pediatrics and Surgery is required. Nursing and allied health personnel must be specially trained. A wide variety of resuscitation and respiratory therapy equipment must be readily available, as well as emergency and frequently used drugs. Some of the more commonly used drugs are listed in Table 1. There must also be sufficient monitoring, with alarm systems, to provide continuous assessment of all basic physiologic parameters. Finally, there must be round-the-clock support by laboratory services and radiology.

Because of the great cost involved in providing pediatric intensive care and the need to provide that care repeatedly in order to remain proficient, pediatric intensive care units (PICUs) should be regionalized. Additionally, because the need for PICU beds for a given population size is less than for adult intensive care beds, these regions should be considered mega-regions, and a sophisticated air and land-based transport system needs to be available to provide transportation of patients from the outlying areas to the regional center. It is only by this means that costly duplication of services and underutilization of units can be avoided.

Monitoring

Until the recent past, PICUs were in fact no more than special monitoring and close observation units. Specific therapy was limited to providing respiratory support with artificial airways and mechanical ventilators. Therapies and techniques available were the same as were practiced in the general pediatric wards. In the early 1970s, however, newer monitoring and treatment techniques became available which could only be provided in a PICU. Most of the monitoring techniques which are currently used in the adult intensive care units are applicable to children, even down to the smallest infant. Techniques for monitoring the *pulmonary system* include continuous respiratory rate and apnea monitors, exhaled tidal volume, inspiratory and expiratory flow rates and inspiratory/expiratory ratios as well as the functional residual capacity of ventilator-dependent patients [3]. *Continuous temperature* monitoring with rectal, esophageal and skin sensors is available, with servocontrol

Table 1. Suggested Stock Medications

General	
Acetazolamide (Diamox)	Pralidoxime (Protopam)
Aminophylline	Prochlorperazine (Compazine)
Atropine	Promethazine
Calcium gluconate	Prostigmine
Chlorpromazine (Thorazine)	Propranolol (Inderal)
Cimetidine	Protamine sulfate
Dextrose −50%	Scopolamine
Diazoxide (Hyperstat)	Sodium bicarbonate
Digoxin (Lanoxin), adult, pediatric	Sodium polystyrene sulfonate (Kayexalate)
Dopamine	Sterile water for injection
Edrophonium	Succinylcholine (Anectine)
Epinephrine	Racemic epinephrine (Vaponephrine) for inhalation
Epinephrine-in-oil (Sus-phrine)	Regular insulin
Ethacrynic acid (Edecrin)	Vitamin K (Aquamephyton)
Furosemide (Lasix)	Antibiotics
Glucagon	Ampicillin
Glycopyrrolate (Robinul)	Carbenicillin (Geopen)
Heparin	Cefazolin (Ancef)
Histamine	Cephalothin (Keflin)
Hydralazine (Apresoline)	Cephapirin (Cefadyl)
Isoetharine (Bronkosol) for inhalation	Chloramphenicol
Isoproterenol (Isuprel)	Clindamycin (Cleocin)
Levarterenol (Levophed)	Erythromycin
Lidocaine (Xylocaine)	Gentamicin
Magnesium sulfate	Kanamycin
Metaraminol (Aramine)	Sulfisoxazole (Gantrisin)
Methyldopa (Aldomet)	Oxacillin
Multiple vitamins (MVI) for injection	Penicillin
Naloxone (Narcan)	Corticosteroids
Nitroprusside (Nipride)	Dexamethasone (Decadron)
Pancuronium bromide (Pavulon)	Hydrocortisone (Solu-cortef)
Paraldehyde	Methylprednisolone (Solu-medrol)
Phenylephrine (Neosynephrine)	Prednisolone
Physostigmine	Prednisone
Potassium phosphate	

mechanisms for automatically adjusting temperature blankets and radiant warmers.

It is in the field of *cardiovascular monitoring* in children where many advances have recently been made. Continuous ECG recording and computer-assisted arrhythmia detection is available, as is continuous vascular pressure recording. Percutaneous insertion of arterial lines can be done at several sites including radial, temporal, dorsalis pedis and posterior tibial arteries. Pulmonary artery catheterization with Swan-Ganz catheters is now available for the pediatric patient. The four-channel catheter available in 5 French sizes permits direct measurement of right atrial, pulmonary artery and pulmonary capillary wedge pressures, and the calculation of cardiac output, cardiac index, shunt fractions and arteriovenous oxygen content differences. The catheter can be inserted percutaneously, most easily from the femoral approach, and usually without the need for fluoroscopic guidance, with confirmation of proper positioning on the basis of pressure wave forms.

Most recently we have developed several techniques which allow us to continuously monitor the *central nervous system*. Radionucleotide imaging of the CNS, including blood flow studies, are now available in the PICU with the use of a portable bedside camera. Continuous electroencephalographic monitors are available from most major manufacturers of bedside monitors and many are available as individual modules which will mate with existing monitoring systems. The most frequently used technique, however, currently remains the continuous measurement of intracranial pressure (ICP).

ICP monitoring requires little additional equipment other than that required for vascular pressure monitoring. The ICP device is connected to standard fluid-filled pressure tubing, which in turn is connected to the transducer via a single-use disposable dome. No Intraflow* is required because there is no fluid infusing through the system. Pressures are recorded in the usual manner.

There are three types of devices available for measuring ICP. A subdural distal orifice catheter [4] can be surgically placed along the arachnoid membrane via burr hole or craniotomy. It should be a thick-walled semirigid catheter to prevent collapsing

---

*Sorenson Research Co.

and thus dampening of the pressure transmitted. This type of system does not permit CSF drainage for relief of pressure and does require placement in the operating room. As such, it offers the pediatric intensivist no advantage over a subarachnoid screw (see below).

The ventricular cannula, long used for acute treatment of hydrocephalus, has frequently been used as a device to allow measurement of ICP. It is inserted at the bedside through a small twist drill hole. It is easier to secure than the subarachnoid screw in smaller infants who have thin cranial tables. It has the advantage of providing a means of draining CSF and thus "venting" the ICP. In children following head trauma, as well as other cerebral insults, however, the ventricles are frequently small when they are first seen and placement of a ventricular cannula may be difficult. An additional disadvantage is that after multiple episodes of "venting" the ventricles may collapse ending the cannula's usefulness as a device to measure pressure, as well as for drainage of CSF.

We favor the Richmond screw or subarachnoid bolt [5]. It is placed by the bedside requiring only a twist drill set. It is a fluid-filled system connected via standard pressure tubing to the same type of transducer as is used for vascular pressure recording. In the past 12 months we have used the Richmond screw 23 times for as long as 13 days. There have been no instances of bacterial contamination, bleeding or cortical damage secondary to the screw or its insertion. It has the disadvantage of not allowing CSF drainage and of being difficult to secure in small infants whose cranial table is thin. We have found the pressures to be reliable with an excellent frequency response, and with appropriate nursing care they rarely, if ever, become obstructed.

PICU Treatment Techniques

Treatment techniques which are currently available to the pediatric intensivist include virtually the entire range available for use with adult patients and beyond the scope of this paper. A few, however, deserve special comment.

Continuous distending pressure (CDP), in one form or another, is used in small infants and children as well as adults. Some form of CDP is indicated in diseases in which there is reduced functional residual capacity, reduced compliance and atelectasis such as with pulmonary edema, drowning and aspiration pneumonitis. It is contraindicated in diseases such as asthma where there is significant air trapping. It can be used in spontaneously breathing patients in whom the airway pressure is kept positive only during the end-expiratory period in which case it is called PEEP or in spontaneously breathing patients in whom sufficient pressure is applied to the airway to maintain greater-than-atmospheric pressure in the airway throughout the entire respiratory cycle (CPAP, continuous positive airway pressure). When CDP is used in conjunction with a mechanical ventilator and the patient is not making any respiratory effort, it is termed CPPB (continuous positive pressure breathing). CPPB and CPAP can be used together in a patient who is making spontaneous, though insufficient effort to breathe by the use of an IMV (intermittent mandatory ventilation) circuit [6]. This allows the patient to inspire fresh gas while maintaining desired end-expiratory pressures when the ventilator is not cycling.

The principles of using *artificial airways* have changed little in recent years, although our understanding of them has improved. Airways currently used in children are made of implant-tested polyvinylchloride, are cuffless and the same diameter throughout their length. The absence of the cuff reduces the likelihood of damage to the tracheal mucosa, while the child's subglottis provides a sufficient seal to permit positive pressure ventilation.

When an endotracheal tube must remain in place for longer than several hours, or when the patient is combative, nasal intubation has several advantages over oral intubation and is the preferred route. Nasotracheal tubes are easier to secure and there is less motion of the tracheal end of the tube with the cycling of the ventilator. The course of the tube is over a less acute angle, thus reducing the airway resistance and consequently the work of breathing. Because the nasotracheal tube is easier to secure, the incidence of accidental extubation is much lower than with the orotracheal tube.

When an artificial airway needs to be in place longer than ten days, it is advisable to use a tracheostomy as the preferred airway. Despite the fact that it requires a surgical procedure, the incidence of postextubation complications from prolonged intubation with a tracheostomy is much less than with nasal or oral intubation. Repair of subglottic stenosis secondary to prolonged endotracheal intubation is difficult and has a higher morbidity and mortality than those associated with elective tracheostomy.

At the present time, support of the *cardiovascular system* in pediatric patients is limited to medical management. The technique of aortic balloon counterpulsation is not generally available for children. Swan-Ganz catheterization, however, has permitted convenient measurement of various parameters of cardiac function which can then be used to guide specific therapy [7]. With the availability of bedside pulmonary artery catheterization in children [8], pediatric intensivists are now able to separate the causes of a decreasing cardiac output into failures related to preload, failures related to problems of afterload and those related to myocardial contractility [9]. A low or decreasing cardiac output coincident with low right atrial pressures indicates an inadequate preload and specific therapy includes expansion of the vascular volume. When the afterload (that is, the stress placed on the ventricular myocardium during systole) is high, the peripheral vessels may be dilated by the use of vasodilators, such as nitroprusside. In those circumstances in which myocardial contractility is the primary cause of a failing cardiac output, inotropic agents, such as dopamine, Isuprel or epinephrine, may be used. For optimal support of the cardiovascular system, management must be directed at the specific factors which are responsible for a failing cardiac output.

The discussion up to this point has been in large measure an extrapolation of techniques of adult medicine to the small child. Children are not simply little adults, however. They are unique and the care they require is more than just smaller doses of adult care.

Differences of Children

One of the greatest differences between adult and pediatric critical care medicine is that in pediatrics one is usually dealing with an acute life-threatening process superimposed on a basically healthy organism, unlike the adult who frequently has had a number of less acute health problems predating the acute life-threatening process. The child, therefore, can tolerate a greater degree of stress both of the disease and the therapy required. For example, one rarely sees a fall in cardiac output from positive end-expiratory pressures in children, although it is relatively common in adults.

Physiologically, one of the more significant differences which must be kept in mind when caring for children is the greater surface area and, therefore, metabolic rate per unit weight. These factors result in a higher maintenance fluid and electrolyte requirement and caloric need. For example, the usual dietary water requirement for a healthy 70 kg man is about 2500 ml or 35 ml/kg. A healthy infant, on the other hand, has an oral water requirement of 130 to 150 ml/kg, approximately four times that of the adult. The factors comprising normal maintenance water requirements are listed in Table 2. Because small infants have a lower heat production per unit surface area than toddlers, and because young children have a greater surface area per unit weight than adults, the caloric expenditure per kilogram of body weight changes with increasing size. If we assume there is a requirement of 100 ml of water for each 100 calories expended, the formula for the calculation of maintenance fluid requirements works out to be 100 ml/kg body weight for the first 10 kg of body weight, 50 ml/kg for the second 10 kg and 20 ml/kg for each kilogram of body weight over 20 kg. Using this formula, a 17 kg child would have 1,350 ml of maintenance fluid requirements per day and a 24 kg child, 1,580 ml per day.

Table 2. Factors Comprising Normal Maintenance
Water Requirements

Component	Water Required (ml/100 cal)
Output	
Insensible water loss	45
Sweat	0-25
Urine	50-75
Stool water	5-10
Intake — water as a byproduct of oxidation	12

Adapted from Winters [10].

It must be remembered that these formulas for calculating maintenance fluid requirements are only guidelines for initiating fluid therapy. The results of that therapy must be monitored closely by following daily weights, total urine output, serum and urine electrolytes and osmolarities, and urine specific gravity. Any clinical circumstance which alters the metabolic rate will alter the basal maintenance fluid requirement. Conditions which cause an increasing metabolic rate and, consequently, fluid requirements include fever and hypermetabolic states, such as salicylism and hyperthyroidism. Circumstances in which there is a decrease in metabolic rate, such as hypothermia, result in a decreased fluid requirement. Additionally, abnormal fluid losses in children, such as vomiting and diarrhea, can be quite significant and must be replaced.

The pulmonary system is another where significant differences between adult and child exist. These differences relate to the airway caliber in both large and small airways. Because the total diameter of each generation of airways is smaller in the child, small reductions of the diameter, such as from mucosal edema or inspissated secretions, will result in large increases in airway resistance and the work of breathing. The airway resistance is inversely related to the fourth power of the radius of the airway. If the total diameter of the airway is 4 mm, 1 mm of mucosal edema will result in an increase of the airway resistance of 16 times! In the small child, the narrowest part of the upper airway is the subglottis and frequently this area will be only 4 to 5 mm in diameter. As a result, postintubation mucosal edema which does not cause significant symptoms in the adult is a common cause of respiratory difficulties in children, even after intubations of only several hours' duration.

Another difference between children and adults is the apparent better outcome following acute cerebral insults in the child as compared to the adult. Bruce et al [11] reported a series of 53 children who had had severe head injuries in whom 90% recovered fully or were only moderately disabled. Contrast this with studies of adults with similar head injuries in whom there was a 49% to 52% mortality. This improved outcome and the diffuse brain swelling commonly noted in children following severe head injury probably relate to differences in pathophysiology. In brief, the swelling appears to be due to cerebrovascular dilation and increased cerebral blood flow. This is manifested as an increase in CT scan density in swollen brain, not the decrease which would be present if the swelling were due to edema alone, and by a diffuse increase in blood flow considerably above normal values, not the decrease in blood flow seen in unconscious adults following head injuries. Bruce et al [11] found that up to 45% of children presenting with absent pupillary light response, abnormal motor posturing and impaired-to-absent caloric response will make a good recovery or be only moderately disabled and that the presence of spontaneous respiratory activity was a good prognostic sign. In our own limited series (Table 3) of 26 patients who had a severe acute cerebral insult, 12 patients presented without any spontaneous respiratory activity and all of these patients died. Of the five patients presenting with normal respiratory activity, regardless of other neurologic defects, all survived neurologically intact, although one subsequently died from pulmonary disease (Table 4). It has become our policy, therefore, to vigorously resuscitate all patients and institute aggressive management with hypothermia and barbiturates (see below) in all patients in whom there is any subsequent respiratory activity or evidence of central neurologic function.

Management of the Acute Cerebral Insult

By the term acute cerebral insult is meant one of nine basic pathophysiologic mechanisms as listed in Table 5 [12]. These

Table 3. Types of Acute Cerebral Insults in
26 Patients Seen at JMH Over 12 Months

Drowning/near drowning		11
Head trauma		6
Meningitis (bacterial)		4
Cardiac arrest		3
Anesthesia mishap	1	
Status epilepticus	1	
Unknown cause	1	
Encephalitis (viral)		1
Reye's syndrome		1

Table 4. Outcome Following Acute Severe Cerebral Insult
vs. Spontaneous Respiration

	Total # Pts.	Spontaneous Respirations		No. Spont. Resp. Effort
		Normal	Abnormal	
Good neurologic outcome	6	4	2	0
Poor neurologic outcome	2	0	2	0
Death	18	1*	5	12

*Two-year-old male — near-drowning — died on 17th hospital day from diffuse necrotizing pneumonitis and ventilatory failure.

are the primary injuries which initiate a series of events which ultimately lead to brain failure. The most frequent of these in pediatrics is global ischemia-anoxia in the form of drowning and cardiac arrest, trauma and infections, such as encephalitis and meningitis.

The basic principle of our aggressive medical management of acute cerebral insults is that the ultimate brain injury which results is a combination of damage which occurs at the time of the primary injury and damage which results from events which follow the primary injury and which could be termed the secondary injury. This secondary injury appears to result from a common mechanism regardless of the type of the primary injury. That is, it results from a fall in intracranial compliance and a rise in intracranial pressure. That the secondary injury occurs at a point in time removed from the primary injury is

Table 5. Basic Pathophysiologic Mechanisms of
Acute Cerebral Insult [12]

Global ischemia-anoxia, i.e., cardiac arrest

Focal ischemia-anoxia, i.e., stroke

Hypoxemia, i.e., severe anemia

Trauma, i.e., cerebral contusion

Hemorrhage, i.e., A-V malformation

Infection, i.e., meningitis

Metabolic failure, i.e., Reye's syndrome

Toxic insults, i.e., poisoning

Mass lesions, i.e., neoplasms

suggested by the ability of barbiturates to ameliorate the ultimate neurologic deficit. This has been demonstrated in cases of trauma [11, 12], ischemic injury [13, 14], hypoxic injury [15], infection [16] and Reye's syndrome [17] and suggests that a significant portion of the ultimate deficit occurs after the circulation and oxygen delivery has been restored.

A sequence of events is initiated by the primary injury, which begins with the loss of autoregulation of cerebral vessels in the area of the injury. This leads to an increase in the local blood volume and results in local cerebral edema. The intracranial pressure rises reducing the cerebral perfusion pressure which furthers the loss of autoregulation. As more edema fluid forms, areas of the brain distant from the original injury become ischemic and the cycle is repeated. Additional factors which can aggravate this cycle include systemic hypotension which amplifies the fall of cerebral perfusion pressure or hypertension which furthers the loss of autoregulation. Hypercarbia causes vascular dilatation increasing the intracranial blood volume and thereby the intracranial pressure [18]. Certain drugs, such as nitroprusside and nitroglycerin, can also cause cerebral vascular dilatation.

The management used in the PICU at the University of Miami is predicated on the principle of the final common pathway of the secondary injury, that is, the fall of intracranial compliance and the rise in ICP. The specific therapeutic maneuvers are based on the Monro-Kellie doctrine, that is, since the cranial vault is a semirigid container, any change in the volume of one of the three components — blood, CSF or brain — must be met by a reciprocal change in the other components if the ICP is to remain constant. When intracranial compliance has reached the steep part of the pressure-volume curve, any therapeutic maneuver which reduces the volume of one of the components will improve the intracranial compliance.

In addition to improving intracranial compliance, we would like to protect and stabilize vascular endothelial membranes to prevent the egress of fluid and cellular membranes to prevent the leakage of osmotically active particles into the interstitium where they promote cerebral edema formation. We are also interested in reducing cerebral metabolism, especially in the injured area, but generally throughout the brain so as to better match available blood supply to the oxygen demand. This will decrease the local hypoxemia and reduce the extent of anaerobic metabolism which is occurring. Finally, we want to reduce the hyperemia which accompanies the injury, especially in children, so as to reduce the blood volume component contributing to the increase in ICP and the fall in intracranial compliance.

There has been much suggestive evidence that for the treatment of the acute brain injury there is a significant therapeutic efficacy in a treatment regimen which includes osmol therapy [19], hyperventilation, steroids [20], hypothermia [12, 21] and barbiturate therapy [13, 22]. The treatment protocol in use in the PICU at the University of Miami incorporates these elements. The basics of the regimen are outlined in Table 6. An acute cerebral insult is defined as having occurred in any child who has evidence of a brain insult and is unresponsive, has abnormal brain stem function or CT evidence of significant cerebral edema following a brain injury. Intracranial pressure is monitored with a subarachnoid bolt unless there is specific indication for a ventricular cannula (i.e., for antibiotic instillation in ventriculitis).

Once the patient has been started on the regimen noted in Table 5, the ICP is used to guide changes in therapy. Any sustained ICP spikes over 20 torr for longer than 30 seconds are acutely treated. Acute therapy used is noted in Table 7 and used sequentially. If these measures are not effective or if the

Table 6. Therapy for Acute Cerebral Insult

Head position – midline, 30° elevation
Controlled intubation (sedation/paralysis)
Antacid therapy
Fluid restriction
Mechanical hyperventilation ($PaCO_2$ = 25-27 torr)
Steroids – dexamethasone (2 mg/kg initially followed by 2 mg/kg/day in four
    doses for duration of elevated ICP)
Paralysis
Mannitol – 1 gm/kg initially followed by 0.25 gm/kg q 4-6 hours; desired
    serum osmolarity 310-320 mOsm/liter
Hypothermia – surface cooling to 34 C
Pentobarbital – initially 3-4 mg/kg over five to ten minutes followed by a
    constant infusion of 1 to 4 mg/kg/hr. Desired serum pentobarbital level
    2.5 to 5.5 mg%

Table 7. Acute Therapy for Sustained
Intracranial Pressure Elevations

1. Manual hyperventilation (2 minutes)
2. Furosemide – 1.0 mg/kg IV
3. Paralysis – pancuronium bromide 0.1 mg/kg
4. Mannitol – 0.25-0.5 gm/kg as *additional* dose

ICP increases to over 20 torr repetitively, the infusion rate of pentobarbital is increased. Additional intravenous fluid and vasopressors are used to maintain the systolic blood pressure over 60 torr and the cerebral perfusion pressure (CPP = mean arterial pressure – intracranial pressure) more than 50 torr.

The treatment is discontinued in a sequential manner after 24 hours have passed in which there have been no spontaneous elevations of the ICP over 20 torr. The sequence of discontinuation is noted in Table 8. The results of this therapy on five patients are summarized in Table 9. Although these data remain anecdotal and not conclusive at this time, it is highly suggestive that combined therapy including moderate hypothermia and pentobarbital infusion is effective in improving the neurologic outcome following an acute brain insult.

Summary

Pediatric critical care medicine has changed a great deal in recent years. No longer is the PICU simply a respiratory care unit. We now have the capability to monitor virtually every organ system and actively intervene with modern aggressive and specific therapy. By far, the most exciting and promising of

Table 8. Discontinuing ACI Therapy

After the third postinjury day therapy shall start being discontinued after 24 hours in which there have been no *spontaneous* elevations of ICP > 20 torr.

Pentobarbital and hypothermia
Hyperventilation
Mannitol
Paralysis and sedation
Mechanical ventilation
Fluid restriction
Steroids

Table 9. Clinical Summary of Five Patients With Acute Cerebral Insults

Patient	Age	Diagnosis	Intracranial Pressure Initial	Peak	Length ACI Rx	Glasgow Coma Score on Admission	Sequelae
I — K.M.	10 mo	Near drowning (Estimated immersion 10-12 min)		—	5 days	3	Pelvic girdle weakness Mild truncal ataxia Motor milestones low-normal Delayed speech development
II — J.B.	11 yr	Near drowning (Estimated immersion 10+ min)	4 torr	27 torr (day 1)	5 days	5	Easy fatigability Bradylalia Expressive aphasia Intention tremor Past pointing Broad based gait Regular classroom
III — P.S.	14 yr	Cerebral & brain stem contusion (MVA)	0-4 torr	40 torr (day 2)	9 days	3	Slurred speech Bradylalia R. hemiparesis R. ankle clonus R. hyperreflexia Special school
IV — T.S.	5 yr	Cerebral contusion	6-15 torr	25 torr (day 1)	11 days	5	Receptive language delay R. hemiparesis Moderate ataxia Past pointing Special instruction
V — G.B.	22 mo	Near drowning (Estimated immersion 8-10 min)	6-10 torr	30 torr (day 2)	5 days	4	Moderately spastic quadriplegia Cortical blindness No verbalization Severely disabled, conscious but totally dependent upon others (Category III — Jennett & Bond *Lancet* 1:480-484, 1975)

these interventions is the medical management of the acute cerebral insult, since it is in this area that we have advanced from simply observing the natural progression of the disease to actively altering that progression. It is in this area that we can make major inroads in reducing the morbidity and mortality in our young patients.

References

1. Downes, J.J. and Raphaely, R.C.: Pediatric intensive care. Anesthesiology 43:238-250, 1975.
2. Guidelines for organization of critical care units. Report of the Committees on Guidelines. JAMA 222:1532-1534, 1972.
3. Geldt, G.P. and Peters, R.M.: A simplified method to determine functional residual capacity during mechanical ventilation. Chest 74:492-496, 1978.

4. Wilkinson, H.A.: The intracranial pressure-monitoring cup catheter: Technical note. Neurosurgery 1:139-141, 1977.

5. Vries, J.K., Becker, D.P. and Young, H.F.: A subarachnoid screw for monitoring intracranial pressure. J. Neurosurg. 39:416-419, 1973.

6. Downs, J.B., Klein, E.F. Jr., Desautels, D. et al: Intermittent mandatory ventilation: A new approach to weaning patients from mechanical ventilators. Chest 64:331-335, 1973.

7. Buchbinder, N. and Ganz, W.: Hemodynamic monitoring: Invasive techniques. Anesthesiology 45:146-155, 1976.

8. Pollack, M.M., Reed, T.D., Holbrook, P.R. et al: Bedside pulmonary artery catheterization in Pediatrics. Crit. Care Med. 7:141, 1979.

9. Ronan, J.A. Jr.: Hemodynamics of the central circulation. In Edwards, J., Lev, M. and Abell, M.R. (eds.): The Heart. Baltimore: Williams and Wilkins, 1974, pp. 17-29.

10. Winters, R.W.: Maintenance fluid therapy. In Winters, R.W. (ed.): The Body Fluids in Pediatrics. Boston:Little Brown & Co., 1973, pp. 113-133.

11. Bruce, D.A., Schut, L., Bruno, L.A. et al: Outcome following severe head injuries in children. J. Neurosurg. 48:679-688, 1978.

12. Shapiro, H.M., Whyte, S.R. and Loeser, J.: Barbiturate - augmented hypothermia for reduction of persistent intracranial hypertension. J. Neurosurg. 40:90-100, 1974.

13. Michenfelder, J.D., Milde, J.H. and Sundt, T.M.: Cerebral protection by barbiturate anesthesia. Arch. Neurol. 33:345-350, 1976.

14. Smith, A.L., Hoff, J.T., Nielson, S.L. and Larson, C.P.: Barbiturate protection in acute focal cerebral ischemia. Stroke 5:1-7, 1974.

15. Michenfelder, J.D. and Theye, R.A.: Cerebral protection by thiopental during hypoxia. Anesthesiology 39:510-517, 1973.

16. Nugent, S.K., Bausher, J.A., Moxon, E.R. et al: Raised intracranial pressure: Its management in Neisseria meningitidis meningo-encephalitis. Am. J. Dis. Child. 133:260-262, 1979.

17. Marshall, L.S., Shapiro, H.M., Rauscher, A. et al: Pentobarbital therapy for intracranial hypertension in metabolic coma: Reye's syndrome. Crit. Care Med. 6:1-5, 1978.

18. Shapiro, H.M.: Intracranial hypertension: Therapeutic and anesthetic considerations. Anesthesiology 43:445-471, 1975.

19. Brown, F.D., Johns, L., Jafar, J.J. et al: Detailed monitoring of the effects of mannitol following experimental head injury. J. Neurosurg. 50:423-432, 1979.

20. Hooshmand, H., Dove, J., Houff, S. et al: Effects of diuretics and steroids on CSF pressure. Arch. Neurol. 21:499-509, 1969.

21. Hendrick, E.B.: The use of hypothermia in severe head injury in childhood. Arch. Surg. 79:362-364, 1959.

22. Shapiro, H.M., Galendo, A., Wyte, S.R. et al: Rapid intraoperative reduction of intracranial pressure with thiopentone. Br. J. Anaesth. 45:1057-1061, 1973.

Self-Evaluation Quiz

1. In large randomized controlled clinical trials, barbiturates have been shown to be of definite efficacy in the treatment of the acute cerebral insult.
   a) True
   b) False

2. An inadequate "preload" as a cause of a low cardiac output is indicated by:
   a) Low right atrial pressure
   b) High right atrial pressure
   c) High pulmonary artery pressure
   d) High pulmonary capillary wedge pressure
   e) None of the above

3. The clinical observation that therapy with barbiturates seems to ameliorate the ultimate neurologic outcome following brain injury seems to indicate that:
   a) The secondary injury occurs at a point in time distant from the primary injury
   b) Barbiturates promote repair of damaged neurons
   c) Part of the secondary injury occurs after the circulation is restored
   d) a and c
   e) b and c

4. Because of the great need, every hospital having an adult intensive care unit should have a pediatric intensive care unit.
   a) True
   b) False

5. Which of the following methods of monitoring intracranial pressure also permits drainage of cerebrospinal fluid as a means of reducing the intracranial pressure?
   a) Subdural distal-orifice catheter
   b) Subarachnoid bolt
   c) Ventricular cannula
   d) a and c
   e) a and b

6. Swan-Ganz catheters permit monitoring of all of the following cardiovascular parameters except:
   a) Right atrial pressure
   b) Pulmonary artery pressure

    c) Pulmonary capillary wedge pressure

    d) Cardiac output

    e) Systemic arterial pressure

7. The narrowest area of the upper airway of a child is the area of the:

    a) Glottis

    b) Vocal cords

    c) Subglottis

    d) Trachea

    e) Carina

8. Mechanical ventilators which incorporate an IMV (intermittent mandatory ventilation) valve permit the patient to breathe spontaneously only while the ventilator is cycling.

    a) True

    b) False

9. The common pathophysiologic mechanism following an acute brain insult which significantly contributes to the ultimate outcome is:

    a) Systemic arterial hypotension

    b) Rising intracranial pressure

    c) Neuronal damage from the primary insult

    d) A rising cerebral blood volume

    e) None of the above

10. Of the requirements for providing intensive care for children, which is not included?

    a) Full-time medical director

    b) Physician availability in all major subspecialties

    c) Pediatric intensive care fellows

    d) Twenty-four-hour laboratory support services

    e) Specially trained respiratory therapists

Answers on page 391.

Pediatric Neurosurgical ICU: Special Issues

Larry K. Page, M.D.

Objectives

To discuss trauma, craniosynostosis, hydrocephalus, cranial-spinal anomalies and brain tuuors in order to illustrate certain special issues that must be dealt with in the pediatric intensive care unit.

It has been pointed out that children are not just small adults. They are often uniquely different. For instance, children are more resilient. They have a better prognosis, in general, in terms of head injury. The child's brain will often recover remarkably well after severe head injury. When an adult has dilated, fixed pupils and is unresponsive, the chance of any useful recovery is practically nil. That is not so with children. Children bounce back and surprise you time after time if one acts quickly to reduce high intracranial pressures. So resilience is more, but reserve is less, especially in terms of blood volume and fluids and electrolytes. In a full-term infant, there is only about 250 or 300 cc of blood volume so that before, during or after operation, if the child is hemorrhaging, there is very much less reserve available and less margin for errors in replacement.

In children, delay in diagnosis is common and can be seen in terms of the size to which a brain tumor will grow before anyone suspects what is occurring. In infants and small children, the nervous system really has not had a chance to develop very well. A frontal brain tumor that would cause an adult to start writing checks carelessly or present with a change in personality

Larry K. Page, M.D., Professor of Neurological Surgery, Department of Neurological Surgery, University of Miami School of Medicine, Fla.

cannot happen in the child who has not yet developed these high order functions. The child does not complain that he has difficulty with vision in one visual field or the other. These are reasons why these tumors grow to tremendous size before they are brought to anyone's attention.

I shall now discuss five types of disease — trauma, craniosynostosis, hydrocephalus, cranial-spinal anomalies and brain tumors — in order to illustrate certain special issues that must be dealt with in the pediatric ICU. Hematomas in children develop in the same areas as in adults. One unique difference is the tremendous edema that can occur diffusely throuuh the brain, sometimes with trivial injury. The ventricles become slitlike and the child rapidly goes into coma when often there is no hematoma involved. Of course, if there is a hematoma, it may be epidural, subdural, intracerebral, in the posterior fossa, or of the petechial variety that occurs in the midbrain. In following a child with head injury, it is useful to obtain serial hematocrits. If an adult patient is in shock with a head injury, one had better look elsewhere for the etiology of the shock, e.g., fractured hip, spleen, etc., if there is no obvious external bleeding. But in a child, subgaleal hematoma or collections of blood inside the calvarium may cause them to become quite anemic and go into shock. This is a valuable parameter that relates to the limited blood volume of children.

Intracranial pressure monitors can be invaluable to the care of the pediatric patient with severe head injury. The location for inserting the ventricular catheter or the subdural screw is the same. The twist drill is placed anteriorly to the coronal suture in the mid-pupillary line. The tools required to place a subdural screw of the Richmond type are a hand drill to go through bone, the bolt and its handle that screws it into the drill hole. We place this about 1 mm below the dura in the subdural space. In order to do that, the dura may be incised or a smaller sized drill bit may be used to penetrate the dura. After the sterile dressing is applied, the lines are filled with saline, and 1 to 2 cc is irrigated into the subdural space. Occasionally, the latter must be repeated when the readings become damped or disappear. In the infant especially, it is usually quite difficult to get the bolt screwed in because the skull is too thin. In such a case, we might use the cup catheter or place a ventricular drain.

Two ways to measure ICP are in current use: millimeters of mercury and millimeters of water. Attempts have been made to convert completely to millimeters of mercury but that will probably never occur because lumbar puncture measurements, which are the more common test, are made via a manometer of cerebrospinal fluid. One should be able to transfer readily from one system to the other. From our experience with hydrocephalus, we feel that if one is dealing with a child with sick neurons, the best milieu for improvement should be a normal or below normal ICP. The goal in the pediatric neuro-ICU is to keep the pressure at 20 mm Hg or below, although we prefer to maintain the ICP at 10 mm Hg or below. The use of mannitol in pediatric patients must be approached with extra caution and only used when absolutely necessary and under carefully controlled and monitored conditions.

Craniosynostosis is a congenital anomaly of the skull — premature closure of one or more of its sutures. The standard method of treatment is to create linear craniectomies lined with plastic film to keep the "iatrogenic fractures" from healing prematurely. Sagittal synostosis is the most common variety. Its correction should be by way of an operation that has almost no morbidity and no mortality. There is one most important point here. The blood volume of the infant on whom you perform this operation is small and critical. The one lethal possibility is mismanagement of blood replacement. These children may postoperatively ooze blood out from the bone and under the scalp. If this goes unrecognized, with a big bandage so it cannot be easily seen, the child can quickly go into profound shock. These patients must be carefully observed postoperatively in the ICU. These postop collections should be tapped percutaneously and measured and the lost volume replaced cubic centimeter for cubic centimeter with whole blood.

In children who have normal cardiovascular systems, and most of the ones who come to neurosurgery do, 10 cc of whole blood per pound of body weight provides a very safe transfusion. If there is any doubt intraoperatively or postoperatively that a child is going into shock, one can immediately give this amount of blood at a rapid rate, with minimal risk of right-heart failure, a complication of greater concern in an older patient population. The more involved these operations, the more blood loss one can expect postoperatively. We often overtransfuse infants to some degree intraoperatively. It is difficult to keep a good intravenous line in place in anticipation of the need for a blood transfusion one to two days later. By staying 10 cc per pound or less ahead of losses at operation, one can often avoid an additional transfusion on the first or second postoperative day. Multiple suture closures, especially the cranio-facial varieties that require combined neurosurgical and plastic procedures, must be very carefully followed in the ICU for airway as well as blood volume complications.

In the normal pediatric patient as well as in the case of hydrocephalus the CSF formation rate is constant. It does not, at least in the acute setting, vary with pressure. The rate of absorption, however, is linearly proportional to ICP. The more pressure, the more CSF is absorbed through the villi into the venous system. The slope of the line when pressure and absorption are measured and plotted in hydrocephalic children is shifted so that more pressure is required to force the same amount of CSF into the venous system through the arachnoid villi. Except in the rare case of choroid plexus papilloma, hydrocephalus occurs because of an increased resistance to CSF absorption.

It is useful to consider hydrocephalus as it occurs in premature infants, full-term infants and children. We have a large premature infant center at our institution. Hydrocephalus in that age group, as more "preemies" survive in the ICU setting, has become more commonplace. It is usually due to intraventricular hemorrhage of indolent onset in children with compromised respiratory systems. They are very heat-dependent and in a generally unstable condition. This physiological instability is so severe at times that one often does not have the luxury of taking them down to the x-ray department to obtain a CT scan. The diagnosis of hydrocephalus is often difficult in premature babies because this condition is not reflected by the size of their head or by the status of their fontanelle. B-scan echo encephalography is a very simple, noninvasive portable scanning test that can show the size of the ventricles quite adequately in the ICU and is currently the diagnostic procedure of choice for hydrocephalus associated with prematurity.

When we are dealing with hydrocephalus, which is a very common problem in pediatric neurosurgery, the issue of whether to put in a subdural pressure monitor or a ventricular catheter is answered easily. The latter, because of the dilated ventricles, is technically easy, more reliable and may be used as a temporary form of treatment as well as a monitoring system. Although there are several commercial produuts available for ventricular drainage one can use any flexible ventricular cannula, an IV tubing set, a plastic blood donor bag and a "T" connector so that the pressure can be monitored or the fluid drained as necessary.

In full-term infants the diagnosis of hydrocephalus can be readily made by increasing head size or the setting sun sign. These children are not usually in desperate straits because their calvaria increases more easily in size and prevents the ICP from becoming too high. Children who are a bit older, however, especially if they are from 6 to 10 years of age, may, when they develop hydrocephalus, whether posttraumatic, postinfectious, congenital, or tumor, become acutely ill. Especially if the sutures are not easily split, these children may present with coma, decerebrate posturing, etc., that develops rapidly over hours. These children should be admitted to the ICU and at the bedside have a ventricular drain inserted. Our experience with drains as well as with subdural monitors has been quite good in terms of infection risk, so that we have no fear of performing the procedure. The child then stabilizes in the ICU and we can proceed more electively with evaluation and treatment.

The Holter shunt is a proximal valve system for shunting the CSF to relieve hydrocephalus. This was the first really effective one-way valved system that was developed in the early 1950s. Today about six manufacturers make CSF shunt systems.

It is important when dealing with the question of shunt malfunction to be able to identify the type apparatus one is confronted with by palpation. The ordinary shunt malfunction is not complete. If the child still has ventricular compliance allowing expansion, he ordinarily will not get into much trouble, except to get a bit sleepy, have headache or vomit. But if the ventricles have been brought back to normal size, are stiff and will not dilate, the patient may develop tremendously high ICP. In those situations, treatment must be initiated immediately, so that it is imperative to be able to identify the kind of shunt that lies under the scalp in order to tap it or to pump it to determine if it is working, and if not, to relieve the pressure expeditiously. In cases when the old records may not be readily available, it is a decided advantage to be familiar with the various kinds of shunt apparatus. The Holter system includes two one-way valves about 1 cm apart and a small reservoir (Rickham) between the burr hole and the valves.

The Cordis (Hakim) pump is similar in size and shape to the Holter model, but instead of the small round reservoir, the tapping area is cylindrical.

All of the other manufacturers use slit valves of silicone rubber. The Cordis Co. uses a ball valve system.

The Denver shunt pump is similar to the Holter and Cordis models in that it is cylindrical in shape, but it lacks the rigid metal valve housings, is soft and completely compressible. There is only one proximal slit valve. Another one is present at the tip of the distal catheter in the heart or abdomen.

We try to avoid operating on shunt malfunctions emergently. If the child can be tided over with intermittent taps or external ventricular drainage, hasty and erroneous decisions are avoided, the child's condition becomes more stable, old records and roentgenograms can be studied and a definitive operation planned. Occasionally, the shunt responds to pumping or irrigation so that operative repair is no longer necessary.

Another system is the Heyer-Schulte shunt. The company makes several different models that may contain an antisiphon device, an occluder, and/or an on-off switch — as well as a soft-domed pump with or without a proximal valve.

The Ames shunt is manufactured by Dow Corning Company which is the supplier of silicone for all of the other shunt manufacturers. Dow Corning is essentially a materials supplier and makes a rather limited production of this finished device. Its distinguishing features are two round plastic domes in series. The only valves are located distally at the tip of the peritoneal or cardiac catheter.

The Codman shunt can either have a proximal pumping device and a distal slit or no proximal pump. The latter is called the "Unishunt" and is essentially one piece of silicone tubing with slit valves at the distal end.

Children with cranial-spinal anomalies sometimes require intensive care pre- and postoperatively. A child about 6 years of age came in with very difficult breathing and was weak in all four extremities. A misdiagnosis of viral myositis had been made in Denver. We found a subluxation at C1-2. The dens was separate from C2 and stuck to the basiocciput. At least half of her canal was compromised unless the head was held in extension. We corrected this by posterior fusion. The child had to have assisted respiration preoperatively and for weeks postoperatively. Finally, a tracheostomy was necessary. In an infant or young child, this often means a year or two years before you can remove it. They have a great tendency to develop tracheal stenosis, so we like to tide these children over for as long as we can with an endotracheal tube to avoid this complication if possible.

As well as subluxation of C1-2, a 12-month-old child had the C2 pedicles congenitally displaced medially, pinching the spinal cord. We corrected this with posterior fusion with excision of the pedicles, but this child, too, had to have assisted respirations for a long time. However, we were able to avoid a tracheostomy and a good deal of the problems that are associated with it by the judicious use of endotracheal intubation and intensive respiratory care.

Ninety percent of children with myelomeningocele have a Chiari II malformation. Occasionally in severe cases, especially thoracolumbar lesions, Ondine's Curse (sleep-induced apnea) may occur, requiring decompression of the Chiari malformation. The arachnoid is removed to show the bayonet deformity of the brainstem and the tonsils down well into the cervical cord. A generous bony decompression is carried out and a dural graft allows for as much additional decompression as possible. These children also must be very carefully observed postoperatively in the ICU.

Brain tumors occur most frequently in children in the posterior fossa. Obstructive hydrocephalus often develops and is the mechanism for production of headaches, somnolence, vomiting and papilledema. Rather than presenting with specific localizing signs for the tumor, they develop diffuse, focal signs and symptoms of hydrocephalus. If a child is in relatively good condition and the pressure symptoms are not severe, we treat with dexamethasone and observe them closely in the ICU. This will often unblock the hydrocephalus, so that we can work them up at leisure and operate electively. If the level of consciousness is depressed or the patient is comatose or bradycardic, then we insert a ventricular catheter, hook him up to a monitor and drain CSF as necessary to keep his pressure at 10 torr or below. We do not use preoperative CSF shunts because many times we can avoid the use of a shunt altogether by excising the tumor and because if the tumor is malignant, it may metastasize through the shunt.

Operative monitoring techniques that are routinely used for children with brain tumors are arterial and central venous pressures and intraventricular pressure. Postoperatively the child should be carefully monitored continuously. Daily lumbar punctures are performed for several days to remove blood from the CSF and to diminish the incidence of post-op hydrocephalus. All children are placed in the ICU following craniotomies for at least the first 48 hours to observe for increased ICP due to hydrocephalus, edema or postoperative hematomas and to provide intensive respiratory care.

The last special pediatric ICU issue to be discussed is that of fluid and electrolytes. A craniopharyngioma is a developmental usually cystic neoplasm, that occurs above or within the sella tursica and that is often amenable to total removal in children. Craniopharyngiomas often arise on the anterior surface of the pituitary stalk. It is not very often that one can remove them without sacrificing the stalk, so that diabetes insipidus is a frequent postoperative complication. This can create extremely critical fluid and electrolyte imbalances in children who, as was previously stated, have a very small margin for error.

During the first few days post-op, one should match the previous hour's urine output with equal volumes of 5% dextrose and water intravenously. We give no additional maintenance fluid. This replacement should match the urine output cubic centimeter for cubic centimeter hourly up to a maximum of 200 cc/hr. If the child is putting out more urine than that, he goes into negative balance, becomes dehydrated and urine output declines. One can allow them to get a bit dehydrated as long as the electrolytes are determined twice a day. We do not replace sodium or potassium during the first 48 hours unless severe deficits are apparent. If the serum sodium falls, the upper limit of replacement is reduced to 100 cc/hr from 200 cc/hr. Usually, sodium titers will soon then approach normal, indicating that this patient had been overhydrated. If the serum sodium rises, diabetes insipidus is almost a certainty. We try to guard against hypernatremia because it is much more difficult to treat than hyponatremia. The options for treatment are to increase the upper limit of fluid replacement to 250 cc/hr, to allow the patient to drink ad libitum fluids or to begin pitressin tannate in oil or nasal spray. We feel that pitressin preparations are dangerous in the first few days, but do not hesitate to use them after the first postoperative week if diabetes insipidus is still a clinical problem.

Self-Evaluation Quiz

1. Craniosynostosis is premature closure of cranial sutures.
   a) True
   b) False
2. Hypernatremia is considerably easier to treat than hyponatremia.
   a) True
   b) False
3. In a child subgaleal or collections of blood inside the calvarium may cause anemia and shock.
   a) True
   b) False

Answers on page 391.

Pediatric Neurology ICU:
Special Issues - Seizure Control

Richard G. Curless, M.D.

Objectives

The evaluation and treatment of seizures in childhood present a number of potential pitfalls which, if not recognized, can result in serious consequences. The discussion will emphasize these special problems, pointing out the high-risk patients. Appropriate drugs and dosages will be described for the management of status epilepticus in the newborn as well as in older children.

The most common neurological problem in the Pediatric ICU is prolonged seizures. Whether or not the child's condition satisfies a diagnosis of status epilepticus, aggressive intravenous therapy is generally initiated promptly. Long ago it became clear that two of the most effective agents, diazepam and phenobarbital, have a dangerously close therapeutic-toxic dosage range in young children. The toxic hazard is central respiratory depression, and this side effect may appear before, during or after the anticonvulsant effects. The equipment and technique required for immediate intubation of an infant is all too often unavailable in a general hospital emergency room. The result may convert an urgent situation into a life-long disaster secondary to hypoxic encephalopathy. For this reason, therapy with these agents should be delayed until the specialist and the equipment are available for intubation.

Similarly, the combination of IV diazepam and phenobarbital is not recommended, since cardiovascular collapse is a potential complication. There is little difference in the mech-

Richard G. Curless, M.D., Associate Professor of Neurology and Pediatrics, University of Miami School of Medicine, Fla.

anism of action of these two drugs; therefore, it is unlikely that one will be effective when the other has failed. Diazepam has a more rapid onset of action and a shorter half life. Administer 0.3 mg/kg (up to 10 mg) of IV diazepam or up to 10 mg/kg of phenobarbital. In both cases inject very slowly to watch for respiratory depression or for cessation of seizures. In the case of phenobarbital, respiratory failure may develop hours later with cumulative doses. In any case, no child under school age should be sent home from the emergency room after receiving these IV medications. At least an overnight hospitalization in a Pediatric ICU is recommended.

There are two alternatives to phenobarbital for initial therapy of status epilepticus or the backup treatment in the advent of treatment failure: phenytoin and paraldehyde. Both can be given intravenously, although there is very little published experience with IV paraldehyde. Phenytoin is a highly effective agent in some patients, and its nonsedating feature is particularly attractive in comatose patients. It has not been used as the initial status drug in large groups of children. This is probably because of the physician's desire to provide aggressive, prompt therapy. In fact, the benefits outweigh the risks if the major concern is a few more minutes of seizure activity. The cardiac toxic effects were overemphasized in past years, and with the aid of a cardiac monitor and slow injection, arrhythmias are very uncommon. This is a relatively safe method for initial therapy of status epilepticus in children, particularly in primary care emergency room settings. A loading dose of 15 mg/kg is recommended for children under 3 years and 10 mg/kg for the older patients.

Parenteral paraldehyde is also highly effective in the treatment of status epilepticus. It can be given IV, deep IM (by "Z" technique) or per rectum in oil. While many proclaim the effectiveness of this mode of therapy, there is no support for its safety in the medical literature or pharmacology textbooks. We are engaged in a study of paraldehyde utilizing a variety of doses and determining blood levels. Our experience has already indicated what appears to be central nervous system respiratory depression from high doses. This is contrary to the published information indicating that the principal risks are pulmonary hemorrhage and edema. Until our study or others like it are complete, the physician (and parent) must accept considerable potential risk with this drug. Accordingly, it is not yet recommended as a modality for initial therapy. However for drug-resistant status it is, in our opinion, appropriate.

Most infants with seizures, whether in status or not, are appropriately admitted to an ICU until the patient is in satisfactory condition. In all cases prompt attention to the correction of the cause is of paramount importance. In young children it may be impossible to stop the seizures without improving the basic pathophysiology. The relatively common problems of meningoencephalitis and electrolyte disturbance will not be mentioned further. However, there are some additional disorders which can present a diagnostic dilemma, particularly in the infant and toddler.

The first is a subdural hematoma. Unlike the adult, infants with acute or chronic subdurals often have multifocal or generalized seizures. In many cases there is no general examination evidence of trauma — old or new. However, the combination of a bulging fontanelle, retinal hemorrhages and seizures represents a subdural hematoma until proven otherwise. Skull translumination may be abnormal with decreased translumination in the acute (hemorrhagic) lesion and increased in the chronic accumulation (hygroma). A CT scan is unnecessary prior to subdural taps in an acutely ill infant with a wide-open anterior fontanelle.

In another example, an infant or school age child presented with a history of a mild upper respiratory infection followed by nausea and vomiting the day before admission. During the ensuing 12 to 18 hours he became lethargic and had a grand mal seizure one hour before arrival in coma without fever or meningismus. The examination failed to indicate a focal neurological deficit, and there were no diagnostic systemic signs. A diagnosis of Reye's acute encephalopathy with fatty infiltration of the viscera was entertained. Blood was drawn in search of hypoglycemia, hyperammonemia and hepatic enzyme elevation, and the patient was promptly given a bolus of hypertonic glucose. An emergency CT scan was negative except for small ventricles and possible cerebral edema. An LP was normal except for high pressure, and the patient was intubated for the purpose of hyperventilation while a subarachnoid bolt was inserted under local anesthesia for continuous intracranial pressure monitoring. Mannitol was added to decrease the pressure further. An elevated PTT prevented a liver biopsy several days later. In the classic example small fat droplets in hepatocytes and mitochondrial abnormalities on electron microscopy would have been demonstrated. The seizures were more responsive to the control of the intracranial pressure than to anticonvulsant therapy.

On another occasion a 4-year-old boy was brought to the emergency room with a headache following a brief focal convulsion. He was a known hemophiliac with less than 5% factor VIII at the time of diagnosis two years earlier. No known trauma was described, but a CT scan verified a 3 cm hematoma in the right parietal lobe. His factor VIII at the time of admission was 15% and treatment with cryoprecipitate was initiated promptly. Anticonvulsant therapy was also initiated and no further seizures developed. The headache cleared and no additional hemorrhage was found on a repeat CT. The important message for this case is that any headache in a hemophiliac, with or without focal neurological symptoms or signs, indicates a strong possibility of intracranial hemorrhage. Replacement therapy is indicated in the patient whether or not CT evidence of hemorrhage is demonstrated. In addition, replacement therapy should be at least initiated before an LP is performed. Extensive brain surgery can be accomplished with adequate factor VIII therapy.

In another case, a 6-year-old black boy with Down's syndrome was brought to the hospital because of several seizures and drowsiness. The patient had a temperature of 102° and was very uncooperative. A heart murmur was heard and the admitting physician noted questionable cyanosis. An LP revealed clear fluid with a mild lymphocytic pleocytosis, normal sugar and a protein of 75. No pressure was recorded and the gram stain was negative. Six hours later the patient was found unresponsive with a left hemiparesis and anisocoria. An emergency CT scan revealed a large right frontoparietal abscess. The patient died despite prompt attempts to lower the intracranial pressure on the way to the operating room.

In this case, the lesson is to avoid lumbar punctures in children with acute neurological symptoms who are at risk for brain abscess. Once the cardiologist for this patient was reached, it was clear that he had cyanotic congenital heart disease. A common cause of acute or subacute focal neurological signs in a child over 2 years of age with cyanotic congenital heart disease is an intracerebral abscess. Children under this age more frequently have strokes as the cause of the neurological dysfunction. Either CT or isotope scanning is satisfactory to diagnose a cerebral abscess. The CT, of course, provides much more information, but if it is not readily available, the isotope study will suffice. Once a negative study is available an LP should be performed, but immediate or delayed herniation syndromes are all too common after a spinal tap in a child with a brain abscess. In the case of a single small abscess without ventricular displacement or multiple abscesses, nonsurgical therapy may be the treatment of choice.

The final case is an 8-year-old girl who was brought to the hospital because of progressive stupor. During the preceding week her teacher complained that she spent too much time daydreaming and sleeping in class. This was uncharacteristic of her usual studious behavior, but before the parents could seek medical advice she developed a dazed, eyes-open appearance with only intermittent response to questions. Examination revealed an afebrile child with a supple neck, generally reduced muscle tone and a fixed, straight-ahead stare. Occasional eyelid flutter was noted. An EEG revealed continuous, diffuse epileptiform discharges. With the EEG running she was given IV diazepam in 2 mg boluses. After the third bolus the EEG converted to 3 cps spike and wave bursts lasting 3 to 4 seconds and occurring once every 15 seconds. The patient was deeply sedated with her eyes now closed. This child had minor motor status epilepticus which required parenteral therapy in the ICU for four days and then began to respond to oral valproate. Other studies were negative and her long-term follow-up was favorable.

Neonatal Problems

Neonatal seizures present a special problem because of the anticonvulsant kinetics in this age group. The bulk of current information involves phenobarbital and phenytoin, and accordingly these are the drugs of choice for the management of neonatal status epilepticus. Phenobarbital has a large volume of distribution, necessitating a high dosage for prompt, adequate blood levels; 20 mg/kg should be given intravenously during prolonged seizure activity. Studies have also pointed out a long half-life of 40 to 100 hours in most newborns. Therefore, subsequent doses should be given in response to blood level monitoring with an eye toward 15 to 25 mg/liter as a therapeutic level. If seizures continue, it may be necessary to give additional doses despite high levels, but respirator assistance may be necessary in view of the central respiratory depression.

Phenytoin may be utilized when phenobarbital fails. Newborn studies also indicate a large volume of distribution of phenytoin so that 10 to 20 mg/kg is required for an initial IV dose in order to reach a therapeutic blood level of 10 to 20 mg/liter. The half-life of this drug is not sufficiently worked out in the newborn. A blood level should be checked six to eight hours after the initial dose and at least daily thereafter. Most newborns require two doses a day beginning with 12 to 24 hours after the initial bolus.

If the seizures continue, the options of paraldehyde or the use of barbiturate coma remain. While there are no specific guidelines for neonatal paraldehyde dosing, 0.3 mg/kg given over 30 minutes has been safe and often effective in our hands. This is probably less dangerous than barbiturate coma although the sparse literature on either treatment leaves the issue open to question.

As with older children, the correction of infection or metabolic disturbance is of paramount importance. The most difficult problems arise when hypoxic encephalopathy is the cause of seizures. Frequently these patients also have hypoxic renal and hepatic damage resulting in defective anticonvulsant metabolism. In this situation it becomes even more important to follow blood levels carefully.

The primary cause of death in premature infants remains intraventricular hemorrhage. The mechanism of this bleeding is uncertain. Earlier concepts of preceding hypoxia and acidosis secondary to respiratory distress syndrome (RDS) now carry reduced significance because of continuous blood gas monitoring techniques. These methods have failed to demonstrate the expected changes in pH and oxygenation. The germinal plate, which lies in the region adjacent to the lateral ventricles, is an area rich in blood supply. It is here that spongioblasts and neuroblasts differentiate into mature glia and neurons and migrate outward to their final location. One theory suggests that increased arterial pressure results in extensive arteriolar bleeding followed by massive venous hemorrhage into the periventricular region. The mechanism of the increased pressure during RDS is unknown. Obviously, it is this type of question which inhibits adequate preventive measures.

The management of these patients has been very unsatisfactory. Fortunately, some infants survive on their own by absorbing the intraventricular blood with or without residual hydrocephalus. In some cases the hydrocephalus recedes spontaneously (without shunting). Aggressive therapy for the acutely ill infant is thus far of uncertain value. The methods include (1) daily spinal taps until the protein is reduced, (2) intraventricular drainage and (3) osmotic diuretics in an effort to reduce the marked cerebral edema. The availability of a sonogram to provide an early diagnosis of hemorrhage without leaving the nursery may facilitate better studies of prompt, aggressive therapy.

Bibliography

Curless, R.G.: Headache in classical hemophilia: The risk of diagnostic procedures. Childs Brain 2:187-194, 1976.

DeVivo, D.C.: Reye's syndrome: A metabolic response to an acute mitochondrial insult? Neurology 28:105-108, 1978.

Painter, M.J., Pippenger, C.: MacDonald, H. and Pttick, W.: Phenobarbital and diphenylhydantoin levels in neonates with seizures. J. Pediatr. 92:315-319, 1978.

Volpe, J.: Neonatal seizures. Clin. Perinatol. 4 (1):43-64, 1977.

Self-Evaluation Quiz

1. Which of the following drugs may produce central respiratory depression? (can be more than one)
   a) Phenytoin
   b) Phenobarbital
   c) Paraldehyde

   d) Diazepam
   e) Dexamethasone

2. The drug least likely to produce sedation in the management of status epilepticus is:
   a) Diazepam
   b) Paraldehyde
   c) Amytal
   d) Phenytoin
   e) Phenobarbital

3. The most likely cause of seizures in a 6-month-old with a normal examination except for retinal hemorrhages is:
   a) Cerebral abscess
   b) Hyponatremia
   c) Aseptic meningitis
   d) Subdural empyema
   e) Subdural hematoma

4. The laboratory abnormality suggestive of Reye's syndrome is:
   a) Hypoglycemia
   b) Hyperammonemia
   c) CSF pleocytosis (greater than 20 WBC's)
   d) Small fat droplet accumulation in hepatocytes
   e) a, b and d

5. An intracranial hemorrhage should be suspected in a hemophiliac with headaches only after a convulsion or a focal deficit develops.
   a) True
   b) False

6. It is advisable to delay doing a spinal tap in a child suspected of having a cerebral abscess until an emergency CT scan or radionucleotide scan can be completed.
   a) True
   b) False

7. An emergency EEG is necessary during the treatment of which one of the following:
   a) Neonatal status epilepticus
   b) Minor motor status epilepticus
   c) Acute cerebral edema
   d) The increased intracranial pressure of Reye's syndrome
   e) Paraldehyde treatment of status epilepticus

8. The most appropriate initial therapy for neonatal status epilepticus is: (can be more than one)
   a) IV paraldehyde
   b) Barbiturate coma
   c) IV phenytoin
   d) IV pyridoxine
   e) IV phenobarbital
9. A reasonable initial dosage for both phenobarbital and phenytoin in the management of neonatal status epilepticus is 15 to 20 mg/kg.
   a) True
   b) False
10. The half-life of phenobarbital in the newborn is so long that a therapeutic blood level may remain for days after a single loading dose.
    a) True
    b) False
11. Hypoxic encephalopathy presents a difficult problem in the management of neonatal seizures because:
    a) Paraldehyde therapy is less effective
    b) Edema prevents the drug from reaching the seizure focus
    c) Other organs (kidney and liver) may also have suffered hypoxic injury
    d) Traumatic lesions usually coexist

Answers on page 391.

Panel Discussion

Moderator: Dr. Marshall

Panelists: Drs. Curless, Holzman and Page

Dr. Curless: (1) In a patient with suspected meningitis, when is it safe to do an LP without a CT scan? (2) What is the incidence of epilepsy in children with febrile seizures?

In high risk situations such as in the child with cyanotic heart disease who might have a cerebral abscess, I would definitely like a scan before an LP is done. Patients with signs of brainstem dysfunction are at risk for cerebellar herniation during or after an LP. Some centers are concerned that Reye's syndrome may have a significant risk for LPs. A children's hospital pediatric neurologist in New England feels that they have reduced their mortality in Reye's because they do not do LPs. I do not quite understand how it is possible to avoid spinal taps in these children because one is still stuck with the problem of possible meningitis. Granted, many Reye's syndrome children do not have meningismus or fever, but I still feel rather comfortable without an LP. Clearly, any child suspected of having meningitis must have a prompt LP without waiting for an LP.

In regard to febrile convulsions and the tendency toward long-term epilepsy, that is a problem that has been addressed at length in the pediatric literature. The risk factor is very low. Less than 0.5% of children with benign febrile convulsions subsequently develop epilepsy. Accordingly the rationale for who is and who is not treated with anticonvulsants is a difficult one. We treat the children with phenobarbital up to 3 years of age after they have had a second febrile convulsion. I do not treat after the first one.

Moderator: Dr. Page, in a child with postoperative diabetes insipidus, what fluid would you use for replacement?

351

Dr. Page: We prefer in the first 48 hours to use 5% dextrose and water to accurately replace the volume of each hour's urinary loss with the next hour's intravenous intake. The logic behind that is that it is much easier to correct a low sodium level than a high one. In a case such as the one I presented with craniopharyngioma and diabetes insipidus, the tendency for a hyperosmolar state is there and can be very difficult to treat. The tumor or the surgeon or both have altered the hypothalamus so that its regulatory mechanism is set too high, and the sodium level tends toward 160 or 170 or higher. It is difficult to treat that. So we try to err in the other direction. We replace just with dextrose and water, at least for the first 48 hours, while monitoring sodium. If, on the other hand, the sodium drops to 125 or 120, then we cut down on the replacement volume. Usually the problem is overhydration. The sodium should then rise toward normal.

With regard to ventricular catheter replacement in children, we like to put that burr hole, as I mentioned earlier, in the midpupil line and anterior to the coronal suture. If we are going to put a drill hole in, we move it up close to the hairline. Occasionally in dire straits when we need a ventricular catheter immediately, an 18-gauge spinal needle is twisted through the suture line itself. We have had no particular problems in terms of motor weakness, although the more central placements have a somewhat higher incidence of epileptogenic foci.

Moderator: Dr. Holzman, please read a question and answer it.

Dr. Holzman: I have a question here about the risk:benefit ratio, if you will, of barbiturate-induced coma versus losing the neurologic assessment.

Moderator: Let me interrupt you to say that I think people should stop using the term barbiturate coma. These patients are comatose and the correct terminology here is high-dose barbiturate therapy or barbiturate therapy. Using the term barbiturate coma has created considerable adverse reaction, particularly in Europe. We never use that term and we have never used that. Since we are responsible for it, in some ways I feel guilty. I would like people to stop using it. It sounds like we are taking people who are awake and making them comatose with barbiturates and that is simply not correct. Now go ahead, Dr. Holzman.

Dr. Holzman: I agree with that. The problem is that with these patients you have a neurologic examination on admission. Then you are confronted with a situation where you really have to either paralyze them and/or use barbiturates and completely lose the neurologic examination. That is why we have uniformly utilized intracranial pressure monitoring prior to the induction of the barbiturate therapy. There is no question that we would like to have a neurologic examination whenever possible but I think the benefit of having the patient with barbiturate levels that are therapeutic or what we feel are therapeutic at least and having the intracranial pressure monitoring device in place far outweighs the risk of losing the neurologic examination. In most cases, we do have preservation of pupillary response. So that has become a very helpful sign.

Moderator: I want to comment about something you said about hypothermia because it sounds different from what I said earlier about hypothermia. Temperature usually falls with barbiturates to about 33 or 34 degrees. That is precisely the point to which Dr. Holzman goes. When people talk about induced hypothermia, they are usually talking about body temperature of 28, 29 or 30 degrees Celsius. As I said earlier, those are the patients in whom I have heard other neurosurgeons and pediatric intensivists who have used barbiturates report problems with hypoxia and lung dysfunction. So there really is not any disagreement between Dr. Holzman and me at all. It is just that he may use a little bit of cooling to get them there faster. I think the combination of barbiturates and hypothermia at least in pediatric management and in a man, not in the laboratory necessarily, has a real potential hazard. We have had ventricular arrhythmias with hypothermia when I was at Philadelphia before I started using barbiturates in patients who had healthy myocardiums previously. So there is not any disagreement between us, since we are going for the same temperatures, and he is just getting there a little bit faster than we are.

Dr. Holzman: I am sure you could visit us in the unit when we are doing this. Frequently, the heating-cooling blanket is heating the patient to keep him at 93 or 94 degrees. So it does not take very much cooling to get him down to that point.

With regard to cuffed endotracheal tubes, we do not use them in any pediatric patient unless we have to go to very high ventilatory pressures, usually in excess of 15 to 18 cm of water. As I mentioned before, the subglottis seals very effectively around the endotracheal tube. There really is very little need for using a cuff in a patient, at least in our experience.

As for the protocol for ICP lines, we do not irrigate our ICP lines when we are using an intracranial bolt and only very rarely when we are using an intraventricular cannula. We use no antibiotic irrigation solutions. It is simply saline that fills the system and then it is left alone. The system is changed every 24 hours.

Metabolic Encephalopathy: A Mechanistic Approach

Alan H. Lockwood, M.D.

Objectives

To review some of the findings on the neurological examination and to provide a framework for an etiological classification that has direct therapeutic implications.

The metabolic encephalopathies are a group of disorders that are characterized by an abnormal mental status. Usually this is the result of a specific disease or organ dysfunction, but intoxications and substrate deficiencies are included as well. Nervous system dysfunction due to metabolic rather than structural disturbances in the brain accounts for about 70% of all examples of coma of unknown etiology.

A disturbance of consciousness is the hallmark of all metabolic encephalopathies. Consciousness can be regarded as having two components: an on-off or quantitative component — alertness vs. deep coma; and a qualitative component, normal cognitive function vs. confusion and inability to perform learned mental tasks. Lesions in the reticular activating system produce coma by affecting the quantitative component and bilateral lesions of the complete cerebral cortex (metabolic or structural) affect the qualitative aspects of consciousness. As a general rule, cortical neuronal function is more sensitive to metabolic disturbances than brain stem neuronal function. Thus, the early signs of metabolic encephalopathy are manifested as confusion, a loss of drive or a blunting of consciousness and difficulty with memory and calculations. As the

Alan H. Lockwood, M.D., Assistant Professor of Neurology and Radiology, University of Miami School of Medicine, Fla.

metabolic disturbances become more severe, the disturbances of cortical and reticular activating system function become severe enough to result in deep coma.

The neuro-ophthalmological examination is of great importance in the differential diagnosis of comatose patients. Patients with metabolic causes of coma almost invariably retain the pupillary light reflex and the eyes move appropriately in response to the oculocephalic test (Doll's eye) or ice-water caloric testing. Structural lesions that cause coma usually eradicate the pupillary light reflex and result in a loss of ocular movement to reflex testing. (Metabolic disturbances associated with loss of a pupillary light reflex include glutethimide (Doridin ®) intoxication, hypoxia and intoxication with anticholinergic agents. Very deep barbiturate coma with isoelectric EEGs may be associated with a loss of the ice-water caloric response as well.

Whereas the motor system response to structural lesions causing coma is often characterized by decorticate or decerebrate posturing and extensor plantar signs, metabolic disturbances may produce a large variety of motor signs. Asterixis is the classic motor sign of metabolic encephalopathy. This finding, a sudden loss of postural tone causing a flapping motion, was originally thought to be pathognomonic for hepatic encephalopathy. Although asterixis is common in hepatic coma, it is also seen in a wide variety of metabolic disorders and is occasionally associated with structural lesions of the brain as well. Other motor signs associated with metabolic encephalopathy include an increase in resistance to passive movement, spasticity, unusual postures, myoclonus and occasionally generalized or multifocal seizures.

Sensory findings in patients with metabolic encephalopathy are usually the result of chronic illness or organ failure. Detailed sensory testing is usually not possible, due to poor patient cooperation.

A mechanistic approach to the differential diagnosis of the cause of metabolic encephalopathy is useful, not only in terms of classification, but in setting priorities for therapy. It is useful to think of coma as the result of *substrate deficiency* (e.g., hypoxia, hypoglycemia), *toxin excess* (e.g., hepatic coma, drug overdose) or *disturbed internal brain environment* (e.g., hyperosmolality and water intoxication).

The brain has a very high metabolic rate. It receives 15% to 20% of the total cardiac output: this high fraction is required to supply the brain with the oxygen and glucose that it requires. Any interruption or compromise in the rate of substrate delivery to the brain may cause unconsciousness within seconds and permanent damage to critical brain regions in minutes. Experimental studies have shown that brain adenosine triphosphate (ATP) levels fall to nearly zero within one minute after complete circulatory arrest. For these reasons the first priority in caring for the comatose patient is to determine that the circulatory and ventilatory status is satisfactory and then to administer glucose, 50 ml of 50% glucose, intravenously. If at all possible, a pretreatment blood sample for glucose testing should be obtained, but the administration of glucose should not be deferred pending a laboratory result. These procedures should be rigorously adhered to, even in hospitalized patients, especially empirical glucose administration. Delay in the administration of glucose risks permanent brain damage. Coma due to hyperglycemia or diabetes ketoacidosis will not be worsened by the relatively small amount of glucose in the test bolus. Thiamine deficiency is another cause of coma that requires prompt therapy. Usually the characteristic eye signs of this syndrome allow the diagnosis to be made with relative ease. It is important to give thiamine parenterally in every questionable case and to remember that giving carbohydrates to an individual who is thiamine deficient will exacerbate the clinical condition, unless thiamine is given concurrently.

Just as the brain is sensitive to substrate deprivation, it also requires rather prompt removal of toxic products of metabolism for normal function. Hepatic encephalopathy (HE) serves as an excellent example of coma due to toxin excess, since a great deal is known about its pathophysiology and treatment.

The liver is a complex metabolic organ and it normally detoxifies a variety of compounds produced by metabolic and catabolic reactions. Ammonia, for example, is produced by colonic bacteria, exercising skeletal muscle and probably to some degree by every body organ. Normally ammonia from the colon, the greatest single source of this toxin, is carried to the liver via the hepatic portal vein where it is converted into urea for excretion by the kidneys. Acute hepatic necrosis, or more commonly shunting of blood from the portal to the systemic circulation, results in ammonia entering the general circulation rather than being converted to urea. Hyperammonemia, in turn, impairs consciousness and produces the clinical syndrome we see as HE. Thus the failure to remove this toxin leads to the development of coma. Therapy consists of restricting dietary protein, removing blood and protein from the gastrointestinal tract by suction and purgation, giving antibiotics such as neomycin to kill colonic ammonia forming bacteria and giving lactulose — all measures designed to reduce the rate of ammonia formation. Other forms of therapy are being evaluated.

This model of coma, i.e., organ failure, toxin buildup and treatment by a reduction in toxin formation, can serve as a basis for considering other specific disorders. Uremic encephalopathy and carbon dioxide narcosis due to chronic lung disease are good examples.

Not all toxins are endogenously formed. Coma may also be due to exogenous toxins, i.e., drug overdose. The accurate diagnosis of these patients requires a knowledge of pharmacology and the ability to recognize the clinical manifestation of various drug intoxications.

The final category is coma due to disturbed body homeostasis, without specific end-organ disease. Water intoxication due to the syndrome of inappropriate antidiuretic hormone (ADH) secretion or hyperosmolality due to hypothalamic disease serve as examples.

Water metabolism is very complex and requires normal renal function, a thirst mechanism, as well as central interaction with ADH, renin, angiotensin and sensors of osmolality. The brain is affected by altered osmolality because of secondary changes in its volume — it swells during hypo-osmolality and shrinks during hyperosmolality. The brain is able to compensate for these stresses by loss of potassium or the gain of osmolality active particles (namely, amino acids), respectively. These changes seek to maintain normal brain volume during periods of stress.

The diagnosis of disordered osmolality can be made clinically but confirmation requires laboratory measurements of osmolality, sodium, glucose and urea, the most important solutes. Treatment is complex and variable and no firm rules can be given. However, it must be remembered that chronically disordered osmolality causes compensatory changes in the brain that tend to maintain normal volume. Treatment that is too rapid or vigorous, e.g., rapid water infusion in a patient with severe dehydration, can cause a paradoxical swelling of the brain and a relative water intoxication. This is the result of water replacement at a rate that exceeds the ability of the brain to rid itself of osmoles it built up during hyperosmolality.

Although some causes of coma do not readily lend themselves to this approach (e.g., meningitis) and some patients may have structured and metabolic causes of coma (e.g., the cirrhotic with a subdural), this classification should provide the clinician with a framework for the diagnosis and treatment of most patients with a metabolic cause for coma. The combination of a careful history, clinical examination and laboratory tests that should include a determination of the blood sugar, urea nitrogen, creatinine, electrolytes, prothrombin time and tests of liver integrity coupled with arterial blood gas determinations and toxicological evaluation of blood and urine should lead to a correct diagnosis and plan for treatment in most cases.

Self-Examination Quiz

1. Asterixis is the classic motor sign of metabolic encephalopathy.
   a) True
   b) False
2. Coma is the result of:
   a) Substrate deficiency
   b) Toxin excess
   c) Disturbed internal brain environment
   d) All of the above
   e) None of the above
3. Asterixis is rare in hepatic coma.
   a) True
   b) False
4. The liver is the greatest single source of ammonia.
   a) True
   b) False

Answers on page 391.

Neuromuscular Crises

author

D. Ram Ayyar, M.D.

Objectives

To present the clinical features, diagnosis and management of five neuromuscular diseases which may present to clinicians as emergencies.

Myasthenia Gravis

Myasthenia gravis is a specific neuromuscular disease manifested by an abnormal amount of muscular weakness and fatigability in voluntary muscles following repetitive or prolonged use. The weakness and fatigability usually recover after a period of rest and after anticholinesterase medication. Myasthenia gravis occurs in all races and affects individuals of all ages. Though the onset may be at any age, there are two ages of peak incidence — the third decade in women and the fifth and sixth decades in men. Women are affected twice as often as men.

Myasthenia gravis is a disorder in which the neuromuscular transmission is at fault, and to understand the nature of the defect some knowledge of normal neuromuscular transmission is necessary. Acetylcholine (ACh), the natural chemical transmitter, is synthesized in the motor nerve terminals and stored in vesicles. Each vesicle or "quantum" contains about 5,000 to 10,000 ACh molecules. Depending upon the ease of their release the vesicles in the nerve terminal can be subdivided into three compartments. The immediately available store contains 1000 quanta, the vesicles being immediately adjacent to the presynaptic membrane of the nerve terminal. These vesicles are

D. Ram Ayyar, M.D., Associate Professor of Neurology, Director EMG Laboratories, University of Miami School of Medicine and Jackson Memorial Hospital, Fla.

most readily available for release. The main store is the largest containing approximately 300,000 quanta which are relatively unavailable for release. The mobilization store is intermediate in availability and contains about 10,000 quanta. ACh is released spontaneously in single quanta and occurs in a random fashion. This results in depolarization of the postsynaptic membrane giving rise to miniature end-plate potentials (MEPPs) which are too small to overcome the muscle fiber threshold. However, when the nerve terminal is invaded by an active potential, there is a marked increase in the number of quanta of ACh released. ACh combines with acetylcholine receptors (AChR) in the end-plate region of the muscle fiber resulting in an end-plate potential (EPP) which easily overcomes the muscle fiber threshold giving origin to the propagated muscle fiber action potential. The amplitude of the EPP depends upon the number of ACh molecules that interact with AChR molecules. Only a small proportion of ACh molecules released interact with AChR molecules and only a small fraction of the millions of acetylcholine receptors are activated at one time. Under normal circumstances, the number of ACh molecule-AChR interactions occurring in response to nerve terminal depolarization is 4 to 12 times more than is necessary to overcome the muscle fiber threshold. This is the "safety margin" of neuromuscular transmission and any disorder that reduces the "safety margin" may result in failure of neuromuscular transmission. The ACh that does not combine with the receptors diffuses away or is hydrolyzed by the enzyme acetylcholinesterase (AChE).

Elmqvist et al [1] found that the amplitude of the MEPPs in myasthenia gravis was reduced and suggested that this was due to a decrease in the number of ACh molecules per quantum. Decreased amplitude of MEPPs due to a decrease in the number of ACh receptors was not thought to be responsible because indirect tests had suggested normal receptor sensitivity. This hypothesis remained in vogue until the demonstration that postsynaptic changes could give rise to all the features of myasthenia gravis. Decrease in the number of ACh receptors per neuromuscular junction [2, 3] and electron microscopic changes of the postsynaptic membrane showing sparse, shallow folds with markedly simplified geometric patterns [4], gave support to the concept of postsynaptic abnormality. Specific pharmacologic blockade of the ACh receptors in experimental animals resulted in models that reproduced the clinical, electrophysiologic and pharmacologic features of myasthenia gravis [5, 6].

While trying to raise antibodies to pure ACh receptors, it was found that rabbits immunized with receptors from electric eel developed profound muscular weakness and respiratory insufficiency [7]. The typical decremental responses and improvement with anticholinesterase agents were noted. Since then, experimental autoimmune myasthenia gravis (EAMG) has been produced in different animals. The presence of IgG and Complement$_3$ (C_3) at the postsynaptic membrane was demonstrated elegantly [8].

It would appear that myasthenia gravis is an autoimmune disorder in which antibodies are produced against ACh receptors. These antibodies impair neuromuscular transmission by accelerated degradation of the ACh receptors and also by receptor blockade. It is not clear how the autoimmune response begins though the thymus gland is considered to be somehow involved in the process.

The characteristic clinical feature in myasthenia gravis is the abnormal weakness and fatigability of some or all voluntary muscles. The weakness increases with repeated or sustained activity and is improved by rest and anticholinesterase drugs. Though any muscle may be involved first external ocular muscles are affected initially in approximately 50% of patients. The external ocular muscles are eventually involved in about 90% of patients. Bulbar muscle weakness heralds the onset of the disease in about 30% of patients. Facial, masticatory, lingual, pharyngeal and laryngeal muscles are commonly involved as are the neck, shoulder-girdle and hip flexor muscles. Proximal limb muscles are usually more severely affected than the distal ones. Involvement of muscles of respiration makes the management of the disorder much more difficult. Symptoms have a tendency to fluctuate not only from day to day but also over much longer periods of time. Spontaneous remissions lasting for varying periods of time do occur particularly in the first three years of the disease. Long and spontaneous remissions are very rare indeed. There are no objective sensory deficits and the deep tendon reflexes are brisk or normally active except when the muscles are markedly weak.

Approximately 10% of patients have thymomas and thymic abnormalities, mainly hyperplasia, are noted in about 75% of patients. Myasthenia gravis tends to affect young women and older men. The syndrome of transient neonatal myasthenia is well recognized and results from the transplacental transfer of circulating anti-acetylcholine receptor antibodies from the myasthenic mother to the fetus [9].

Diagnosis

The diagnosis of myasthenia gravis is based on the clinical history, physical findings, electrophysiological and pharmacological studies and determination of the serum anti-AChR antibody titer. Under special circumstances in vitro microelectrode studies of neuromuscular transmission and ultrastructural studies of the motor end-plate may be required.

When the history and physical findings are typical, diagnosis of myasthenia gravis is easy. However, the disease can present in unusual ways and the diagnosis may be missed. Patients may present with weakness of several extraocular muscles or just with laryngeal muscle weakness. A high index of suspicion will facilitate the diagnosis in these patients.

Edrophonium (Tensilon) is a short-acting acetylcholinesterase (AChE) inhibitor and acts within a few seconds when given intravenously. Its effects last for only a few minutes. Two milligrams of the drug is injected intravenously over 15 seconds. If there is no response, an additional 8 mg is given. Dramatic and unequivocal objective improvement in muscle strength is diagnostic of myasthenia gravis [10]. A placebo injection before the test increases the validity of the test.

Electrophysiologic studies are useful in the diagnosis of myasthenia gravis. Supramaximal stimuli are applied to a motor nerve and the evoked compound muscle action potential is recorded with surface electrodes. At slow rates of repetitive stimulation (3 Hz), maximal decrement usually occurs with the fifth response. In normal subjects, the decrement is not greater than 7%. Examining the proximal and distal muscles gives a positive response in at least one of the muscles in 95% of the patients [11]. The test is positive in 50% if only one small hand muscle is tested. The sensitivity of the test in the small hand muscles can be improved by combining it with the regional curare test [12], by heating of the limb [13] and by observing the decremental response and postactivation exhaustion under normal and then ischemic conditions [14].

Single fiber electromyography (SFEMG) is used to study the action potentials generated by adjacent muscle fibers belonging to the same motor unit. The mean interpotential interval between two muscle fibers is called the jitter. In myasthenia gravis the jitter is increased compared to normal and a certain proportion of impulses fail to generate an action potential at one of the two fibers [15]. SFEMG requires special equipment and training.

Determination of anti-AChR antibody titer in the serum is quite helpful in diagnosing myasthenia gravis. It is positive in 87% of patients with myasthenia gravis [16]. False-positive results have not been reported.

Differential diagnosis should include botulism where the defect is presynaptic. The clinical features and diagnosis are discussed later in this paper. Though Lambert-Eaton syndrome is a disorder where neuromuscular transmission is at fault, the clinical and electrophysiologic features are quite different from those of myasthenia gravis [17]. A new myasthenic syndrome associated with end-plate AChE deficiency, small nerve terminals and reduced ACh release has been described. The patient had fluctuating ptosis, generalized weakness increased by exertion and decremental response at low as well as high frequencies of stimulation. Though the disorder may resemble myasthenia gravis, the various differences have been well characterized [18].

Treatment

Anticholinesterase drugs, prednisone, thymectomy, immunosuppressive drugs other than prednisone and plasmapheresis are the forms of therapy most frequently used to treat myasthenia gravis.

The most commonly used anticholinesterase drug is pyridostigmine bromide (Mestinon). The effect begins in 10 to 30 minutes after oral administration, reaches a peak in about two hours and is over at approximately four hours. The only way to determine the appropriate dosage of Mestinon is by the subjective responses of the patient and by the objective improvement as noted by the physician. The usual adult starting dose is 60 mg and this can be adjusted according to the response. Neostigmine bromide (Prostigmin) and ambenonium chloride (Mytelase) are the other anticholinesterase drugs sometimes used. Mestinon timespan 180 mg is available and is usually given at bedtime because its effects last about eight to ten hours.

Thymectomy is being increasingly used in the treatment of myasthenia gravis. The presence of thymoma is an indication for thymectomy though myasthenic patients with thymoma do not fare as well as those myasthenics who do not have a thymic tumor. The indications for thymectomy vary in different centers. Some would recommend thymectomy to only those myasthenics who do not respond to medical treatment including prednisone therapy, whereas some would favor early thymectomy in all patients with generalized myasthenia. Though many believe in the efficacy of thymectomy its value has not really been proven and a prospectively controlled study is warranted. Transsternal thymectomy is the most popular method though some favor transcervical operation.

In recent years it has become customary to use prednisone in patients who do not respond satisfactorily to anticholinesterase medication and thymectomy. Many would start prednisone therapy even before thymectomy. The dose of prednisone varies from 50 mg daily or 100 mg on alternate days to an initial alternate day dose of 25 mg raised in steps of 12.5 mg every six days until reaching 100 mg on alternate days or maximal benefit. Though some reports claim no complications from prednisone therapy, there are several reports documenting the well-known complications such as Cushing's syndrome, vertebral collapse, congestive heart failure, gastric hemorrhage, psychosis, cataracts and aseptic necrosis of the bone. Despite numerous papers attesting to the effectiveness of prednisone therapy in myasthenia gravis, it is still not clear as to how long the full dosage should be used before deciding that the patient will not respond or how long the full dosage should be continued when there is significant improvement. It is the general impression among physicians treating myasthenia gravis that prednisone therapy is quite helpful. The rationale for prednisone therapy is the immunologic nature of the disease though the precise nature of action of the drug is far from clear.

Immunosuppressives other than prednisone have been used to treat myasthenia gravis [19]. Azathioprine 100 mg/day or purinethol 75 mg/day has been found to be effective. It takes 4 to 15 months before the optimal improvement is reached. Azathioprine may stabilize the disease even in those who do not respond to prednisone therapy. Bone marrow suppression and severe infection are among the complications of this form of treatment.

Plasmapheresis was reported to be beneficial in the treatment of myasthenia gravis in 1978 [20]. Since then this procedure has been used in several centers and has been found to be quite effective in most of the patients. One cannot predict which patients will respond on clinical ground or on the basis of the presence or absence of high levels of AChR antibodies. Indications for plasmapheresis include those patients who are seriously disabled and do not respond to the other measures, myasthenic crisis, prior to thymectomy and in patients who fail to improve after thymectomy, prednisone and immunosuppressive therapy. The procedure is expensive and influenza-like syndromes are more common after plasmapheresis. Subacute bacterial endocarditis and one fatality have also been reported.

Myasthenic crisis has become relatively uncommon in recent years because of better understanding of the nature of the disease and advances in management. However, one still sees crisis in an undiagnosed or newly diagnosed myasthenic. Infections and failure to take the drugs may precipitate an attack of crisis in a well-established myasthenic. Patients with myasthenic crisis or muscarinic crisis present with increasing weakness and respiratory insufficiency. Though bradycardia, increased intestinal motility and miosis are features of muscarinic crisis, very often when patients present with respiratory insufficiency it may be impossible to differentiate myasthenic from muscarinic crisis and no time should be wasted trying to differentiate one from the other. All anticholinesterase medication should be stopped. The management of respiratory insufficiency is the single most important aspect of treatment. When the vital capacity falls below 10 to 15 ml/kg of body weight or the patient is unable to generate an inspiratory force of at least -25 cm $H_2O(-0.2$ kPa), tracheal intubation is indicated. The patients should be managed in an intensive care unit. The modern endotracheal tubes have soft, large capacity

high-compliance balloons and these tubes may be left in place
for as long as 21 days. Tracheotomy is indicated for long-term
care and this has the advantage of comfort and ease of
suctioning. Mechanical ventilation plays a most important role
in the management. The pattern of breathing is adjusted to suit
the needs of each patient. The tidal volume is based on the
formula of 10 to 14 ml/kg and a slow rate of 10 to 12 per
minute is usually ideal. The adjustments of ventilator are carried
out by keeping an eye on the patient to make sure that the
patient is comfortable with the patterns of breathing controlled
by the ventilator.

Infections should be promptly treated with appropriate
antibiotics. Some antibiotics such as neomycin, streptomycin,
gentamicin, kanamycin, polymyxin, bacitracin and colistin are
known to impair neuromuscular transmission in some but not
all patients. These agents can be given without hesitation since
the patients have respiratory support. Attention should be paid
to electrolyte balance, particularly to hypokalemia since it may
increase the weakness.

Plasmapheresis is helpful in the management of myasthenic
crisis and is indicated in difficult problems not responding
satisfactorily. High-dose alternate day prednisone therapy may
be initiated while the patient is still intubated, since worsening
of muscle strength that sometimes occurs in the initial period
will pose no problem. If anticholinesterase medication is to be
started, it is wise to begin with very small doses since the
patient may become extremely sensitive to the drugs.

The patient can be weaned when he no longer requires
external mechanical respiratory support. Precautions should be
taken to prevent pulmonary embolism. Attention should be
paid to the nutritional status of the patient. Psychosocial
support is a very important aspect of the management of these
patients but is beyond the scope of this review.

Botulism

Botulism is caused by the action of the exotoxin of
Clostridium botulinum, an anaerobic gram-positive, spore-forming rod. Botulinum toxin is the most deadly toxin known to
man. The toxin is heat labile, but the spores of *Clostridium
botulinum* are heat resistant. When the spores are present in the

food, the bacilli multiply, actively producing the toxin at room temperature under anaerobic conditions at a pH of 6 or more [21].

Ingestion of contaminated home processed food is responsible for the vast majority of cases. Symptoms usually occur within 12 to 36 hours after ingestion of the contaminated food. Occasionally the onset of the symptoms may be delayed for a week. The neurologic picture is one of progressive muscle weakness beginning in the cranial nerve territory. Ptosis, diplopia, dysarthria and dysphagia occur early. Marked extraocular muscle weakness is invariably present. Although weakness is bilateral, it is often asymmetric. Weakness of the face, tongue and pharyngeal muscles is followed by weakness of neck muscles and, to a lesser extent, of the limb muscles. Respiratory paralysis is the most dangerous aspect of the disease and is fatal if not dealt with promptly. Deep tendon reflexes are hypoactive and sensation and mentation are normal. Weakness reaches a plateau in four or five days. Recovery takes weeks or months. Dryness of the mouth and eyes, hypoperistalsis, obstipation and retention of urine may be present and are due to parasympathetic dysfunction [22].

Malaise, dizziness, nausea, vomiting, substernal and epigastric distress, abdominal cramps and diarrhea are the initial complaints in most patients.

Pupils are usually normal though in some they may be dilated and fixed.

Eight immunologically distinct toxins have been identified $(A,B,C_1,C_2,D,E,F$ and $G)$. The vast majority of human botulism is due to the A,B and E types.

Diagnosis is confirmed by detecting the toxin in the contaminated food or in the patient's serum or stool.

The clinical picture of botulism is the result of impaired acetylcholine (ACh) release from the nerve terminals caused by the toxin. Therefore, electrophysiological studies may be expected to be abnormal and indeed this has been shown to be so [23]. The findings consist of decreased amplitude of the evoked muscle action potential to supramaximal nerve stimulation, potentiation of the muscle action potential in response to rapid, repetitive stimulation or following ten seconds of isometric muscle contraction, and small short duration motor unit potentials on electromyography. The facilitation seen in botulism is not as marked as in Eaton-Lambert syndrome. Several nerves may have to be stimulated before one finds the characteristic defect. The defect tends to evolve with time, being present in some limbs but not in all.

Patients with botulism should be hospitalized immediately. Early administration of antitoxin may be helpful, particularly in cases of type E botulism. Specific typing of the toxin is done, but the treatment is started with trivalent ABE antitoxin. The antitoxin is horse serum; therefore, skin testing and precautions to deal with anaphylactic reactions are essential. Ten thousand units of antitoxin is administered intravenously. Minor allergic reactions may occur and may require treatment with antihistamines or corticosteroids.

Maintenance of respiratory function is the most important aspect in treating cases of botulism. Patients who appear to have mild symptoms may progress rapidly to respiratory failure. Therefore, it is essential to frequently monitor respiratory function in all patients until signs of improvement appear. If the vital capacity falls to 1,000 ml, elective intubation is indicated. Severe dysphagia is not uncommon and will require a nasogastric tube or endotracheal intubation to prevent aspiration. Recovery of spontaneous ventilation may occur in two weeks, but often it takes much longer and tracheotomy and positive pressure respiratory support are often necessary in these patients. Other important aspects of management include maintenance of fluid and electrolyte balance, gastric antacid therapy, injections of penicillin to eliminate any Clostridia and supportive management of adynamic ileus which is frequently seen in severe cases of botulism.

Guanidine hydrochloride has been found to be of benefit in patients with botulism [24]. However, there are also reports of patients who do not benefit from guanidine therapy. The usual dose is 15 to 45 mg/kg of body weight in divided doses. 4-Aminopyridine (4-AP) has been found to be effective in experimental botulism in animals [25], but it remains to be seen if it will be of help in human botulism. In botulism the transmitter release mechanism appears to be intact, but a reduced sensitivity to calcium has been shown [26]. Guanidine and 4-AP increase the level of free calcium inside the nerve terminal and this may be the mechanism by which these drugs restore evoked transmitter release in botulism poisoning [27].

Though the majority of cases of human botulism follow ingestion of food contaminated with botulinum toxin, human botulism may follow infection of wounds by *Clostridium botulinum* [28]. While outbreaks of food-borne botulism involve more than one person, in wound botulism characteristically only one person is affected. The clinical features of wound botulism are similar to those of food-borne botulism. However, there are some differences. Fever may be present in wound botulism, whereas it is absent, at least at the onset, in the food-borne type. If the wound is severe in an extremity, trauma and local infection may result in sensory findings. Moreover, the patients with wound botulism are due to infection with type A organisms. Gastrointestinal symptoms are not part of the clinical picture of wound botulism because they are less common in type A botulism than in types B and E.

Electrophysiologic studies may reveal similar defects of neuromuscular transmission as in food-borne botulism. Management is identical to treatment of food-borne botulism. In addition, surgical debridement and medical treatment of the wound are necessary.

In recent years, a new syndrome of infantile botulism has been recognized [29]. Infantile botulism appears to be more common than is recognized. The infants appear healthy at birth and for the next few weeks. Over a period of a day or two, the healthy infants lose their ability to suck and swallow and become hypotonic and profoundly weak. The cry becomes feeble and there is loss of head control. Many infants become constipated. Cranial nerve signs are reminiscent of adult botulism with ptosis, decreased extraocular motility, facial weakness and decreased gag reflexes. Pupils are normal or may react sluggishly to light. Stretch reflexes are decreased. Respiratory arrest is the most dangerous aspect of the disease. Fortunately, these infants seem to recover with appropriate management. Electrophysiologic studies are helpful in diagnosis in many but not in all cases.

Since no common source of toxin has been identified, it is believed that the disorder results from sporulation and toxin production by *Clostridium botulinum* from the gut. In infant botulism, the toxin may be found in the stool and not in the serum.

The most important aspect of therapy is respiratory support. Cathartics may be helpful in getting rid of the toxin from the gut. Since the disease appears to be a self-limited one, antitoxin is probably not indicated.

Guillain-Barré Syndrome

Guillain-Barré syndrome (GBS) is an acute or subacute polyradiculoneuropathy of unknown etiology occurring in all parts of the world and in persons of all ages. Diagnostic criteria for GBS have been established by an ad hoc NINCDS (National Institute of Neurological and Communicative Disorders and Stroke) Committee [30]. The disorder may follow various viral infections, surgery, inoculations and mycoplasma infections. GBS also seems to occur more frequently in Hodgkin's disease, lymphoma and lupus erythematosus. The presence of preceding events is not essential to the diagnosis of GBS though it is frequent. The most striking feature of the illness is a progressive motor weakness of more than one limb. The weakness may be severe resulting in paralysis of all four extremities and trunk, bulbar and facial paralysis and external ophthalmoplegia, but in some patients only mild weakness is noted. Maximum weakness is reached by two weeks but in some weakness may progress as long as four weeks. Both sides are involved but one side may be weaker than the other. Areflexia or hyporeflexia is a constant feature. Though sensory symptoms may be present, it is unusual to find profound sensory changes. Cranial nerve involvement is common, facial weakness occurring in about 50% of patients. Facial weakness is frequently bilateral. The cranial nerves innervating the tongue and muscles of deglutition may be involved and in some the disease manifests with external ophthalmoplegia. Recovery begins two to four weeks after the weakness reaches the nadir, functional recovery being noted in the vast majority of patients. Patients with GBS are afebrile at the time of onset of the neurologic symptoms. Autonomic dysfunction is not uncommon and is manifested by tachycardia, arrhythmias, postural hypotension, hypertension and vasomotor symptoms. Hypo- or hyperactivity of the sympathetic and parasympathetic systems may be noted in the same patient at different times. Occasionally a subacutely evolving disorder with sympathetic dysfunction is seen without involvement of the peripheral nerves either clinically or electrophysiologically. The cerebrospinal fluid protein may be increased and the illness may follow an upper respiratory tract infection [31].

Cerebrospinal fluid (CSF) protein is increased after the first week of symptoms. If the CSF protein is normal, serial examinations will show an increase. The CSF contains ten or less mononuclear leukocytes per cubic millimeter.

Electrophysiologic studies are abnormal in the majority of patients. Diffuse slowing of conduction is the most common abnormality, the slowing often being pronounced at common sites of nerve compression. In some patients, the slowing of conduction is confined to these sites [32]. "F" wave latencies may be increased confirming slowing of conduction in the proximal segments of the nerve despite normal conduction in the peripheral segments [33].

The pathologic changes are inflammatory in nature with lymphocytic cellular infiltration of peripheral nerve and de-struction of myelin [34]. Some of the lymphocytes are in the process of blast transformation. The pathologic features of GBS are identical to those found in experimental allergic neuritis; therefore, cell-mediated immunological reaction has been thought to be responsible for GBS. Activation of peripheral blood lymphocytes on exposure to peripheral nerve protein in vitro has been shown using different techniques [35, 36]. The presence of circulating antibodies directed against the peripheral nervous system has been demonstrated raising the possibility that humoral processes may play a part in the pathogenesis of GBS.

The diagnosis of a typical case of GBS is easy. Acute intermittent porphyria may mimic GBS but the other features discussed later in this paper help to differentiate the disorder from GBS. When the disorder is confined to the extraocular muscles or other cranial nerves, botulism and myasthenia gravis have to be considered in the differential diagnosis. Nerve conduction studies of the facial nerve are likely to be abnormal in GBS and abnormal neuromuscular transmission studies are to be expected in botulism and myasthenia gravis.

Management

There is no specific therapy for GBS. The main problems are respiratory failure and autonomic dysfunction. Seriously ill patients must be managed in an intensive care unit where it will be easier to monitor respiratory function and the blood gases. The indications for artificial ventilation are vital capacity of less than 15 ml/kg of body weight, an inspiratory force numerically less than -25 cm $H_2O(-0.25$ KPa) or evidence of decrease in blood oxygen saturation. Tracheal intubation is soon followed by tracheotomy. Mechanical ventilation is employed as has been mentioned in the section on myasthenia gravis. Particular attention is paid to respiratory toilet and chest physical therapy.

Dysphagia may be troublesome and feeding by nasogastric tube is required. Footboards to prevent foot drop and wrist splints to prevent wrist drop are helpful.

Autonomic dysfunction may create difficult problems in management. Hypertension is not uncommon but the blood pressure usually returns to normal without the use of hypotensive agents. Hypotension seems to be more common and more dangerous. It can be brought on by turning the patient quickly. Sinus tachycardia is common and may be interrupted by bradycardia which may occur spontaneously or be provoked by tracheal suction, ocular compression [37] or carotid sinus stimulation [38]. Tracheal aspiration should be preceded by a five-minute period of oxygen administration and the aspiration should be terminated if bradycardia or extrasystoles appear.

The role of corticosteroids is far from clear. Some patients show a dramatic improvement within a day or two, but many others continue to worsen. The results of a multicenter, randomized trial of prednisolone in GBS indicated that steroid treatment was not beneficial and could be detrimental [39]. It is indeed difficult to assess the effectiveness of the corticosteroids in a disorder where there is so much variation from one series of patients to another.

Plasmapheresis has been tried in some patients and there are conflicting reports as to its efficacy. Larger series of patients have to be treated before any meaningful conclusion can be arrived at.

Modern intensive care techniques and equipment have improved the outlook for patients with GBS. One such advance has been the use of Kinetic Therapy and the Roto Rest Treatment Table for the intensive care of these patients with multiple problems associated with their paralysis and respiratory insufficiency. Many of these patients make a good functional recovery although some may be left with sequelae.

Porphyrias

The porphyrias are a group of genetically determined disorders caused by defects in the synthesis of heme and associated with overproduction and excretion of porphyrins and porphyrin precursors. Porphyrias are divided into two general groups. Erythropoietic porphyrias primarily involve the erythropoietic tissue and are characterized by marked photosensitivity and do not concern the neurologist. Hepatic porphyrias primarily involve the metabolism of porphyrin in the liver and include acute intermittent porphyria (AIP), variegate porphyria (VP), hereditary coproporphyria (HC) and porphyria cutanea tarda (PCT) or symptomatic porphyria. The first three are dominantly inherited and are characterized by acute attacks separated by latent phases. Porphyria cutanea tarda is not inherited and acute attacks do not occur and will not be discussed further.

Pathogenesis

Amino acid glycine and succinyl CoA condense to form δ-aminolevulinic acid (ALA). This is catalyzed by ALA synthetase and is the rate-limiting step in porphyrin and heme synthesis. Heme feeds back to inhibit the condensation of glycine and succinyl CoA. Two molecules of ALA condense to form porphobilonogen (PBG) which undergoes polymerization to form uroporphyrinogens (UP) III and I. Uroporphyrinogen III leads to protoporphyrin and heme. The further metabolic pathway of uroporphyrinogen I comes to a dead end. Most porphyrins are secreted in the bile and excreted in the feces except for ALA and PBG which are excreted in the urine because of their greater solubility in water. High levels of ALA and PBG are associated with acute attacks of porphyria.

AIP is more common in persons of Scandinavian or English origin. Women are more frequently affected and seem to have more acute attacks. The clinical features of AIP can be divided into three main categories — abdominal, psychologic and neurologic. The typical patient is a young to middle-aged woman who has a history of recurrent attacks of abdominal pain, has a bizarre personality and has neurologic signs. The abdominal pain is usually severe suggestive of an abdominal emergency or it may mimic an attack of renal colic. It is not uncommon to see evidence of previous laparotomies. Constipation is common though some patients may have diarrhea. Nausea and vomiting are often present and fever may be noted occasionally. If barbiturates are given to sedate the patient, symptoms worsen. A wide variety of emotional disturbances may be seen. Restlessness, insomnia, crying and nightmares may be present or the patient may be clearly psychotic. The neuropathy usually begins with weakness and may be preceded or be accompanied by pain in the muscles or back. The upper limbs are more frequently involved than the lower limbs and the proximal muscles are usually weaker. The weakness is usually symmetric but can be quite asymmetric. The weakness progresses steadily reaching its nadir in one to four weeks. Respiratory impairment and arrest are not uncommon.

Cranial nerves are frequently involved. Vagus and facial nerve involvement is common and there may be bilateral facial paralysis. The 3rd, 5th, 11th and 12th cranial nerve may also be involved.

Sensory symptoms may be the presenting feature in some patients. Unpleasant paresthesiae may be felt not only in the limbs but in any part of the body. Hypalgesia may be in a "glove and stocking" distribution or it may be noted only in a proximal distribution. Sometimes the distribution is peculiar and "bathing trunk" and "long johns" distribution may be seen.

Deep tendon reflexes are usually diminished or absent but variations to this theme occur. Reflexes may be preserved despite weakness or reflexes may be absent except for the presence of normal ankle jerks.

Bladder involvement is not uncommon and seizures are noted in about 25% of patients.

Hyponatremia may be present secondary to inappropriate secretion of antidiuretic hormone. Sympathetic overactivity may pose a problem in management and may contribute to fatality.

Recovery from an acute attack usually begins two to three weeks after the neuropathy has reached its peak but in some improvement may be delayed for months. Further attacks may occur with or without neuropathy. The intervals between the attacks are highly variable. Fatality is not infrequent, 10 out of 29 patients dying according to one report [40].

Diagnosis

Diagnosis is made by demonstrating an increase in urinary ALA or PBG. Watson-Schwartz test can be used to detect lower levels of PBG in the urine. Hoesch test utilizes only one reagent [41]. Two drops of urine are added to this reagent and if PBG is present the mixture immediately turns red. Between the acute episodes ALA and PBG may be normal. However, a definitive biochemical diagnosis can be made by demonstrating deficient levels of uroporphyrinogen synthetase in red blood cells [42].

Axonal degeneration appears to be the primary mechanism of nerve damage in porphyric neuropathy [43] with some degree of secondary demyelination. Nerve conduction velocities are normal or near normal with evidence of denervation on electromyography.

Management

Fasting and dehydration may initiate an attack and therefore hydration including intravenous administration of glucose is useful. This may abort the attack in some patients. Chlorpromazine is helpful in controlling the abdominal pain. Propranolol will decrease the heart rate and blood pressure and sometimes alleviate abdominal pain [44, 45]. Seizures may be treated with intramuscular or rectal paraldehyde. Bromides or clonazepam may be started later. Respiratory paralysis should be treated by tracheotomy and controlled ventilation. It usually takes two to eight weeks for respiratory function to show evidence of recovery. Administration of heme or hematin has shown encouraging results. There may be long-lasting improvement with reduction in the number and severity of attacks [46, 47].

Prophylaxis is very important as several drugs are known to provoke an attack of AIP. Barbiturates are the most frequent offending agents. Sulfonamides, estrogen and griseofulvin are among the long list of drugs that can precipitate an acute attack and these drugs should not be used.

VP has clinical features similar to AIP in addition to cutaneous manifestations. Between acute episodes ALA, PBG and urinary porphyrins are normal. However, fecal levels of coproporphyrin and protoporphyrin remain high. Diagnosis is confirmed by quantitative analysis of porphyrin in the stool.

HC is not much different from VP. Between attacks high levels of fecal coproporphyrin and low levels of protoporphyrin are noted. During acute attacks excretion of coproporphyrin is markedly increased in the urine and stool.

The above two disorders are managed in the same fashion as AIP.

Tetanus

Tetanus is a life-threatening disease caused by the exotoxin of *Clostridium tetani* which is a gram-positive anaerobic spore-forming rod commonly found in the soil and in the intestines of domestic animals. The organism is commonly introduced by a laceration or puncture wound usually sustained outdoors. In 20% of cases there is neither a history of injury nor a detectable wound. The organism has been known to multiply in unexpected sites such as decubitus ulcers, burns, blisters, insect bites and chronically infected middle ears. Cases of tetanus have occurred following abortions, abdominal operations and vaccinations.

Clostridium tetani exists in two forms. The spores are highly resistant to heat and many chemical agents and can survive for many years. The second form is the vegetative rod which is anaerobic. The rods germinate and multiply under suitable conditions.

Tetanolysin and tetanospasmin are the two toxins released by the organism. The neurologic symptoms are produced by tetanospasmin which is a water-soluble protein with a molecular weight of about 67,000. Intra-axonal transport from peripheral nerve endings into the spinal cord [48] and vascular spread are the two mechanisms that have been proposed to explain the transport of the toxin to the central nervous system. After reaching the motor neurons by retrograde axonal transport the toxin migrates transynaptically across the synaptic clefts and binds to presynaptic nerve terminals ending on motor neurons. Once tetanospasmin binds to nerve terminal membranes it

cannot be neutralized by antitoxin. The toxin acts presynaptically and blocks the release of the spinal inhibitory transmitters
from interneurons disrupting the normal spinal inhibitory
control mechanisms. This results in the typical clinical picture
of tetanus consisting of a background of muscle hypertonia
with cocontraction of all muscles about a joint and with
superimposed muscle spasms. Tetanospasmin acts on the motor
end-plates, brain and sympathetic nervous system in addition to
the spinal cord [49-53].

Clinical presentation can take three forms — generalized,
cephalic and local. The incubation period is usually between 3
and 21 days but may be as short as one day or as long as several
months. The shorter incubation period is usually associated
with severe forms of tetanus.

Generalized tetanus is the most common form of tetanus.
Trismus is the most common presenting feature and, when
persistent, results in a fixed, sneering expression, the so-called
risus sardonicus. Many muscles develop stiffness giving rise to
neck stiffness, rigidity of abdominal muscles and dysphagia.
Tonic spasms produce sudden, severe, painful contractions of
agonist and antagonist muscles resulting in opisthotonus,
boardlike abdomen, rigid extension of lower extremities and
flexion of the upper extremities. During the painful spasms
consciousness is fully retained. Laryngospasm obstructs the
upper respiratory passages and can cause cyanosis and asphyxia
if not promptly relieved. The intense muscle contractions
during the spasms may result in elevation of body temperature.
The severity and frequency of the spasms vary.

Overactivity of the sympathetic nervous system contributes
significantly to the mortality. Hypertension is sometimes
followed by profound hypotension. Peripheral vasoconstriction,
excessive sweating, tachycardia and arrhythmias may occur.

The average mortality is 45% to 55%. There are two types
of tetanus that carry a poor outlook. One of these is tetanus
occurring in heroin addicts and the other is tetanus neonatorum. In some countries tetanus neonatorum is common and
is due to the contaminated agents that are employed to sever
the cord at birth [54].

The diagnosis of fully developed generalized tetanus is easy.
In the initial stages other causes of trismus such as peritonsilar

abscess, dental lesions and phenothiazine-induced trismus have to be excluded. Neck stiffness may be suggestive of meningitis but there is no pleocytosis in the cerebrospinal fluid.

The 3rd, 4th, 7th, 9th, 10th and 12th cranial nerves are involved either singly or in various combinations. Facial nerve is most often involved. In the absence of a wound diagnosis may be extremely difficult. Generalized tetanus may follow cephalic tetanus in some cases [55].

Local tetanus [56] is a relatively benign condition, persistent hypertonia being confined to a group of muscles. Any group of muscles may be involved. Intermittent spasms of these muscles may occur. Sometimes generalized tetanus may follow local tetanus after a few days.

Treatment

There are several aspects to the treatment of a severe case of tetanus. Although antitoxin cannot neutralize the toxin that is already bound to the receptors, the unbound toxin should be neutralized before it binds itself to the receptors. Human tetanus immune globulin is best for this purpose and is given intramuscularly or intravenously in a dose of 3000 to 10,000 units. If it is unavailable, equine antitoxin may be used but only after prior skin tests for hypersensitivity are done. The usual dose is 50,000 units intramuscularly followed by 50,000 units in a slow intravenous infusion. Further toxin production should be eliminated by debridement of the wound and by the intramuscular administration of Procaine penicillin 1.2 million units daily for ten days. If the patient is allergic to penicillin, tetracycline 2 gm/day may be used.

Control of tetanic spasms is crucial to the successful management of tetanus. Of the numerous drugs that have been tried, diazepam, chlorpromazine, phenobarbital and pentobarbital are the most helpful. Diazepam is given intravenously in a dose of 2 to 20 mg every two to eight hours [57]. It acts at supraspinal and spinal locations by potentiating the postsynaptic action of gamma-aminobutyric acid (GABA) at its receptor sites, thereby facilitating the inhibition mediated by GABA. In addition, diazepam depresses fusimotor activity and diminishes mono- and polysynaptic reflexes. Chlorpromazine in doses of 200 to 300 mg per day is effective in controlling the rigidity and spasms. Phenobarbital and pentobarbital are also highly useful drugs and may be given in doses of 30 to 60 mg every four hours. The daily requirement has to be adjusted according to response. A combination of two drugs is much more efficacious than administration of a single compound.

If drugs and sedatives are not helpful in controlling spasms, neuromuscular blocking agents and mechanical ventilation are indicated. If a patient has an attack of laryngospasm, it should be terminated immediately with a neuromuscular blocking agent and tracheostomy performed without delay. Most patients with severe tetanus will need tracheostomy. The neuromuscular blocking agents d-tubocurarine 6 to 12 mg IV every hour, pancuronium 0.5 to 2 mg IV every hour or succinylcholine 500 mg intramuscularly every hour are the most helpful. The dose is adjusted to maintain the minimal level required to prevent spasms.

Overactivity of the sympathetic nervous system contributes significantly to the mortality of the disease and suppression of the symptoms by effective treatment is most important. A combination of propranolol and bethanidine satisfactorily controls hypertension, tachycardia and cardiac arrhythmias [58].

Particular attention should be paid to care of the skin, mouth and sphincters in tetanus. Proper calorie intake and maintenance of the water and electrolyte balance are also essential.

Clinical tetanus does not establish clinical immunity. Prior to discharge from the hospital, the patient should be given the first dose of tetanus toxoid.

References

1. Elmqvist, D., Hofman, W.W., Kugelberg, J. et al: An electrophysiological investigation of neuromuscular transmission in myasthenia gravis. J. Physiol. (Lond) 174:417-434, 1964.
2. Fambrough, D.M., Drachman, D.B. and Satyamurti, S.: Neuromuscular junction in myasthenia gravis: Decreased acetylcholine receptors. Science 182:293-295, 1973.
3. Drachman, D.B., Kao, I., Pestronk, A. et al: Myasthenia gravis as a receptor disorder. Ann. N.Y. Acad. Sci. 274:226-234, 1976.
4. Engel, A.G. and Santa, T.: Histometric analysis of the ultrastructure of the neuromuscular junction in myasthenia gravis and in the myasthenic syndrome. Ann. N.Y. Acad. Sci. 183:46-63, 1971.

5. Satyamurti, S., Drachman, D.B. and Slone, F.: Blockade of acetylcholine receptors: A model of myasthenia gravis. Science 187:955-957, 1975.
6. Chang, C.C. and Lee, C.Y.: Electrophysiological study of neuromuscular blocking action of cobra neurotoxin. Br. J. Pharmacol. Chemother. 28:172-181, 1966.
7. Patrick, J. and Lindstrom, J.: Autoimmune response to acetylcholine receptor. Science 180:871-872, 1973.
8. Engel. A.G., Lambert, E.H. and Howard, F.M. Jr.: Immune complexes (IgG and C_3) at the motor end-plate in myasthenia gravis. Mayo Clin. Proc. 52:267-280, 1977.
9. Keesey, J., Lindstrom, J., Cokeley, H. and Herrmann, C. Jr.: Anti-acetylcholine receptor antibody in neonatal myasthenia gravis. N. Engl. J. Med. 296:55, 1977.
10. Osserman, K.E. and Teng, P.: Studies in myasthenia gravis — a rapid diagnostic test. Further progress with edrophonium (Tensilon) chloride. JAMA 160:153-155, 1956.
11. Özdemir, C. and Young, R.R.: Electrical testing in myasthenia gravis. Ann. N.Y. Acad. Sci. 183:287-302, 1971.
12. Horowitz, S.H., Genkins, G., Kornfeld, P. and Papatestas, A.E.: Electrophysiological diagnosis of myasthenia gravis and the regional curare test. Neurology (Minneap) 26:4-1-417, 1976.
13. Desmedt, J. and Borenstein, S.: Diagnosis of myasthenia gravis by nerve stimulation. Ann. N.Y. Acad. Sci. 274:174-188, 1976.
14. Desmedt, J.E. and Borenstein, S.: Double-step nerve stimulation for myasthenic block: Sensitization of postactivation exhaustion by ischemia. Ann. Neurol. 1:55-64, 1977.
15. Stalberg, E.J., Trontelj, V. and Schwartz, M.S.: Single muscle-fiber recording of the jitter phenomenon in patients with myasthenia gravis and in members of their families. Ann. N.Y. Acad. Sci. 274:189-202, 1976.
16. Lindstrom, J.M., Seybold, M.E., Lennon, V.A. et al: Antibody to acetylcholine receptor in myasthenia gravis. Neurology (Minneap) 26:1054-1059, 1976.
17. Lambert, E.H. and Elmqvist, D.: Quantal components of end-plate potentials in the myasthenic syndrome. Ann. N.Y. Acad. Sci. 183:183-199, 1971.
18. Engel, A.G., Lambert, E.H. and Gomez, M.R.: A new myasthenic syndrome with end-plate acetylcholinesterase deficiency, small nerve terminals and reduced acetylcholine release. Ann. Neurol. 1:315-330, 1977.
19. Mertens, H.G., Balzereit, F. and Leipert, M.: The treatment of severe myasthenia gravis with immunosuppressive agents. Europ. Neurol. 2:321-339, 1969.
20. Newsom-Davis, J., Pinching, A.J., Vincent, A. and Wilson, S.G.: Function of circulating antibody to acetylcholine receptor in myasthenia gravis; Investigation by plasma exchange. Neurology 28:266-272, 1978.

21. Finegold, S.F.: Intoxications due to anaerobic bacteria. *In* Anaerobic Bacteria in Human Disease. New York-San Francisco-London:Academic Press, 1977, pp. 472-487.

22. Cherington, M.: Botulism: Ten year experience. Arch. Neurol. 30:432-437, 1974.

23. Cherington, M.: Botulism: Electrophysiologic and therapeutic observations. *In* Desmedt, J.E. (ed.): New Developments in Electromyography and Clinical Neurophysiology 1:375-397, 1971.

24. Cherington, M. and Ryan, D.W.: Treatment of botulism with guanidine: Early neurophysiologic studies. N. Engl. J. Med. 282:195-197, 1970.

25. Harvey, A.L. and Marshall, I.G.: The actions of three diaminopyridines on the chick biventer cervicis muscle. Eur. J. Pharmacol. 44:303-309, 1977.

26. Cull-Candy, S.G., Lundh, H. and Thesleff, S.: Effects of botulism toxin on neuromuscular transmission in the rat. J. Physiol. (Lond) 260:177-203, 1976.

27. Lundh, H., Leander, S. and Thesleff, S.: Antagonism of the paralysis produced by botulinum toxin in the rat: The effects of tetraethylammonium, guanidine and 4-aminopyridine. J. Neurol. Sci. 32:29-43, 1977.

28. Merson, M.H. and Dowell, V.R.: Epidemiologic, clinical and laboratory aspects of wound botulism. N. Engl. J. Med. 289:1005-1010, 1973.

29. Pickett, J., Berg, B., Chaplin, E. and Brunstetter-Shafer, M.: Syndrome of botulism in infancy: Clinical and electrophysiological study. N. Engl. J. Med. 295:770-772, 1976.

30. Asbury, A.K., Arnason, B.G.W., Karp, H.R. and McFarlin, D.E.: Criteria for Guillain-Barré diagnosis. Arch. Neurol. 35:623-624, 1978.

31. Thomashefsky, A.J., Horowitz, S.J. and Feingold, M.H.: Acute autonomic neuropathy. Neurology (Minneap) 22:251-255, 1972.

32. Lambert, E.H. and Mulder, D.W.: Nerve conduction in the Guillain-Barré syndrome. Am. Assoc. Electromyogr. Electrodiag. 10:13, 1963.

33. Kimura, J. and Butzer, J.F.: F-wave conduction velocity in Guillain-Barré syndrome — Assessment of nerve segment between axilla and spinal cord. Arch. Neurol. 32:524-529, 1975.

34. Asbury, A.K., Arnason, B.G.W. and Adams, R.D.: The inflammatory lesion in idiopathic polyneuritis. Medicine (Baltimore) 48:173-215, 1969.

35. Caspary, E.A., Currie, S., Walton, J.N. and Field, E.J.: Lymphocyte sensitization to nervous tissues and muscle in patients with Guillain-Barré syndrome. J. Neurol. Neurosurg. Psychiatry 34:179-181, 1971.

36. Currie, S. and Knowles, M.: Lymphocyte transformation in the Guillain-Barré syndrome. Brain 94:109-116, 1971.

37. Goulon, M., Nouailhat, F., Babinet, P. et al: La dysantonomie des polyradiculonevrites aigues primitives. Rev. Neurol. (Paris) 131:95-119, 1975.

38. Lichtenfeld, P.: Autonomic dysfunction in the Guillain-Barré syndrome. Am. J. Med. 50:772-780, 1971.

39. Hughes, R.A.C., Newsom-Davis, J.M., Perkin, G.D. and Pierce, J.M.: Controlled trial of prednisolone in acute polyneuropathy. Lancet 2:750-753, 1978.

40. Ridley, A.: The neuropathy in acute intermittent porphyria. Q. J. Med. 38:307-333, 1969.

41. Lamon, J., With, T.K. and Redeker, A.G.: The Hoesch test: Bedside screening for urinary porphobilinogen in patients with suspected porphyria. Clin. Chem. 20:1438-1440, 1974.

42. Magnussen, C.R., Levine, J.B., Doherty, J.M. et al: A red cell enzyme method for the diagnosis of acute intermittent porphyria. Blood 44:857-868, 1974.

43. Cavanagh, J.B. and Mellick, R.S.: On the nature of peripheral nerve lesions associated with acute intermittent porphyria. J. Neurol. Neurosurg. Psychiatry 28:320-327, 1965.

44. Bealtie, A.D., Moore, M.R., Goldberg, et al: Acute intermittent porphyria: Response of tachycardia and hypertension to propranolol. Br. Med. J. 3:256-260, 1973.

45. Atsmon, A. and Blum, I.: Treatment of acute porphyria variegate with propranolol. Lancet 1:176-197, 1970.

46. Treatment of acute hepatic porphyria (editorial). Lancet 1:1024-1026, 1978.

47. Lamon, J.M., Bennett, M., Frykholm, B. and Tschudy, D.: Prevention of acute porphyric attacks by intravenous haematin. Lancet 2:492-496, 1978.

48. Price, D.L., Griffin, J., Young, A. et al: Tetanus toxin: Direct evidence for retrograde intra-axonal transport. Science 188:945-947, 1975.

49. Brooks, V.B., Curtis, D.R. and Eccles, J.C.: Mode of action of tetanus toxin. Nature 175:120-121, 1955.

50. Brooks, V.B. and Asanuma, H.: Action of tetanus toxin in the cerebral cortex. Science 137:674-676, 1962.

51. Carrea, R. and Lanari, A.: Chronic effect of tetanus toxin applied locally to the cerebral cortex of the dog. Science 137:342-343, 1962.

52. Kaeser, H.E. and Saner, A.: Tetanus toxin: A neuromuscular blocking agent. Nature 223:842, 1969.

53. Kerr, J.H., Corbett, J.L., Prys-Roberts, C. et al: Involvement of the sympathetic nervous system in tetanus: Studies on 82 cases. Lancet 2:236-241, 1968.

54. Friedlander, F.C.: Tetanus neonatorum: Report on eight cases with two recoveries. J. Pediatr. 39:448-454, 1951.

55. Bagratuni, L.: Cephalic tetanus with report of a case. Br. Med. J. 1:461-463, 1952.

56. Struppler, A., Struppler, E. and Adams, R.D.: Local tetanus in man. Its clinical and neurophysiological characteristics. Arch. Neurol. 8:162-178, 1963.

57. Cordova, A.B.: Control of the spasms of tetanus with diazepam (Valium): Evaluation of clinical usefulness based upon observation of three childhood cases. Clin. Pediatr. 8:712-716, 1969.

58. Prys-Roberts, C., Kerr, J.H., Corbett, J.L. et al: Treatment of sympathetic overactivity in tetanus. Lancet 1:542-546, 1969.

Self-Evaluation Quiz

1. Which of the following is not common to both Guillain-Barré syndrome and acute intermittent porphyria^
   a) Weakness of the extremities
   b) Cranial nerve involvement
   c) Significantly slowed nerve conduction
   d) Depressed or absent deep tendon reflexes
2. A patient with myasthenia gravis is seen because of increasing weakness and respiratory difficulty with a vital capacity of 600 ml. Which of the following is most appropriate?
   a) Differentiate clinically myasthenic from cholinergic crisis
   b) Do immediate Tensilon test
   c) Increase anticholinesterase medication to improve respiration
   d) Stop anticholinesterase medication, intubate and give assisted respiration
3. External ophthalmoplegia may be seen in myasthenia gravis, botulism and Guillain-Barré syndrome.
   a) True
   b) False
4. Neuromuscular transmission is impaired in myasthenia gravis, botulism and tetanus.
   a) True
   b) False
5. For plasmapheresis to be effective in myasthenia gravis serum levels of AChR antibodies should be very high.
   a) True
   b) False
6. The botulinum toxin acts presynaptically whereas tetanospasmin acts postsynaptically.
   a) True
   b) False

Answers on page 391.

Panel Discussion

Moderator: Dr. Marshall

Panelists: Drs. Ayyar and Lockwood

Moderator: Dr. Lockwood, why is it so difficult for house officers to give glucose to unconscious patients after having drawn a blood sugar?

Dr. Lockwood: I do not know the answer, but I can say that it is crucial that this be done in every instance. That applies to children as well as to adult patients, even in the absence of diagnosis of diabetes, since there are many disorders, ranging from ketotic hypoglycemics of childhood to alcoholics of adulthood, which may present with hypoglycemia. The administration of glucose promptly is essential to prevent catastrophic neurologic deficit. Perhaps in some emergency rooms where physicians are not present all the time this should be incorporated into the nursing protocols, just as intensive care unit nurses initiate cardiopulmonary resuscitation. I think it is very important.

Moderator: How soon and how rapidly should potassium be replaced in diabetic ketoacidosis?

Dr. Lockwood: I do not think there is a hard and fast answer to that question. These patients almost always require potassium replacement. In planning the management of these individuals, I think it is appropriate to bear in mind that too much potassium is worse than not enough, since hyperkalemia causes cardiac arrhythmias and may cause death as a result of that. These patients usually will require potassium, but I think you need to know what the renal status of these patients is and how severe their ketoacidosis is before you can make that decision.

Moderator: If one inhales ammonia, what are the consequences and what, if any, are the treatments?

387

Dr. Lockwood: Ammonia is a refrigerant that is used in some very large walk-in supermarket freezers and coolers. I suppose individuals may be exposed to this in industrial accidents as well as freight cars being derailed and things of that nature. If you have ever cleaned windows with ammonia, you know what it smells like. It is a very irritating toxic substance to the lungs. Although I have not personally seen a case of ammonia gas intoxication, the clinical syndrome I am sure is one of pulmonary edema and very severe pulmonary difficulties. The ammonia that actually gets into the body is eliminated very quickly. Ammonia clearance half-times in blood are on the order of several minutes. Any ammonia that gets into the body from an exogenous source would be very rapidly metabolized and be gone by the time you could get the patient to the emergency room.

Moderator: Is there an adult variant of Reye's syndrome causing coma?

Dr. Lockwood: Reye's syndrome is usually limited to children, usually young children, but there have been a few recent well-documented cases occurring in teenagers and one in a 23-year-old individual. In young adults, one should certainly keep this diagnosis in mind when evaluating a patient with coma of unknown origin.

Moderator: Dr. Ayyar, what has been your experience with the effectiveness of plasmaphoresis in the diagnosis of Guillain-Barré syndrome?

Dr. Ayyar: We do not use it for diagnosis and treatment of Guillain-Barré syndrome, but for treatment of several other disorders.

Moderator: Please comment on the value of plasmaphoresis as a treatment modality for acute Guillain-Barré syndrome.

Dr. Ayyar: It was reported in 1978 that plasmaphoresis may be an effective treatment for Guillain-Barré syndrome. There are a few reports in the literature evaluating the effect of plasmaphoresis in GBS. Many patients improved but some did not. A large series of patients have to be treated before one can form definite conclusions, but at the moment it appears that plasmaphoresis will benefit some, if not all, with GBS.

Moderator: Do you sedate botulism and myasthenia gravis patients for intubation?

Dr. Ayyar: We do not usually sedate these patients for intubation. If you have a physician who is experienced, sedation is seldom necessary. However, there are some patients who will be anxious and apprehensive and in these patients mild sedation may be helpful.

Moderator: How do you intubate a patient with tetanus without provoking tetanic spasms?

Dr. Ayyar: Ideally a patient with tetanus should not be allowed to have generalized spasms or opisthotonos. Tracheostomy should be performed after the onset of the first generalized seizure. Asphyxia may result from spasm of the glottis and larynx, the spasm often developing suddenly and without warning. In moderate cases of tetanus, if one is concerned about the upper airway, endotracheal intubation followed by tracheotomy is carried out. Neuromuscular blocking agents are quite helpful in the management of these patients. My experience with several hundred patients with tetanus has taught me to resort to tracheotomy in almost all the patients with severe tetanus.

Moderator: Is acute porphyria mainly a disease of Mediterranean countries?

Dr. Ayyar: Acute intermittent porphyria (AIP) occurs all over the world, as far as I know. The incidence of porphyria in the United States is approximately 1 in 1,000 but its occurrence in blacks is extremely rare. AIP is transmitted as an autosomal dominant trait.

Moderator: What causes the abdominal pain in AIP? How does hematin help patients with AIP?

Dr. Ayyar: I do not know the answers to these questions. During an acute attack there is a marked increase in the amounts of δ-aminolevulinic acid (ALA) and porphobilinogen (PBG) excreted in the urine. This increase is due, at least in part, to enhanced activity of ALA synthetase. Heme inhibits the activity of ALA synthetase and administration of hematin, which is a heme pathway end-product, results in decrease in the urinary excretion of ALA and PBG presumably due to decreased production. This may have something to do with amelioration of symptoms.

Answers to Self-Evaluation Quizzes

Page 17:   1(d); 2(e); 3(c); 4(b); 5(a); 6(d); 7(c); 8(b); 9(d); 10(d).

Page 29:   1(b); 2(e); 3(e); 4(b).

Page 45:   1(b); 2(b); 3(a); 4(b); 5(a,d); 6(a,b,d); 7(b); 8(a,b); 9(b); 10(e).

Page 58:   1(d); 2(b); 3(b); 4(d); 5(c); 6(d); 7(e); 8(e).

Page 67:   1(c); 2(b); 3(b,c,d); 4(d); 5(e); 6(b); 7(d,e); 8(b).

Page 74:   1(b); 2(b); 3(d); 4(b); 5(e); 6(a); 7(e); 8(b).

Page 92:   1(a,d,e,f); 2(b), 3(a,d,e); 4(a); 5(b); 6(a,c); 7(a).

Page 115:   1(d); 2(b); 3(b); 4(b); 5(e); 6(c); 7(a); 8(b); 9(d,e).

Page 124:   1(b); 2(a); 3(b); 4(a); 5(a).

Page 128:   1(d); 2(a).

Page 153:   1(a); 2(b); 3(a); 4(b); 5(b).

Page 168:   1(d); 2(a); 3(d); 4(d); 5(a); 6(a); 7(b); 8(c); 9(e); 10(d).

Page 199:   1(c); 2(b); 3(c); 4(d); 5(a); 6(b); 7(e); 8(c); 9(d); 10(b); 11(a).

Page 214:   1(a); 2(b); 3(a).

Page 226:   1(b); 2(a,d); 3(a).

Page 247: 1(a); 2(d); 3(d); 4(a); 5(b); 6(a); 7(d); 8(c); 9(e).

Page 269: 1(d); 2(c); 3(c); 4(c); 5(b); 6(a); 7(d); 8(d); 9(a); 10(c).

Page 290: 1(b); 2(b); 3(b); 4(b); 5(c); 6(b); 7(b); 8(b); 9(c); 10(c).

Page 301: 1(a); 2(a); 3(b); 4(a); 5(b).

Page 329: 1(b); 2(a); 3(d); 4(b); 5(c); 6(e); 7(c); 8(b); 9(b); 10(c).

Page 339: 1(a); 2(b); 3(a).

Page 347: 1(b,c,d); 2(d); 3(e); 4(e); 5(b); 6(a); 7(b); 8(c,e); 9(a); 10(a); 11(c).

Page 359: 1(a); 2(d); 3(b); 4(b).

Page 385: 1(c); 2(d); 3(a); 4(a); 5(b); 6(b).

Author Index

Subject Index